Vaccines in Veterinary Medicine

Vaccines in Veterinary Medicine

Edited by Isabel Myers

SYRAWOOD
PUBLISHING HOUSE
New York

Published by Syrawood Publishing House,
750 Third Avenue, 9th Floor,
New York, NY 10017, USA
www.syrawoodpublishinghouse.com

Vaccines in Veterinary Medicine
Edited by Isabel Myers

International Standard Book Number: 978-1-64740-257-0 (Hardback)

Cataloging-in-Publication Data

Vaccines in veterinary medicine / edited by Isabel Myers.
p. cm.
Includes bibliographical references and index.
ISBN 978-1-64740-257-0
1. Veterinary vaccines. 2. Veterinary medicine. 3. Vaccination of animals. I. Myers, Isabel.
SF918.V32 V33 2022
636.089 537 2--dc23

TABLE OF CONTENTS

PREFACE

Veterinary medicine is the branch of medicine which focuses on the treatment of disease, injury and disorder in animals. It is also concerned with the diagnosis and prevention of these ailments. Veterinary science benefits human health by monitoring and controlling infectious diseases which can be transmitted from animals to humans. One of the approaches through which this is accomplished is through vaccination. Veterinary vaccines seek to improve the health and welfare of companion animals and prevent animal-to-human transmission for both domestic animals and wild animals. There are different approaches to the development of veterinary vaccines such as molecularly defined subunit vaccines, whole pathogen preparations, genetically engineered organisms, and naked DNA injections. The various advancements in veterinary vaccines are glanced at and their applications as well as ramifications are looked at in detail in this book. It is meant for students who are looking for an elaborate reference text on vaccines in veterinary medicine.

After months of intensive research and writing, this book is the end result of all who devoted their time and efforts in the initiation and progress of this book. It will surely be a source of reference in enhancing the required knowledge of the new developments in the area. During the course of developing this book, certain measures such as accuracy, authenticity and research focused analytical studies were given preference in order to produce a comprehensive book in the area of study.

This book would not have been possible without the efforts of the authors and the publisher. I extend my sincere thanks to them. Secondly, I express my gratitude to my family and well-wishers. And most importantly, I thank my students for constantly expressing their willingness and curiosity in enhancing their knowledge in the field, which encourages me to take up further research projects for the advancement of the area.

Editor

1

Efficacy of *Mycoplasma hyopneumoniae* vaccination before and at weaning against experimental challenge infection in pigs

Ioannis Arsenakis[1*], Luca Panzavolta[1], Annelies Michiels[1], Rubén Del Pozo Sacristán[1], Filip Boyen[2], Freddy Haesebrouck[2] and Dominiek Maes[1]

Abstract

Background: Commercial bacterins are widely used at weaning to control *Mycoplasma hyopneumoniae* infections in pigs. However, it is not known whether the efficacy of vaccinating against *M. hyopneumoniae* can be influenced by the weaning process when vaccination is applied at the day of weaning. The present study assessed the efficacy of a single *M. hyopneumoniae* vaccination (Ingelvac MycoFLEX®) three days before weaning (V1) or at weaning (V2) against experimental challenge infection. Four weeks after vaccination, groups V1 and V2 ($n = 20$ pigs each) and a non-vaccinated, positive control group (PCG) ($n = 20$) were endotracheally inoculated with a virulent *M. hyopneumoniae* field strain. Five pigs were used as a negative control group. All pigs were euthanized 5 weeks after challenge. The main parameters investigated included macroscopic and histopathological lung lesions at necropsy, immunofluorescence (IF) staining and quantitative real-time PCR (qPCR) on broncho-alveolar lavage (BAL) fluid for quantifying *M. hyopneumoniae.*

Results: The average macroscopic lung lesion scores in groups V1, V2 and PCG were 0.54, 0.88 and 1.04, respectively ($P > 0.05$). The average lymphohistiocytic infiltration scores in groups V1, V2 and PCG were 2.95, 3.16 and 3.61, respectively ($P < 0.05$). The average IF scores were: V1 = 1.13, V2 = 1.19 and PCG = 1.25 ($P > 0.05$), the qPCR values were: V1 = $10^{2.94}$, V2 = $10^{2.76}$ and PCG = $10^{3.23}$ ($P > 0.05$). All pigs of the negative control group remained negative throughout the study.

Conclusions: Both vaccinated groups had lower numbers of macroscopic and histopathological lung lesions, and lower numbers of *M. hyopneumoniae* organisms in the BAL fluid compared to the PCG. However, no firm conclusions could be made on whether weaning negatively influences the efficacy of *M. hyopneumoniae* vaccination, since significant differences between the treatment groups were only obtained for the histopathological lung lesions. This could be attributed to the fact that milder macroscopic lung lesions were produced in the inoculated pigs, when compared to previous trials conducted by the same group. Further research under field conditions is warranted to assess possible differences between the two vaccination strategies.

Keywords: Weaning, *Mycoplasma hyopneumoniae*, Vaccination, Efficacy, Strain

* Correspondence: Ioannis.Arsenakis@UGent.be
[1]Porcine Health Management Unit, Department of Reproduction, Obstetrics & Herd Health, Faculty of Veterinary Medicine, Ghent University, Salisburylaan 133, Merelbeke 9820, Belgium
Full list of author information is available at the end of the article

Background

Mycoplasma hyopneumoniae is the etiological agent of enzootic pneumonia (EP), a chronic respiratory disease affecting mainly grow-finishing pigs [1, 2]. *M. hyopneumoniae* infections have been detected in almost all countries with intensive production systems and are responsible for major economic losses in the pig industry [1, 3]. These economic losses are due to pig growth retardation, higher feed conversion ratios, increased antimicrobial use and increased susceptibility to other respiratory pathogens such as *Pasteurella multocida, Actinobacillus pleuropneumoniae, Trueperella pyogenes* and *Streptococcus suis* [4]. *M. hyopneumoniae* is also an important pathogen involved in the porcine respiratory disease complex (PRDC) [5, 6].

Control of *M. hyopneumoniae* infections can be achieved in a number of ways, such as optimizing management and housing conditions, antimicrobial medication and vaccination. In many countries, more than 70 % of pig herds are vaccinated against *M. hyopneumoniae* in an effort to control the disease [7]. Vaccination with commercial bacterins has been extensively proven to reduce performance losses, the severity of clinical signs and lung lesions [8–12]. Different vaccination schemes can be implemented, depending on the type of herd, the production system, the infection pattern and the preference of the farmer.

Currently, both double and single vaccination strategies are widely practiced. Single vaccination is often administered either at 1 week of age or at weaning. Vaccination is often done at weaning because the piglets are handled then anyway, so vaccination can easily be included in routine farm management practices [12, 13]. On the other hand, weaning is one of the most stressful events in the pig's life [14, 15]. The piglets are then experiencing the abrupt separation from the sow, they are being handled, they are being moved to other facilities, they are usually being mixed with other pigs, and they are receiving a different type of feed [14, 15]. Stress may interfere with an optimal response to vaccination, and therefore it is generally recommended not to vaccinate animals that are severely stressed [16].

Consequently, one important question that remains to be answered, and whose answer could contribute to the optimization of existing vaccination schemes, is whether the efficacy of vaccinating against *M. hyopneumoniae* can be influenced by the weaning process when vaccination is applied at the day of weaning. The objective of this trial was to investigate the efficacy of a one-shot vaccination applied either at weaning or three days before weaning in pigs experimentally infected with a virulent *M. hyopneumoniae* field strain.

Results

Clinical and performance parameters

In total, two pigs died during the trial, after receiving the endotracheal challenge infection (one in the V2 group and one in the PCG group). These pigs were not included in the analysis. In groups V1, V2 and PCG, coughing started approximately six days after challenge and continued to increase towards the end of the trial. In groups V1 and V2, coughing peaked between 66 and 70 days of age, whereas in the PCG, the peak was noticed at 80 days of age. The respiratory disease score (RDS) values for the period before challenge and the period after challenge, as well as for the overall period, are shown in Table 1. There were no significant differences between the groups ($P > 0.05$).

The average daily weight gain (ADG) results of groups V1, V2 and PCG during the period before challenge and during the period after challenge, as well as during the overall period, are presented in Table 2. There were no significant differences ($P > 0.05$) between the groups.

Macroscopic and histopathological lung lesions, and IF testing for *M. hyopneumoniae*

Only numerical differences in macroscopic lung lesions ($P > 0.05$) were found between groups V1, V2 and PCG (Table 3). The lowest average macroscopic lung lesion score was given to group V1 (0.54). The average lung lesion scores of the pigs in groups V2 and PCG were 0.88 and 1.04, respectively. There were no macroscopic lung lesions in the negative control group.

Statistically significant differences ($P < 0.05$) in histopathological lung lesions were present between groups V1, V2 and PCG (Table 3). The average lymphohistiocytic infiltration score was lower in group V1 (2.95) when compared with groups V2 (3.16) and PCG (3.61). The V1 group had the highest average percentage of air in the lung tissue (44.28), followed by group V2 (37.47) and PCG (31.46).

The results from the IF testing that was used to semi-quantitatively assess the load of *M. hyopneumoniae* organisms in the lung tissue, namely 1.13 (group V1),

Table 1 Average (± standard deviation) of the daily RDS of the pigs for the three different periods

Age range (days)	V1 ($n = 20$)	V2 ($n = 19$)	PCG ($n = 19$)	P value
29–47	0.07 ± 0.26	0.28 ± 0.69	0.11 ± 0.37	0.108
48–83	0.79 ± 1.30	0.62 ± 1.20	0.65 ± 1.19	0.626
29–83	0.54 ± 0.94	0.50 ± 1.03	0.47 ± 0.91	0.852

Scores ranged from 0 (no coughing) to 6 (severe coughing undisturbed) (Halbur et al. [29]). Treatment groups: V1 (vaccinated before weaning, at 18 days of age), V2 (vaccinated on the day of weaning, at 21 days of age) and PCG (non-vaccinated). Overall and pairwise comparisons did not reveal any significant differences between groups for the three different periods. D48: experimental infection, D83: euthanasia

Table 2 ADG (± standard deviation SD) of each treatment group during the three different periods

	ADG (±SD) (g/pig/day)			
Age range (days)	V1 ($n = 20$)	V2 ($n = 19$)	PCG ($n = 19$)	P value
20–48	293 ± 41	299 ± 42	303 ± 55	0.491
48–83	701 ± 116	681 ± 129	718 ± 140	0.442
20–83	519 ± 56	511 ± 66	533 ± 71	0.461

Treatment groups: V1 (vaccinated before weaning, at 18 days of age, challenge infected), V2 (vaccinated on the day of weaning, at 21 days of age, challenge infected) and PCG (non-vaccinated, challenge infected). Overall and pairwise comparisons did not reveal any significant differences between the groups for the three different periods. D48: experimental infection, D83: euthanasia

1.19 (group V2) and 1.25 (PCG), were not significantly different ($P > 0.05$) between groups (Table 3). All pigs of the negative control group were negative for IF staining.

qPCR assay and bacteriological examination

The number of *M. hyopneumoniae* organisms quantified by qPCR in the BAL fluid was not significantly different ($P > 0.05$) between groups V1, V2 and PCG (Table 3). Lower numbers of organisms were detected in groups V1 and V2 ($10^{2.94}$ and $10^{2.76}$ copies/mL, respectively) compared to group PCG ($10^{3.23}$ copies/mL). No *M. hyopneumoniae* DNA was detected in pigs of the negative control group.

Several bacteria were isolated from BAL fluid. In groups V1 and V2, *Bordetella bronchiseptica* (V1: 3/20 pigs; V2: 1/20 pigs) and polybacterial cultures (V1: 4/20 pigs; V2: 2/20 pigs) were obtained. In the PCG, *Haemophilus parasuis* (1/20 pigs), *S. suis* (1/20 pigs) and polybacterial cultures (1/20 pigs) were obtained. The bacteriological culture remained negative for all pigs in the negative control group.

Serology

The serological results for *M. hyopneumoniae* at 21, 48 and 83 days of age are presented in Table 4. At 21 days of age, all the piglets were serologically negative for *M. hyopneumoniae*. At 48 days of age, 40 % of the pigs in each of the vaccinated groups V1 and V2 had seroconverted. None of the pigs in the PCG had seroconverted to *M. hyopneumoniae* at that time. At 83 days of age, all the pigs in groups V1 and V2 were seropositive, while 95 % of the pigs in the PCG had seroconverted. All pigs in the negative control group were serologically negative at all time-points.

Discussion

The present experimental trial investigated whether the efficacy of one-shot vaccination is influenced by the weaning process. Differences between V1 (vaccination three days before weaning), V2 (vaccination at weaning) and the PCG (no vacination) were small and mostly statistically not significant, except for the microscopic lung lesions, which were lower in V1.

Apart from the transport related to the weaning process, the piglets in the present study were also transported to the experimental facilities, a trip that lasted anywhere from one-half to two hours. In fact, age- and site-segregated pork production is a complex process that involves movement of the piglets from the farrowing house to the nursery facilities, which are situated in different locations [17]. It can be expected, though, that the stress imposed on the piglets in our study may have been greater than when the piglets remain on the same site and are not transported (e.g. in single site farrow-to-finish pig herds) [18].

Vaccination at the moment of weaning, when the piglets are being handled anyway, is a common practice, as it can be implemented easily in the daily management of a pig herd. The pigs of V1 were vaccinated three days before weaning. This vaccination strategy is also commonly practiced by some pig producers in order to avoid any possible negative effects of the weaning process, and/or to avoid too much handling or interventions on the same day [19]. A difference of three days between

Table 3 Average (± standard deviation SD) values of macroscopic and histopathological lung lesion scores, IF scores, and qPCR

Parameter[a]	V1 ($n = 20$)	V2 ($n = 19$)	PCG ($n = 19$)	P value
Macroscopic lung lesions	0.54 ± 0.67^{A}	0.88 ± 1.45^{A}	1.04 ± 2.45^{A}	0.777
Lymphohistiocytic infiltration	2.95 ± 0.50^{A}	3.16 ± 0.58^{B}	3.61 ± 0.59^{C}	0.002
Percentage of air in lung tissue	44.28 ± 14.68^{A}	37.47 ± 17.76^{B}	31.46 ± 14.51^{C}	0.000
IF	1.13 ± 0.54^{A}	1.19 ± 0.79^{A}	1.25 ± 0.70^{A}	0.896
qPCR on BAL fluid	$10^{2.94} \pm 10^{1.24A}$	$10^{2.76} \pm 10^{1.48A}$	$10^{3.23} \pm 10^{1.33A}$	0.616

Treatment groups: V1 vaccinated before weaning, at 18 days of age, challenge infected, V2 vaccinated at weaning, at 21 days of age, challenge infected, and PCG positive control group i.e. non-vaccinated, challenge infected

Values with different superscript (A-C) in capital letter within a row are significantly different ($P \leq 0.05$)

[a] Macroscopic lung lesion scoring based on Hannan et al. [30]

Lymphohistiocytic infiltration score based on Morris et al. [31]

Percentage of air in lung tissue measured by means of automatic image analysis system (Optimas® 6.5, Media Cybernetics, Silver Spring, USA)

IF scoring based on Kobisch et al. [32]

Values from qPCR on BAL fluid expressed as copies of *M. hyopneumoniae*/mL

Table 4 Percentage of seropositive pigs in the different groups at different time-points during the trial

Days of age	V1 ($n = 20$)	V2 ($n = 19$)	PCG ($n = 19$)
21[a]	0	0	0
48[b]	40	40	0
83[c]	100	100	95

Treatment groups: V1 (vaccinated before weaning, at 18 days of age, challenge infected), V2 (vaccinated on the day of weaning, at 21 days of age, challenge infected), PCG (non-vaccinated, challenge infected) and NCG (non-vaccinated, non-challenge infected)

[a] Day of weaning and transport to the animal facilities of the Faculty of Veterinary Medicine, Ghent University

[b] Inoculation time

[c] Necropsy

the two vaccination groups most probably allowed sufficient time for the development of the first and most critical steps of the immune response prior to the stress of weaning [20]. At the same time, too great a difference in age at vaccination was avoided between the piglets in the V1 and V2 groups. In this sense, the two vaccination schemes are relevant for the situation in many pig herds.

The experimental infection model used for *M. hyopneumoniae* was similar to that used in previous trials [21–24]. Challenge infection proved to be successful since the vast majority of the infected pigs had positive qPCR values, exhibited the presence of *Mycoplasma*-like macroscopic lung lesions at necropsy and were positive for IF staining. However, the macroscopic lung lesions observed in the present trial were milder compared to trials that had been previously conducted using the same inoculation dose of *M. hyopneumoniae* F7.2C field strain, experimental facilities and way of allocation [23–25]. The precise reasons for this difference are not known. Based on the macroscopic lung lesion scores, serology, qPCR testing and IF staining, all the pigs in the negative control group were negative for *M. hyopneumoniae* throughout the trial, thus confirming that the study piglets were free of *M. hyopneumoniae.*

The RDS values in the PCG were similar to those mentioned in other experimental trials [22, 24]. Compared with the vaccinated groups V1 and V2, the only differences found in the PCG were numerical. There were no significant differences in ADG between the groups. This is mainly due to the high standard deviations observed and the limited numbers of pigs. ADG was measured, but it was not considered an important parameter for this experimental study. In vaccination trials under field conditions however, in which many more animals can be included, ADG is an important parameter.

Group V1 had the lowest numbers of macroscopic and histopathological lung lesions, and the lowest IF scores when compared to groups V2 and PCG. Nevertheless, significant differences between groups V1, V2 and PCG were only obtained for the histopathological lung lesions. This was confirmed by the results of the percentage of air parameter in the lung tissue measured by means of an automatic image analysis system. The statistically significant differences between groups V1, V2 and PCG proved that *M. hyopneumoniae* vaccination is effective in reducing lymphohistiocytic infiltration and increasing the percentage of air in the lung. This reduction of the lymphohistiocytic infiltration scores in the vaccinated groups is in accordance with previous experimental trials [22, 24]. The less severe histopathological lesions may be due to a modulation of the immune response in vaccinated animals. It has been shown that vaccination with a bacterin against *M. hyopneumoniae* reduces the infiltration of macrophages in the lung tissue [26].

Although lower qPCR values were recorded in the vaccinated groups when compared to the PCG, it was not possible to conclude whether vaccination was associated with the reduced bacterial load in the lungs, since the differences between the groups were only numerical. However, the detection of *M. hyopneumoniae* in the BAL fluid of groups V1 and V2 confirms that vaccination alone is not able to prevent colonization of the pig's respiratory tract [4, 22, 24].

The pigs of groups V1, V2 and PCG were seronegative for *M. hyopneumoniae* on the day of transportation to the experimental facilities. At the time of inoculation, 40 % of the pigs in each of the vaccinated groups V1 and V2 had seroconverted. This is in agreement with other studies which have reported that vaccination with commercial bacterins induces seroconversion rates ranging from 30 to 100 % [4, 27]. At necropsy, all the pigs in groups V1 and V2 were seropositive, while the percentage of pigs that had seroconverted in group PCG was 95 %.

Overall, no firm conclusions could be made as to whether group V1 performed better than groups V2 and PCG, since only the microscopic lung lesions were significantly lower in the pigs in group V1. Further research under field conditions is necessary to elucidate the possible effect of weaning on the efficacy of one-shot *M. hyopneumoniae* vaccination. Field trials make it possible to include more animals and to study the entire course of *M. hyopneumoniae* infections up to the time of slaughter.

Conclusions

In conclusion, the differences between the vaccinated groups V1 and V2 were small and mostly statistically not significant. Thus, no firm conclusions could be made as to whether the process of weaning had a negative impact on the efficacy of vaccinating against *M. hyopneumoniae.* A future field trial could possibly provide further insight on the same topic.

Methods

Animals

Sixty-five cross-bred piglets (Topigs 20 sows and Pietrain boars) were purchased from a herd that was free of *M. hyopneumoniae* and PRRSV. Sows and fattening pigs of different age groups in the herd had been repeatedly monitored clinically and serologically, and then by means of macroscopic pneumonia lung lesions at slaughter, and no evidence for the presence of *M. hyopneumoniae* or PRRSV in the herd was found at 3 weeks of age (day seven), the piglets were weaned and transported for one-half to two hours to the animal facilities of the Faculty of Veterinary Medicine, Ghent University, Belgium. From this point onwards, all the pigs received *ad libitum* a commercial, antibiotic-free feed.

Experimental design and *M. hyopneumoniae* inoculation

At 14 days of age, prior to purchase, piglets from 20 different litters were individually ear-tagged and randomly allocated to four different groups. The three main treatment groups were: V1 (vaccinated before weaning, at 18 days of age and while still on the farm; $n = 20$), V2 (vaccinated during weaning, at 21 days of age and before being transported to the experimental facilities; $n = 20$) and a non-vaccinated positive control group (PCG; $n = 20$). Five pigs were used as a negative control group, to verify that they remained free of *M. hyopneumoniae*. They were not vaccinated. The pigs in groups V1 and V2 received a single-shot intramuscular (i.m.) injection (1 mL) of a commercial *M. hyopneumoniae* bacterin vaccine (Ingelvac MycoFLEX®, Boehringer Ingelheim Vetmedica). The pigs in PCG were left untreated and were not injected with a placebo to simulate field conditions. Upon arrival at the Faculty of Veterinary Medicine, each group was housed in a different experimental room equipped with a high efficiency particulate air filter to avoid possible transmission of the pathogen between groups.

At 48 days of age, the two vaccinated groups, V1 and V2, as well as the PCG were challenge infected endotracheally with a 7 mL inoculum containing 10^7 color changing units per mL of the virulent *M. hyopneumoniae* F7.2C field strain as described previously [28]. The pigs in the negative control group were inoculated with 7 mL of sterile culture medium. For the inoculations, the pigs were anaesthetized by administering a mixture of Xyl-M® 2 % and Zoletil 100® i.m. at a dose rate of 0.3 mL/kg bodyweight.

All animals were euthanized and necropsied at 83 days of age. Deep anesthesia was induced by administering i.m. 0.3 mL/kg of a mixture of Xyl-M® 2 % and Zoletil 100®, followed by exsanguination. The study was approved by the ethical committee for animal experiments of the Faculty of Veterinary Medicine, Ghent University (EC2013/35).

Parameters of comparison

Clinical and performance parameters

Each treatment group was examined daily for a minimum of 15 min for the presence of clinical signs throughout the entire trial period. Coughing severity was evaluated in a blinded manner by means of an RDS on a scale from 0 to 6 [29]. According to that scale: 0 (no coughing), 1 (mild coughing after being encouraged to move), 2 (mild coughing while at rest), 3 (moderate coughing after being encouraged to move), 4 (moderate coughing while at rest), 5 (severe coughing after being encouraged to move), and 6 (severe coughing while at rest). The daily RDS values were averaged for the three following periods: from day 29 until day 47, from day 48 (day of inoculation) until day 83 (day of necropsy), and from day 29 until day 83.

Individual bodyweights were measured at 20, 48 and 83 days of age to determine the ADG of each treatment group during the three following periods: from day 20 until day 48, from day 48 until day 83 and from day 20 until day 83.

Macroscopic and histopathological lung lesions, and IF testing for M. hyopneumoniae

After necropsy, *Mycoplasma*-like macroscopic lung lesions were quantified in a blinded manner using a lung lesion score diagram [30]. Theoretically, the total lung lesion scores could range between 0 (absence of lesions) and 35 (entire lung affected).

Two lung tissue samples per lobe (apical, cardiac and diaphragmatic) were collected from the right lung of each pig for histopathology and IF testing. Samples were collected from the edges of the lung lesions, if present [24].

For histopathology, the tissue was fixed in 10 % neutral buffered formalin and routinely processed and embedded in paraffin. One slide was made per lobe sample. Using light microscopy, the severity of peribronchiolar and perivascular lymphohistiocytic infiltration and nodule formation consistent with *M. hyopneumoniae* lesions were scored on a scale from 1 to 5 [31]. Scores 1 and 2 were classified as lesions not related to *Mycoplasma* infections. Scores 3, 4 and 5 were considered to be associated with *Mycoplasma* infections (mild, moderate and severe lesions characteristic of broncho-interstitial (cuffing) pneumonia, surrounding the bronchioles but extending to the interstitium, with lymphofollicular infiltration and mixed inflammatory cell exudates). After three lobes per pig were investigated, the average score per treatment group was calculated.

The percentage of lung area occupied by air (percentage air) was examined by means of an automatic image analysis system (Optimas® 6.5, Media Cybernetics, Silver Spring, USA). This percentage is inversely proportional to the severity of peribronchiolar and perivascular lymphohistiocytic infiltration in the lung tissue and the amount of intrabronchiolar – intrabronchial exudate. An average percentage per treatment group was calculated [28].

A direct IF assay was performed to assess the presence of *M. hyopneumoniae* in the lungs. The scores given could range from 0 to 3: 0 (no IF), 1 (limited IF), 2 (moderate IF), and 3 (intense IF) [32].

qPCR and bacteriological examination

During necropsy, BAL fluid was collected from the left part of the lungs before the tissue samples for histopathology and IF were taken [21]. The recovered fluid was divided into two aliquots, immediately cooled to 4 °C, and then stored at −70 °C until analysis. The first aliquot was used to quantify *M. hyopneumoniae* organisms by qPCR [33]. DNA was extracted (Qiagen, Blood and tissue kit, Belgium) and qPCR was performed using the CFX96 real-time PCR detection system (Bio-Rad). The analysis was done in a double-replicate single setting. To convert the threshold values to the number of organisms, a tenfold dilution series of *M. hyopneumoniae* DNA was used. Values below the last dilution were considered as negative.

The second aliquot of BAL fluid was used for routine bacteriological culture to detect the presence of *Actinobacillus* and *Haemophilus spp.*, and other pathogens which may affect the respiratory tract, such as *S. suis, B. bronchiseptica, P. multocida* and *T. pyogenes* [24].

Serology for M. hyopneumoniae

Blood samples were collected from all pigs at 21, 48 and 83 days of age to measure antibodies against *M. hyopneumoniae*, using a blocking ELISA (IDEIA, *M hyopneumoniae* EIA kit, Oxoid, UK) [12]. Sera with optical density (OD) values < 50 % of the $OD_{buffer\text{-}control}$ were considered positive, while sera with OD values ≥ 50 % of the $OD_{buffer\text{-}control}$ were considered negative.

Statistical analysis

The statistical analysis was performed on groups V1, V2 and PCG. Pigs of the negative control group ($n = 5$) were not included, as they were only employed to ensure that the animals remained free of *M. hyopneumoniae* throughout the experiment. The RDS data were analyzed using repeated measures analysis of variance (ANOVA). Levene's test was used to assess the homogeneity of the variances between the different groups. The ADG, macroscopic and histopathological lung lesions, percentage of air in the lungs, IF testing and qPCR were analyzed with a non-parametric Kruskal-Wallis ANOVA. These five continuous variables did not fulfill the criteria for homogeneity of variances. Statistical results were considered significant when the *P*-values were ≤ 0.05 (two-sided test). The statistical package SPSS 21.0 for Windows (SPSS 21, SPSS Inc., IL, USA) was used to analyze the data.

Competing interests
The authors declare that they have no competing interests.

Authors' contributions
JA performed the lab work and the statistical analyses, interpreted the data and wrote all the drafts of the manuscript. LP was involved in the lab analyses and the trial. AM and RDPS were involved in the performance of the trial and the review of the final manuscript. FB, FH and DM contributed to the development of the protocol, the planning of the study, the review of the final manuscript and the approval for publication. All the authors read and approved the final manuscript.

Acknowledgements
The study was financially supported by Boehringer-Ingelheim Vetmedica GmbH, Ingelheim am Rhein, Germany. The authors are grateful to Ria Spiessens and Els De Fré for their technical assistance in numerous arrangements of the trial.

Author details
[1]Porcine Health Management Unit, Department of Reproduction, Obstetrics & Herd Health, Faculty of Veterinary Medicine, Ghent University, Salisburylaan 133, Merelbeke 9820, Belgium. [2]Department of Pathology, Bacteriology and Avian Diseases, Faculty of Veterinary Medicine, Ghent University, Salisburylaan 133, Merelbeke 9820, Belgium.

References

1. Vicca J, Maes D, Thermote L, Peeters J, Haesebrouck F, Kruif AD. Patterns of *Mycoplasma hyopneumoniae* infections in Belgian farrow-to-finish pig herds with diverging disease-course. J Vet Med. 2002;B49:49–353.
2. Sibila M, Bernal R, Torrents D, Riera P, Llopart D, Calsamiglia M, et al. Effect of sow vaccination against *Mycoplasma hyopneumoniae* on sow and piglet colonization and seroconversion, and pig lung lesions at slaughter. Vet Microbiol. 2008;127:165–70.
3. Thacker EL. Mycoplasmal disease. In: Straw BE, Zimmermann JJ, D'Allaire S, Taylor DJ, editors. Diseases of swine. Ames: Wiley-Blackwell Publishing; 2006. p. 701–17.
4. Maes D, Segales J, Meyns T, Sibila M, Pieters M, Haesebrouck F. Control of *Mycoplasma hyopneumoniae* infections in pigs. Vet Microbiol. 2008;126:297–309.
5. Fablet C, Marois C, Kuntz-Simon G, Rose N, Dorenlor V, Eono F, et al. Longitudinal study of respiratory infection patterns of breeding sows in five farrow-to-finsh herds. Vet Microbiol. 2011;147:329–39.
6. Del Pozo Sacristán R, Rodríguez AL, Sierens A, Vranckx K, Boyen F, Dereu A, et al. Efficacy of in-feed medication with chlorotetracycline in a farrow-to-finish herd against a clinical outbreak of respiratory disease in fattening pigs. Vet Rec. 2012;171:22–9.
7. Villarreal I, Vranckx K, Duchateau L, Pasmans F, Haesebrouck F, Jensen JC, et al. Early *Mycoplasma hyopneumoniae* infections in European suckling pigs in herds with respiratory problems: detection rate and risk factors. Vet Med-Czech. 2010;55:318–24.
8. Maes D, Deluyker H, Verdonck M, Castryck F, Miry C, Lein A, et al. Effect of vaccination against *Mycoplasma hyopneumoniae* in pig herds with a continuous production system. J Vet Med. 1998;B45:495–505.
9. Maes D, Deluyker H, Verdonck M, Castryck F, Miry C, Vrijens B, et al. Effect of vaccination against *Mycoplasma hyopneumoniae* in pig herds with an all-in/all-out production system. Vaccine. 1999;17:1024–34.
10. Jensen CS, Ersboll AK, Nielsen JP. A meta-analysis comparing the effect of vaccines against *Mycoplasma hyopneumoniae* on daily weight gain in pigs. Prev Vet Med. 2002;54:265–78.

11. Wilson S, Van Brussel L, Saunders G, Taylor L, Zimmermann L, Heinritzi K, et al. Vaccination of piglets at 1 week of age with an inactivated *Mycoplasma hyopneumoniae* vaccine reduces lung lesions and improves average daily gain in body weight. Vaccine. 2012;30:7625–29.
12. Del Pozo Sacristán R, Sierens A, Marchioro SB, Vangroenweghe F, Jourquin J, Labarque G, et al. Efficacy of early *Mycoplasma hyopneumoniae* vaccination against mixed respiratory disease in older fattening pigs. Vet Rec. 2013;174:197–202.
13. Alacron P, Wieland B, Mateus ALP, Dewberry C. Pig farmers' perceptions, attitudes, influences and management of information in the decision-making process for disease control. Prev Vet Med. 2013;116:223–42.
14. Pié S, Lallés JP, Blazy F, Laffitte J, Sève B, Oswald IP. Weaning is associated with an upregulation of expression of inflammatory cytokines in the intestine of piglets. J Nutr. 2004;134:641–47.
15. Campbell JM, Crenshaw JD, Polo J. The biological stress of early weaned piglets. J Anim Sci Biotechnol. 2013;4:19.
16. Chase CCL, Lunney JK. Immune system. In: Zimmerman JJ, Karriker L, Ramirez A, Schwartz K, Stevenson G, editors. Diseases of swine. Ames, IA: Wiley-Blackwell Publishing; 2012. p. 227–50.
17. Whiting TL, Brandt S. Minimum space allowance for transportation of swine by road. Can Vet J. 2002;43:207–12.
18. Lambooij E. Transport of pigs. In: Grandin T, editor. Livestock handling and transport. Wallingford, UK: CAB International; 2012. p. 228–45.
19. Gillespie JR, Flanders FKB. Modern livestock and poultry production. 8th ed. New York: Delmar; 2010.
20. Kick AR, Tompkins MB, Hammer JM, Routh PA, Almond GW. Evaluation of peripheral lymphocytes after weaning and vaccination for *Mycoplasma hyopneumoniae*. Res Vet Sci. 2011;91:68–72.
21. Villarreal I, Maes D, Meyns T, Gebruers F, Calus D, Pasmans F, et al. Infection with a low virulent *Mycoplasma hyopneumoniae* isolate does not protect piglets against subsequent infection with a highly virulent *M. hyopneumoniae* isolate. Vaccine. 2009;27:1875–79.
22. Villarreal I, Maes D, Vranckx K, Calus D, Pasmans F, Haesebrouck F. Effect of vaccination of pigs against experimental infection with high and low virulence *Mycoplasma hyopneumoniae* strains. Vaccine. 2011;29:1731–35.
23. Del Pozo Sacristán R, Thiry J, Vranckx K, Rodríguez AL, Chiers K, Haesebrouck F, et al. Efficacy of florfenicol injection in the treatment of *Mycoplasma hyopneumoniae* induced respiratory disease in pigs. Vet J. 2012;194:420–22.
24. Villarreal I, Vranckx K, Calus D, Pasmans F, Haesebrouck F, Maes D. Effect of challenge of pigs previously immunized with inactivated vaccines containing homologous and heterologous *Mycoplasma hyopneumoniae* strains. BMC Vet Res. 2012;8:2.
25. Meyns T, Dewulf J, De Kruif A, Calus D, Haesebrouck F, Maes D. Comparison of transmission of *Mycoplasma hyopneumoniae* in vaccinated and non-vaccinated populations. Vaccine. 2006;24:7081–86.
26. Vranckx K, Maes D, Marchioro SB, Villarreal I, Chiers K, Pasmans F, et al. Vaccination reduces macrophage infiltration in bronchus-associated lymphoid tissue in pigs infected with a highly virulent *Mycoplasma hyopneumoniae* strain. BMC Vet Res. 2012;8:24.
27. Thacker EL, Thacker BJ, Boettcher T, Jayappa H. Comparison of antibody production, lymphocyte stimulation, and protection induced by four commercial *Mycoplasma hyopneumoniae* bacterins. J Swine Health Prod. 1998;6:107–12.
28. Vicca J, Stakenborg T, Maes D, Butaye P, Peeters J, de Kruif A, et al. Evaluation of virulence of *Mycoplasma hyopneumoniae* field isolates. Vet Microbiol. 2003;97:177–90.
29. Halbur PG, Paul PS, Meng XJ, Lum MA, Andrews JJ, Rathje JA. Comparative pathogenicity of nine US porcine reproductive and respiratory syndrome virus (PRRSV) isolates in a five-week-old cesarean-derived, colostrum-deprived pig model. J Vet Diagn Invest. 1996;8:11–20.
30. Hannan P, Bhogal B, Fish J. Tylosin tartrate and tiamutilin effects on experimental piglet pneumonia induced with pneumonic pig lung homogenate containing mycoplasmas, bacteria and viruses. Res Vet Sci. 1982;33:76–8.
31. Morris CR, Gardner IA, Hietala SK, Carpenter TE. Enzootic pneumonia: comparison of cough and lung lesions as predictors of weight gain in swine. Can J Vet Res. 1995;59:197–204.
32. Kobisch M, Tillon JP, Vannier P, Magueur S, Morvan P. Pneumonie enzootique á *Mycoplasma suipneumoniae* chez le porc: diagnostic rapide et recherché d' anticorps. Rec Med Vet Ec Alfort. 1978;154:847–52.
33. Marois C, Dory D, Fablet C, Madec F, Kobisch M. Development of a quantitative Real-Time TaqMan PCR assay for determination of the minimal dose of *Mycoplasma hyopneumoniae* strain 116 required to induce pneumonia in SPF pigs. J Appl Microbiol. 2010;108:1523–33.

2

Prime-boost vaccination with attenuated *Salmonella* Typhimurium *ΔznuABC* and inactivated *Salmonella* Choleraesuis is protective against *Salmonella* Choleraesuis challenge infection in piglets

Giovanni Loris Alborali[1*†], Jessica Ruggeri[1†], Michele Pesciaroli[2,3], Nicola Martinelli[1], Barbara Chirullo[2], Serena Ammendola[4], Andrea Battistoni[4], Maria Cristina Ossiprandi[5], Attilio Corradi[5] and Paolo Pasquali[2*]

Abstract

Background: *Salmonella enterica* serovar Choleraesuis (*S.* Choleraesuis) infection causes a systemic disease in pigs. Vaccination could represent a solution to reduce prevalence in farms. In this study, we aimed to assess the efficacy of an attenuated strain of *Salmonella enterica* serovar Typhimurium (*S.* Typhimurium *ΔznuABC*) against *S.* Choleraesuis infection. The vaccination protocol combined priming with attenuated *S.* Typhimurium *ΔznuABC* vaccine and boost with an inactivated *S.* Choleraesuis vaccine and we compared the protection conferred to that induced by an inactivated *S.* Choleraesuis vaccine.

Methods: The first group of piglets was orally vaccinated with *S.* Typhimurium *ΔznuABC* and boosted with inactivated *S.* Choleraesuis, the second one was intramuscularly vaccinated with *S.* Choleraesuis inactivated vaccine and the third group of piglets was unvaccinated. All groups of animals were challenged with a virulent *S.* Choleraesuis strain at day 35 post vaccination.

Results: The results showed that the vaccination protocol, priming with *S.* Typhimurium *ΔznuABC* and boosted with inactivated *S.* Choleraesuis, applied to group A was able to limit weight loss, fever and organs colonization, arising from infection with virulent *S.* Choleraesuis, more effectively, than the prime-boost vaccination with homologous *S.* Choleraesuis inactivated vaccine (group B).
(Continued on next page)

* Correspondence: giovanni.alborali@izsler.it; paolo.pasquali@iss.it
†Equal contributors
[1]Istituto Zooprofilattico Sperimentale della Lombardia e dell'Emilia Romagna [Experimental Zooprophylactic Institute of Lombardy and Emilia Romagna], 25124 Brescia, Italy
[2]FAO Reference Center for Veterinary Public Health, Department of Veterinary Public Health and Food Safety, Istituto Superiore di Sanità, 00161 Rome, Italy
Full list of author information is available at the end of the article

(Continued from previous page)

Conclusion: In conclusion, these research findings extend the validity of attenuated *S.* Typhimurium Δ*znuABC* strain as a useful mucosal vaccine against *S.* Typhimurium and *S.* Choleraesuis pig infection. The development of combined vaccination protocols can have a diffuse administration in field conditions because animals are generally infected with different concomitant serovars.

Keywords: Attenuated and inactivated vaccines, Mucosal vaccine, *Salmonella* Choleraesuis, Piglets, Salmonellosis, IFN-gamma

Background

Salmonella enterica serovar Typhimurium (*S.* Typhimurium) and *Salmonella enterica* serovar Choleraesuis (*S.* Choleraesuis) are the main etiological agents of salmonellosis in pigs. The former is responsible for enterocolitis in pigs [1] and zoonotic infections through consumption of contaminated pork products [2]. Conversely, *S.* Choleraesuis induces septicemia, pneumonia, enterocolitis, hepatitis, meningo-encephalitis and abortion in pigs [3], causing significant economic losses in pig industries [1, 4].

The principal tools for controlling typhoid-*Salmonella* are antimicrobials, vaccines, farm management and biosecurity plans. Differently, clinical cases of non-typhoid *Salmonella* are rare and, generally, pigs are sub-clinically infected [5, 6]. Recent monitoring programs had demonstrated that number of *Salmonella* multi-drug-resistant strains (typhoid and non-typhoid) has been incrementing. Antimicrobials are generally used for metaphylaxis or treatment of enterocolitis or other diseases caused by several pathogens in post-weaning phase. This activity has also determined an increment of multidrug strains frequently present in herds without clinical evidence (included *Salmonella* strains). It is also well recognized the ability of these bacteria to acquire drug-resistance from other bacteria by plasmid-transfer. However, due to the diffusion of multi-drug-resistant strains, the further uses of antibiotics is highly discouraged [7]. In alternative, vaccines could be an efficacious solution in reducing shedding of *Salmonella* spp., especially when vaccination is combined with biosecurity strategies [8, 9]. Unfortunately, safe and immunogenic live *Salmonella* attenuated vaccines are limited on the market and their efficacy against heterologous challenge is still not completely known [6, 10].

In recent years we have shown that mutant strains of *S.* Typhimurium, deleted of *znuABC* genes (*S.* Typhimurium Δ*znuABC*) are drastically attenuated and have significant potential as live vaccine [11]. In fact, we have demonstrated that this strain is attenuated and protective in both mouse and pig models of infections, against challenges with *Salmonella* Typhimurium wild type [12–16].

The aim of this study was to assess whether *S.* Typhimurium Δ*znuABC*, boosted with the inactivated *S.* Choleraesuis, is able to exert protective effects versus wild type *S.* Choleraesuis and to compare its efficacy related to that induced by an inactivated *S.* Choleraesuis prime-boost vaccine. We boosted an attenuated *S.* Typhimurium vaccine with an inactivated *S.* Choleraesuis because attenuated vaccines favor T-cell response, which is very highly protective against intracellular bacteria as *Salmonella.* However, it is only partially protective against a typhoid *S.* Choleraesuis infection. For this reason, we boosted with a homologous inactivated vaccine, favoring maturation of affinity of the immune response and, in particular, of B cell, to complete immune response. In this way, antibodies versus all epitopes of this strain were generated, ensuring protection against extracellular bacteria which systemically spread during typhoid-infection.

Methods

Salmonella spp. cultures

As a vaccine strain, we used an attenuated *S.* Typhimurium *ΔznuABC* strain containing a cassette for chloramphenicol resistance inserted in the *znuABC* locus made resistant also to streptomycin by P-22 mediated transduction of *hsdR::spec* allele. Briefly, a fragment containing chloramphenicol resistance cassette was amplified from plasmid pKD3 and electroporated in a *S.* Typhimurium virulent strain (ATCC 14028). Correct insertion was confirmed by inability to grow in a zinc-poor medium and by PCR. Phage P-22 was used to transduce the mutation into a *S.* Typhimurium strain also resistance for streptomycin (transduction of *hsdR::spec* allele) [11].

S. Choleraesuis was cultivated in BHI broth (Reparto produzione Terreni, IZSLER, Brescia) at 37 °C overnight in a fermenter (Sartorius, Biostat Cplus, Italy) and then was inactivated with formaldehyde 0.8% (*v*/v). The final concentration of 2 × 10^{10} CFU/ml was determined by a Cell Density Meter (WPA CO 8000 Biowave Cell Density Meter, Biochrom Ltd., Cambridge, UK) and then absorbed in 10 mg/ml of Aluminum hydroxide. Complete inactivation was confirmed by cultivating an aliquot of prepared vaccine in BHI agar at 37 °C for 48 h. (Vaccine and Reagent Preparation Laboratory of the "Experimental Zooprophylactic Institute of Lombardy and Emilia Romagna", IZSLER).

S. Typhimurium *ΔznuABC* and virulent *S.* Choleraesuis were grown overnight at 37 °C in Brain Heart Infusion (Oxoid Ltd., UK), harvested by centrifugation and then washed twice in ice-cold phosphate buffer solution (PBS) (Sigma–Aldrich, Italy).

Experimental design

Experiments were authorized by the national authorities in accordance with Italian and European regulations (D.lgs 116/1992 implementing the European directive n° 86/609/CEE) and were conducted under the supervision of certified veterinarians.

Eighteen weaned piglets (28 days-old) were housed in the animal facility of the IZSLER, acclimatized for one week before the experiment and checked to be *Salmonella*-free using microbiological and serological analysis. The health-status of the native farm was monitored during last years. Particularly, sows were negative because they did not produce antibodies against a broad range of serogroups (IDEXX Herd-check Swine Salmonella Antibody test kit) and fecal samples, collected during last weeks of pregnancy, were negative for *Salmonella* culture performed in accordance with ISO 6579:2002. Similarly, serum and feces of their piglets, enrolled in this study, were collected a week before movement to test seroconversion and presence of positive culture. Piglets were divided into three groups (6 animals per group).

Vaccines were administered a week after their arrival (35 days-old) following a protocol described below. Group A, vaccinated by oral gavage, with 5×10^7 CFU of *S.* Typhimurium *ΔznuABC* dissolved in 20 ml of sodium bicarbonate buffer, and boosted after two weeks with an intramuscular administration of inactivated *S.* Choleraesuis at the dose of 2×10^9 CFU/ml. Group B was intramuscularly vaccinated with *S.* Choleraesuis inactivated vaccine and boosted after two weeks at the dose of 2×10^9 CFU/ml. Group C was maintained as an unvaccinated naïve control. Fecal samples were collected at 1, 5, 13, 18 and 33 days after vaccination to determine the amount of *S.* Typhimurium *ΔznuABC* attenuated strain.

All groups were challenged, by gavage, with 5×10^8 CFU of *S.* Choleraesuis virulent strain dissolved in 20 ml of sodium bicarbonate buffer, at day 35 from first vaccination. Temperature was measured at 3, 4, 5 and 7 days after infection. Animals were weighed at first vaccination and before necropsy (day 47 from first vaccination). Tonsils, ileocecal lymph nodes, spleen, liver, intestinal content of ileum, cecum, colon and jejunum were collected during necropsy for microbiological analyses and gross lesions of organs were recorded.

Microbiology

Fecal shedding and organ colonization of *S.* Choleraesuis and *S.* Typhimurium *ΔznuABC* were determined using the ISO 6579: 2002/ Amendment 1: 2007 protocol. Samples were weighed and homogenized in 9 parts of Buffered Peptone Water (BPW) (Oxoid Ltd., UK). This solution was first used to perform a Serial Dilution in BPW. All BPW samples (diluted or not) were incubated at 37 °C for 18 ± 3 h. Afterwards, 0.1 ml of BPW cultures were seeded on modified semisolid Rappaport-Vassiliadis agar (MSRV) plates (Oxoid Ltd., UK) and incubated at 41.5 °C for 48 h for selection and enrichment of *Salmonella.* A loopful of culture from an MSRV plate was streaked onto Xylose-Lysine-Deoxycholate Agar (Oxoid Ltd., UK) and Brillant Green Agar (Oxoid Ltd., UK) plates and then incubated at 37 °C overnight. Suspect *Salmonella* colonies were subjected to biochemical identification by BBL Enterotube II (BD Franklin Lakes, NJ USA) and serological identification using *Salmonella* group-specific antisera. XLD agar allows a primary distinction of H_2S+ and H_2S- *Salmonella* strains. This is a semi-quantitative approach consisting in application of the qualitative approach to each ten-fold dilution.

The semi-quantitative approach allows us to establish a range of concentration of *Salmonella* in a sample. This method limits enumeration of *Salmonella* in a sample, but it reduces presence of concomitant bacteria and favors isolation of *Salmonella*. Results express a range of concentration in each sample as reported in Table 1.

Interferon-γ production

At necropsy, ileocecal lymph nodes, draining the site of inoculum, were collected from animals of groups A-C to compare IFN-γ concentration after challenge. Lymph nodes were homogenized by a mortar in fetal calf serum (Gibco Life Technologies, Paisley, UK) + 5% DMSO (Sigma-Aldrich, St.Louis, MO, USA) and filtered with gauze to retain coarse particles. An aliquot of cell suspension was then stored at −80 °C using a proteinase inhibitor (Protease Inhibitor Cocktail kit, Thermo Scientific, Rockford, IL., USA), until use. IFN-γ production was assessed by a sandwich ELISA (Pig Interferon-γ; –IFN-γ, ELISA Kit, Cusabio, P.R. China), in accordance with the manufacturer's instructions. The exact amount of IFN-γ production was then calculated by normalizing the result using total protein content. Total protein content was determined by application of Lambert-Beer Law

Table 1 Semi-quantitative approach for count of *Salmonella*-colonies

Ten-fold dilution positive	results express in	
	LOG_{10}	CFU/g
Negative	0	Negative also after enrichment
$1{:}10^1$	1	1–10 CFU/g
$1{:}10^2$	2	11–100 CFU/g
$1{:}10^3$	3	101–1000 CFU/g
$1{:}10^4$	4	1001–10,000 CFU/g
$1{:}10^5$	5	10,001–100,000 CFU/g
$1{:}10^6$	6	100,001–1,000,000 CFU/g
$1{:}10^7$	7	1,000,001–10,000,000 CFU/g

Results of positive ten-fold dilution are expressed as LOG_{10} and correspond to a range of CFU/g. They represent a semi-quantitative approach to establish concentration in a sample

[17]. In particular, The amount of the tissues after homogenization was standardized by total protein concentration and a specific volume of each homogenate was analyzed by ELISA kit. In conclusion, results were determined by the concentration of cytokine per ng of total protein (pg of IFN-g/ng of total protein).

Serology

The serological examination was performed using a commercial indirect ELISA test capable of detecting antibodies against *Salmonella* serogroups B, C1 and D (Herd-Check Swine Salmonella Antibody Test Kit, IDEXX Laboratories Inc., Switzerland). The test was carried out in accordance with the manufacturer's instructions and analyzed at an optical density of 450 nm. Results were expressed as a sample to positive ratio [S:P ratio = (OD of sample – OD of negative control)/(OD of positive control – OD of negative control)].

Statistical analysis

All statistical analyses were performed using GraphPad Prism (vers. 4.0) software (GraphPad Inc., San Diego, CA, USA). Data related to temperature and antibody titers were analyzed using Two-Way ANOVA and completed with the Bonferroni post-test. Data related to organ colonization were analyzed using the Kruskal–Wallis test (non-parametric one-way analysis of variance – ANOVA) and completed with the Dunn's Multiple Comparison post-test. A *P*-value <0.05 was considered to indicate statistically significant differences.

Results

S. Typhimurium *ΔznuABC* strain is not detectable in feces 18 days after vaccination

Firstly, we wanted to reconfirm the safety and the limited environmental contamination of attenuated *S.* Typhimurium *ΔznuABC*. For this reason, fecal samples were weekly collected after vaccination in animals of group A, to estimate the amount of *S.* Typhimurium *ΔznuABC* (Fig. 1). Fecal samples were also collected in animals of groups B and C, but these animals did not shed *Salmonella* spp. (data not shown). The attenuated strain was shed up to 18 days after vaccination and the number of shedder pigs and the concentration of bacteria sharply decreased from vaccination and thereafter.

Combined vaccination protocol reduces clinical symptoms induced by *S.* Choleraesuis infection

We analyzed the efficacy of vaccination, considering the clinical, microbiological and immunological parameters influenced by a *S.* Choleraesuis infection.

The mean temperatures of the three groups are shown in Fig. 2. Overall, irrespective to the treatment, piglets challenged with the wild-type strain of *Salmonella* Choleraesuis showed a raise of body temperature which tend to drop back down to baseline one week after infection.

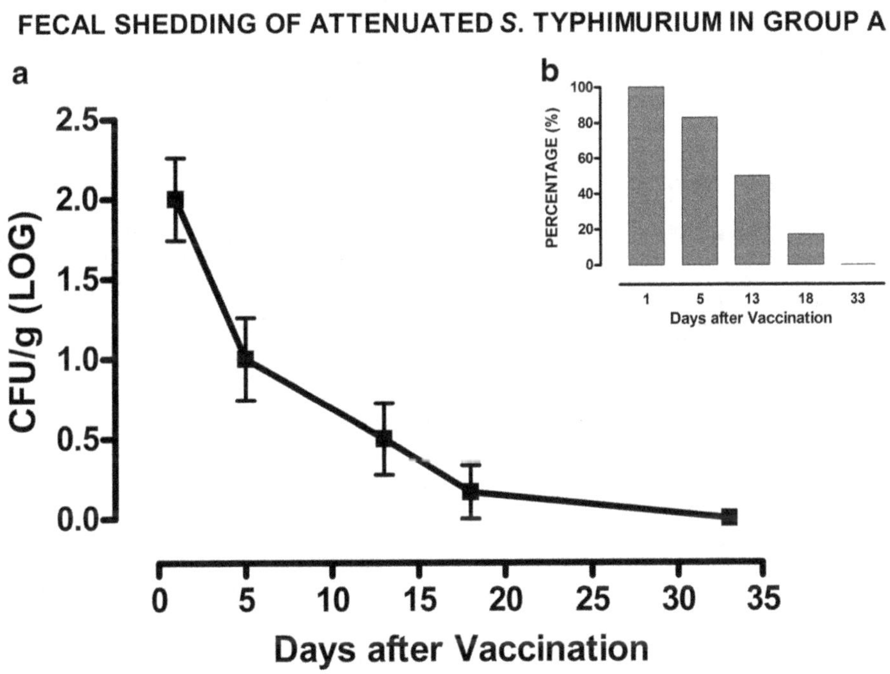

Fig. 1 Attenuated *S.* Typhimurium *ΔznuABC* is not detectable from day 18 after vaccination. In **a**, symbols depict the mean concentration of *S.* Typhimurium *ΔznuABC* (expressed as LOG_{10} CFU/g) in group A at different time points (day 1, 5, 13, 18, 33 after vaccination). Bars represent the standard deviation. In **b**, columns represent the percentage of shedder piglets of group A at different time-points. *S.* Typhimurium *ΔznuABC* is not detectable from day 18 after vaccination. Group B and C are not shown because negative. Depicted microbiological results derived from the semi-quantitative approach

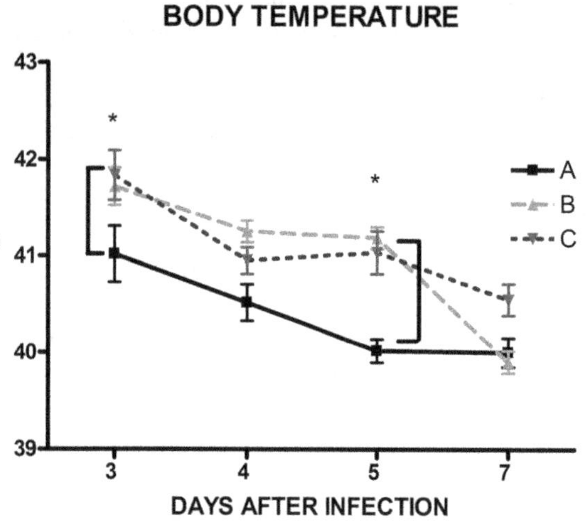

Fig. 2 Vaccination with attenuated *S.* Typhimurium Δ*znuABC* prevents fever. Body temperature of groups A, B and C is shown at different time points (day 3, 4, 5 and 7 after challenge). Symbols represent mean and bars standard deviation. Symbols (*) represent differences statistically significant among groups with $p < 0.01$

Nevertheless, we observed that the raise of body temperature of group B and C was higher than that of group A, especially at 3 and 5 days after infection ($p < 0.05$).

We further compared the weight gain from vaccination to the killing to assess if different protocols of vaccination could influence the weight gain. As depicted in Fig. 3, we did not record any difference among groups throughout the observation in terms of weight gain.

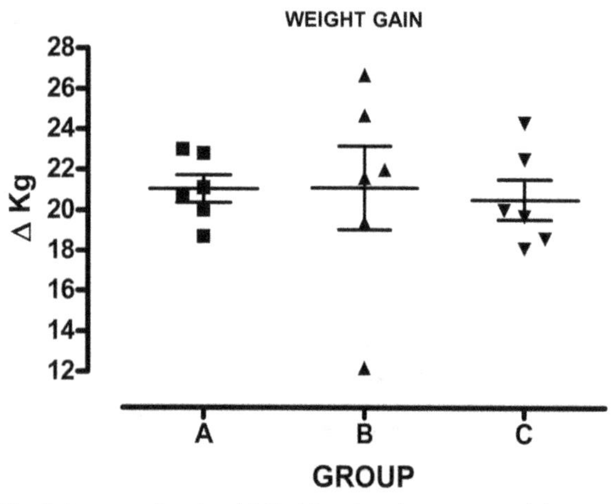

Fig. 3 Attenuated strain of *S.* Typhimurium does not retard the weight gain of piglets. Symbols represent the weight gain of eighteen animals, divided into groups A, B and C, while vertical bars represent the standard deviation from the beginning to the end of the study (day 0 and 47). No differences are recorded. The weight of animals vaccinated with the attenuated strain of *S.* Typhimurium is not different from other groups

Combined vaccination protocol significantly reduces organ colonization after challenge infection with virulent *S.* Choleraesuis

Organ colonization tested at 12 days after challenge was low and barely detectable in many organs. Tonsils, spleen, liver and intestinal content of jejunum were colonized only in a very limited percentage (data not shown). Organs which showed the most reliable colonization were cecum and ileocecal lymph nodes (Fig. 4). Overall, we observed that piglets of group A, treated with combined vaccination protocol (oral administration of attenuated *S.* Typhimurium Δ*znuABC* vaccine boosted after two weeks with an intramuscular injection of inactivated *S.* Choleraesuis), showed a reduction of *Salmonella* Choleraesuis colonization and that inactivated vaccine, administered to piglets of group B, did not exert an analogous effect. In particular, cecum colonization of group A was statistically different from group B and C, and ileocecal lymph nodes colonization of group A was significantly lower than group B.

Combined vaccination protocol induces both innate and humoral immunity in response to a *S.* Choleraesuis challenge infection

We estimated the response induced by vaccination and infection, by analyzing IFN-γ and humoral response. At day 47 after the first vaccination (i.e. 12 days after the challenge infection), IFN-γ was produced in a higher concentration in the ileocecal lymph nodes from piglets of group C compared to those from piglets of vaccinated groups (Fig. 5). In particular, IFN-γ concentration was approximately 0.02 ng/ml in group C and the difference was statistically significant when compared to the concentration in group A. On the contrary, the concentration of IFN-γ in leukocytes of group B was not statistically different from that in group C.

Antibody response was monitored after vaccination and after challenge in all groups of piglets enrolled in this study. Vaccinated piglets of group A and B had a humoral response starting from the first week after vaccination, with an increasing of s/p ratio (OD) thereafter; in group C, on the other hand, the response started after infection. Humoral responses were similar between the two vaccinated groups and the differences observed were statistically significant when comparing the group A to C (Fig. 6).

Discussion

Salmonellosis is a public health problem primarily caused by consumption of pork products contaminated with *S.* Typhimurium [2]. On the contrary, *S.* Choleraesuis, a host-adapted serovar in pigs, causes a typhoid-like disease in piglets, which is characterized by reduced growth and, in the most severe cases, a high mortality rate, and hence mainly representing an economic problem [1, 18]. *S.* Choleraesuis is not considered to be a major agent of zoonotic

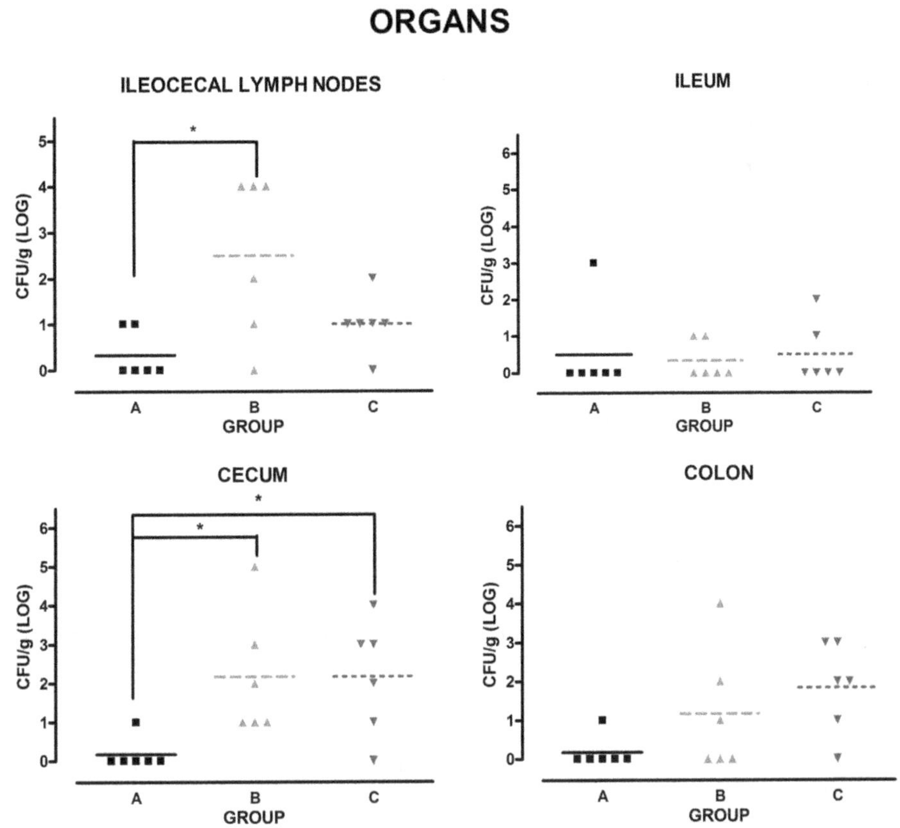

Fig. 4 S. Typhimurium Δ*znuABC* vaccine reduces organ colonization. Amount of S. Choleraesuis in lymph nodes, ileum, cecum and colon of group A-C piglets was determined 12 days after challenge. Depicted microbiological results derived from the semi-quantitative approach. Each symbol represents microbiological results obtained from each animal and each bar represents mean concentration. Differences are statistically significant in cecum between group A and the other groups ($p < 0.05$) and in lymph nodes between group A and B

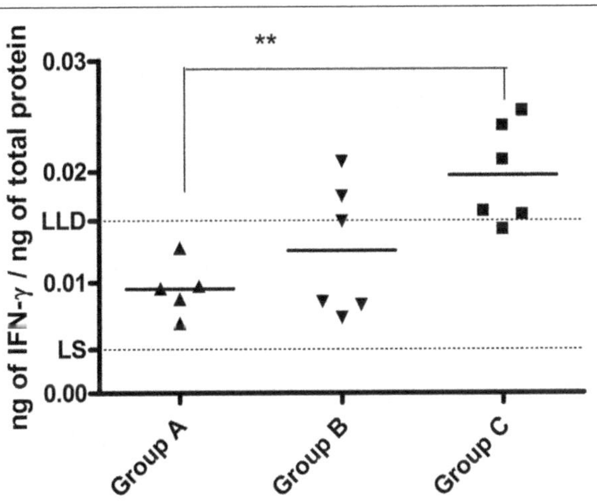

Fig. 5 S. Choleraesuis challenge infection induces IFN-ɣ production. Symbols and bars represent piglets and IFN-ɣ mean concentration, respectively. Concentration of IFN-ɣ was normalized in relation to total protein content. Difference was statistically significant between the unvaccinated group (C) and group A vaccinated with the attenuated strain ** ($p < 0.05$). LLD indicates Lower Limit of Detection (15.6 pg/ml); LS indicates Limit of Sensitivity (minimum detectable dose, 3.9 pg/ml)

infections, although some cases of human infection have been recorded, especially in Asia [8].

Vaccination of pigs could represent a valid control system in countries with a high prevalence of salmonellosis in animals. Attenuated vaccines are more effective than inactivated ones in protecting against enteric diseases, due to their ability to induce cell-mediated and mucosal immunity [19]. To address this issue, in previous study we assessed the safety and efficacy of S. Typhimurium *ΔznuABC* strain in different models of infection [11 16]. In the current work, an attenuated S. Typhimurium *ΔznuABC* boosted with an inactivated S. Choleraesuis vaccine was compared to an inactivated S. Choleraesuis vaccine in providing immune-based protection against a S. Choleraesuis challenge infection.

The cross-protection had already been investigated in a mouse challenge infection [12], suggesting that S. Typhimurium *ΔznuABC* is able to induce partial protection against heterologous challenge with S. Choleraesuis. We therefore set up a new vaccination protocol based on an oral vaccination with attenuated S. Typhimurium

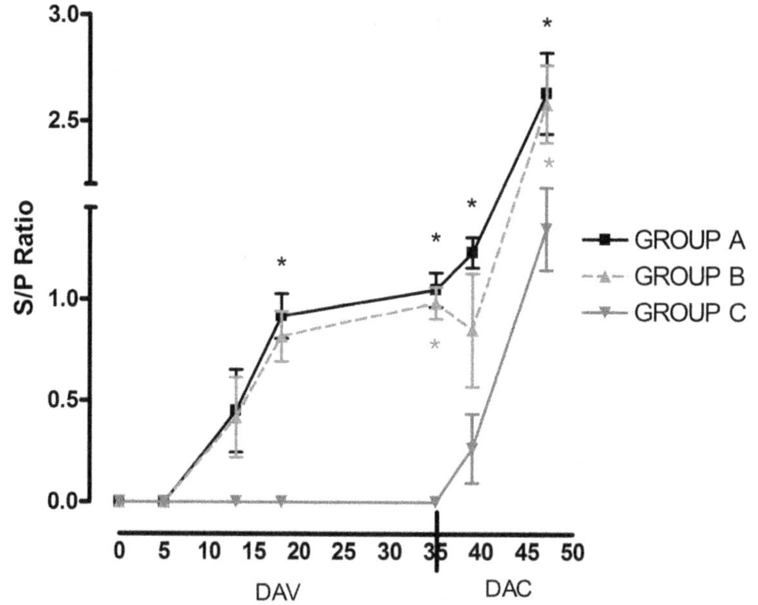

Fig. 6 Attenuated *S.* Typhimurium Δ*znuABC* vaccine and inactivated *S.* Choleraesuis vaccine induce antibody production. Symbols and bars represent mean and standard deviation of s/p ratio in 3 groups, respectively. The pattern of humoral immunity is similar between group A (vaccinated with Attenuated *S.* Typhimurium Δ*znuABC*) and in group B (vaccinated with killed *S.* Choleraesuis). The X-axis is divided into two segments to differentiate between antibody response after vaccination (DAV) and challenge (DAC). Differences are statistically significant between vaccinated piglets with attenuated strain and unvaccinated piglets from day 18 after vaccination. On the contrary, differences are statistically different between vaccinated piglets with inactivated strain and unvaccinated piglets only at day 35 and 47 after vaccination. Gray star indicates significant difference between groups B and C, while black star indicates significant difference between group A and C

ΔznuABC followed by an intramuscular boost with an inactivated *S.* Choleraesuis vaccine after two weeks.

As control groups, piglets were vaccinated and boosted with inactivated *S.* Choleraesuis vaccine or were kept as naïve unvaccinated ones. Attenuated vaccines induce a more effective T-cell involvement against facultative intracellular bacteria, such as *Salmonella* [20, 21]. We hypothesized that, a boost with an inactivated vaccine may favor the maturation of affinity of the immune response and the production of mucosal and serum antibodies against somatic antigens, thus completing the host immune response and enhancing the efficacy of the attenuated strain. The shedding pattern of *S.* Typhimurium *ΔznuABC* was characterized by a sharp decline within few days and then it was not detectable in feces after five weeks. Those data corroborate findings and data previously published that showed a limited and self-limiting persistence of *S.* Typhimurium *ΔznuABC* [14–16]. We found that, when challenged with virulent *S.* Choleraesuis, piglets vaccinated with the prime-boost protocol with attenuated *S.* Typhimurium *ΔznuABC* and inactivated *S.* Choleraesuis vaccine showed a lower increase in body temperature compared to the other groups. In this study, we observed a modest colonization of organs which suggests that the employed *Salmonella* Choleraesuis strain is not highly virulent and/or that it needs more time or different condition to develop the acute form. Nonetheless, cecum colonization of group A was lower than colonization of groups B and C, whilst ileocecal lymph nodes colonization was lower only in comparison to group B.

These findings suggest that this combined vaccination protocol is able to exert protection, while prime-boost vaccination with inactivated *S.* Choleraesuis vaccine does not curb the progression of infection and organ colonization. These data support the hypothesis that vaccination with the attenuated *S.* Typhimurium *ΔznuABC*, previously investigated as safe and effective against *S.*Typhimurium [14–16], followed by boost with inactivated *S.* Choleraesuis vaccine could decrease the number of pigs carrying different serovars of *Salmonella* in field conditions.

Studies focused on the heterologous protection have previously been published. Schwarz et al. [22] demonstrated that an attenuated strain of *S.* Choleraesuis reduced the prevalence of *Salmonella* in carrier pigs at the slaughterhouse. This attenuated strain was used on a farm infected with *S.* Brandenburg, *S.*Typhimurium and *S.* Agona. Moreover, cross-protection was also documented between host-specific strains. House et al. [23] demonstrated that an attenuated *S.* Choleraesuis vaccine, licensed for swine, was more efficacious than an autogenous *Salmonella* bacterin in pregnant cows infected with *S.* Montevideo. We can infer that there is an overlap between antigenic determinants that induce protection. Other studies, however, should be performed to identify the common virulence factors of different serovars involved in animal salmonellosis. This knowledge is necessary to develop an efficacious multivalent *Salmonella* vaccine.

To better understand the protection induced by vaccination, we analyzed host response after challenge, considering IFN-γ and antibody production. IFN-γ was chosen as a paradigmatic cytokine for a Th1 cell mediated immune response which is known to be involved in the control of *Salmonella* infection. Particularly, IFN-γ is an important cytokine produced by natural killer cells (NK) and T-cells, in response to phagocytosis of *Salmonella* by macrophages and other antigen presenting cells (APC) during the earlier phase of its systemic dissemination [19, 24]. In our study, the concentration of IFN-γ in groups A and B was lower than that of group C, at day 12 after infection suggesting that IFN-γ production is a marker of the host response, as reported previously [15]. Moreover, we obtained a seroconversion of piglets one week after vaccination that significantly increase after challenge with virulent *S.* Choleraesuis. These results are in line with the study of Husa et al. [25] that compared the safety, cross-protection and serological response of two commercial live *S.* Choleraesuis in response to experimental challenge infection with *S.* Typhimurium. *S.* Choleraesuis vaccines, indeed, induced a humoral response characterized by an increase in antibody titers after vaccination, which rapidly rose after challenge with the heterologous strain.

Conclusion

In conclusion, we produce scientific evidence that a vaccination protocol, characterized by combination of attenuated and inactivated vaccines of *S.* Typhimurium and *S.* Choleraesuis, is effective against challenge infection with *S.* Choleraesuis. In perspective, these data suggest that it is could be possible to develop new effective vaccine strategies for the treatment of animals simultaneously infected by different serovar of *Salmonella*, a condition that commonly occurs in field conditions.

Abbreviations

ANOVA: Analysis of variance; BPW: Buffered peptone water; CFU: Colony Forming Unit; DMSO: DiMethyl sulfoxide; IFN-γ: Interferon-gamma; IZSLER: Istituto Zooprofilattico Sperimentale della Lombardia e dell'Emilia Romagna [Experimental Zooprophylactic Institute of Lombardy and Emilia Romagna]; ml: milliliter; MSRV: Modified semisolid rappaport vassiliadis agar; ng: nanogram; NK: Natural killer cells; OD: Optical density; PBS: Phosphate buffer solution; XLD: Xylose-lysine-deoxycholate agar

Acknowledgements

Special thanks to Staff of the animal facilities for their dedication and to Studio Moretto for the English writing assistance. The research by Pesciaroli Michele was partly supported by a PICATA postdoctoral contract of the Moncloa Campus of International Excellence (UCM-UPM, Campus Moncloa, VISAVET).

Funding

The research study was supported by internal funding of IZSLER.

Authors' contributions

GLA: Designed experimental approach; performed experimental design; analyzed data. JR: Performed experimental design and microbiological and serological analyses; analyzed results; drafted manuscript. MP: Performed experimental design and analyses; analyzed results; drafted manuscript. NM: Performed experimental design. BC: Performed serological and immunological analyses; analyzed results; contributed to draft manuscript. SA: Performed experimental design and analyses; contributed to draft manuscript. AB: Designed experimental approach; analyzed results; contributed to draft manuscript. MCO: Designed experimental approach; performed experimental design. AC: Designed experimental approach; performed experimental design. PP: Designed experimental approach; performed experimental design; analyzed data, contributed to draft manuscript. All authors read and approved the final manuscript.

Consent for publication

Not applicable.

Competing interests

The authors declare that they have no competing interests.

Author details

[1]Istituto Zooprofilattico Sperimentale della Lombardia e dell'Emilia Romagna [Experimental Zooprophylactic Institute of Lombardy and Emilia Romagna], 25124 Brescia, Italy. [2]FAO Reference Center for Veterinary Public Health, Department of Veterinary Public Health and Food Safety, Istituto Superiore di Sanità, 00161 Rome, Italy. [3]UCM-UPM, Campus Moncloa, Madrid, Spain. [4]Department of Biology, Università di Roma Tor Vergata, 00133 Rome, Italy. [5]Department of Veterinary Sciences, University of Parma, Parma, Italy.

References

1. Foley SL, Lynne AM, Nayak R. *Salmonella* challenges: prevalence in swine and poultry and potential pathogenicity of such isolates1,2J Anim Sci. Apr. 2008;86:E149–62. Epub 2007 Oct 2. Review
2. EFSA. Trends and sources of zoonoses and zoonotic agents and food-borne outbreaks in the European Union in 2008. EFSA J. 2010;8(1):1496.
3. Ku YW, McDonough SP, Palaniappan RU, Chang CF, Chang YF. Novel attenuated *Salmonella enterica* serovar Choleraesuis strains as live vaccine candidates generated by signature-tagged mutagenesis. Infect Immun. 2005;73:8194–203.
4. Selke M, Meens J, Springer S, Frank R, Gerlach GF. Immunization of pigs to prevent disease in humans: construction and protective efficacy of a *Salmonella enterica* serovar Typhimurium live negative-marker vaccine. Infect Immun. 2007;75:2476–83.
5. Wales AD, Cook AJ, Davies RH. Producing *Salmonella*-free pigs: a review focusing on interventions at weaning. Vet Rec. 2011;168:267–76.
6. De Busser EV, De Zutter L, Dewulf J, Houf K, Maes D. *Salmonella* control in live pigs and at slaughter. Vet J. 2013;196:20–7.
7. Glenn MN, Lindsey RL, Frank JF, Meinersmann RJ, Englen MD, Fedorka-Cray PJ, Frye JG. Analysis of antimicrobial resistance genes detected in multidrug-resistant *Salmonella enterica* serovar Typhimurium isolated from food animals.. Crit rev Microbiol. 2013; 39:57-69. Microb Drug Resist. 2011;17(3):407–18.
8. Haneda T, Okada N, Kikuchi Y, Takagi M, Kurotaki T, Miki T, Arai S, Danbara H. Evaluation of *Salmonella enterica* serovar Typhimurium and Choleraesuis slyA mutant strains for use in live attenuated oral vaccines. Comp Immunol Microbiol Infect Dis. 2011;34:399–409.
9. Wilhelm B, Rajic A, Parker S, Waddell L, Sanchez J, Fazil A, Wilkins W, McEwen S. Assessment of the efficacy and quality of evidence for five on-farm interventions for *Salmonella* reduction in grow-finish swine: a systematic review and meta-analysis. Prev Vet Med. 2012;107:1–20.
10. Foss DL, Agin TS, Bade D, Dearwester DA, Jolie R, Keich RL, Lohse RM, Reed M, Rosey EL, Schneider PA, Taylor LP, Willy MS. Protective immunity to

Salmonella enterica is partially serogroup specific. Vet Immunol Immunopathol. 2013;155:76–86.
11. Ammendola S, Pasquali P, Pistoia C, Petrucci P, Petrarca P, Rotilio G, Battistoni A. High-affinity Zn2+ uptake system ZnuABC is required for bacterial zinc homeostasis in intracellular environments and contributes to the virulence of *Salmonella enterica*. Infect Immun. 2007;75:5867–76.
12. Pasquali P, Ammendola S, Pistoia C, Petrucci P, Tarantino M, Valente C, Marenzoni ML, Rotilio G, Battistoni A. Attenuated *Salmonella enterica* serovar Typhimurium lacking the ZnuABC transporter confers immune-based protection against challenge infections in mice. Vaccine. 2008;26:3421–6.
13. Pesciaroli M, Aloisio F, Ammendola S, Pistoia C, Petrucci P, Tarantino M, Francia M, Battistoni A, Pasquali P. An attenuated *Salmonella enterica* serovar Typhimurium strain lacking the ZnuABC transporter induces protection in a mouse intestinal model of *Salmonella* infection. Vaccine. 2011;29:1783–90.
14. Pesciaroli M, Gradassi M, Martinelli N, Ruggeri J, Pistoia C, Raffatellu M, Magistrali CF, Battistoni A, Pasquali P, Alborali GL. *Salmonella* Typhimurium lacking the ZnuABC transporter is attenuated and immunogenic in pigs. Vaccine. 2013;31:2868–73.
15. Gradassi M, Pesciaroli M, Martinelli N, Ruggeri J, Petrucci P, Hassan WH, Raffatellu M, Scaglione FE, Ammendola S, Battistoni A, Alborali GL, Pasquali P. Attenuated *Salmonella enterica* serovar Typhimurium lacking the ZnuABC transporter: an efficacious orally-administered mucosal vaccine against salmonellosis in pigs. Vaccine. 2013;31:3695–701.
16. Ruggeri J, Pesciaroli M, Gaetarelli B, Scaglione FE, Pregel P, Ammendola S, Battistoni A, Bollo E, Alborali GL, Pasquali P. Parenteral administration of attenuated *Salmonella* Typhimurium Δ*znuABC* is protective against salmonellosis in piglets. Vaccine. 2014;32:4032–8.
17. Rodger A. Concentration Determination Using Beer-Lambert Law. In: Roberts GCK, editor. Encyclopedia of Biophysics. Berlin: Springer Berlin Heidelberg; 2012. p. 360–1.
18. Schwartz KJ. Salmonellosis. In: Straw BE, D'Allaire S, Mengeling WL, Taylor DJ, editors. Diseases of swine. 8th ed. Ames, Iowa: Iowa State University Press; 1999. p. 535–51.
19. Mastroeni P, Chabalgoity JA, Dunstan SJ, Maskell DJ, Dougan G. *Salmonella*: Immune response and vaccines. Vet J. 2000;161:132–64.
20. Wallis TS. *Salmonella* pathogenesis and immunity: we need effective multivalent vaccines. Vet J. 2001;161:104–6.
21. Haesebrouck F, Pasmans F, Chiers K, Maes D, Ducatelle R, Decostere A. Efficacy of vaccines against bacterial diseases in swine: what can we expect? Vet Microbiol. 2004;100:255–68.
22. Schwarz P, Kich JD, Kolb J, Cardoso M. Use of an avirulent live *Salmonella* Choleraesuis vaccine to reduce the prevalence of *Salmonella* carrier pigs at slaughter. Vet Rec. 2011;169:553.
23. House JK, Ontiveros MM, Blackmer NM, Dueger EL, Fitchhorn JB, McArthur GR, Smith BP. Evaluation of an autogenous *Salmonella* bacterin and a modified live *Salmonella* serotype Choleraesuis vaccine on a commercial dairy farm. Am J Vet Res. 2001;62:1897–902.
24. Lalmanach AC, Lantier F. Host cytokine response and resistance to *Salmonella* infection. Microbes Infect. 1999;1:719–26.
25. Husa JA, Edler RA, Walter DH, Holck JT, Saltzman RJ. A comparison of the safety, cross-protection, and serologic response associated with two commercial oral *Salmonella* vaccines in swine. J Swine Health Prod. 2009;17:10–21.

3

DISCONTOOLS: a database to identify research gaps on vaccines, pharmaceuticals and diagnostics for the control of infectious diseases of animals

Declan O'Brien[1*], Jim Scudamore[2], Johannes Charlier[3] and Morgane Delavergne[1]

Abstract

Background: The public and private sector in the EU spend around €800 million per year on animal health and welfare related research. An objective process to identify critical gaps in knowledge and available control tools should aid the prioritisation of research in order to speed up the development of new or improved diagnostics, vaccines and pharmaceuticals and reduce the burden of animal diseases.

Method: Here, we describe the construction of a database based on expert consultation for 52 infectious diseases of animals.

Results: For each disease, an expert group produced a disease and product analysis document that formed the basis for gap analysis and prioritisation. The prioritisation model was based on a closed scoring system, employing identical weights for six evaluation criteria (disease knowledge; impact on animal health and welfare; impact on public health; impact on wider society; impact on trade; control tools). The diseases were classified into three groups: epizootic diseases, food-producing animal complexes or zoonotic diseases.

Discussion: The highly ranked diseases in the prioritisation model comprised mostly zoonotic and epizootic diseases with important gaps identified in vaccine development and pharmaceuticals, respectively. The most important outcome is the identification of key research needs by disease. The rankings and research needs by disease are provided on a public website (www.discontools.eu) which is currently being updated based on new expert consultations.

Conclusion: As such, it can become a reference point for funders of research including the European Commission, member states, foundations, trusts along with private industry to prioritise research. This will deliver benefits in terms of animal health and welfare but also public health, societal benefits and a safe and secure food supply.

Keywords: Prioritisation, Animal disease, Research needs, EU

Background

Animal diseases are estimated to reduce the production of animal products by at least 20% according to the World Organisation for Animal Health (OIE) [1]. As such, the prevention and control of animal diseases has benefits in terms of animal health and welfare but also human health where zoonoses are concerned and broad societal benefits in terms of companion animal health and the security of a safe food supply.

In terms of funding, it is estimated that the public sector spends €400 million per year in Europe on animal health and welfare related research [2, 3] and the private sector spends €400 million per year on animal health research [4]. With about €800 million being spent per year, the added value of an objective process to prioritise critical research can be appreciated. By focusing a proportion of this expenditure on critical gaps in priority diseases, it will be possible to speed up the development and delivery of new and improved disease control tools including diagnostics, vaccines and pharmaceuticals to reduce the burden of disease on animals. Given that the current value of animal based products at producer prices in the E.U. is €154 billion per year [5], every percentage

* Correspondence: declanjobrien@hotmail.com
[1]International Federation for Animal Health Europe, Avenue de Tervueren 168, box 81150 Brussels, Belgium
Full list of author information is available at the end of the article

reduction in the impact of animal disease on production would be of major economic importance.

During the work of the European Technology Platform for Global Animal Health (ETPGAH)[1] from 2004 to 2012, it was recognised that disease prioritisation was one of the most important initiatives that needed to be undertaken to focus and prioritise research [6]. This work necessitates the identification of gaps in knowledge as well as control tools – diagnostics, vaccines and pharmaceuticals.

The DISCONTOOLS project was funded under the EU 7th framework programme from 2008 to 2013 and originated from the Action Plan of the ETPGAH. The general objective of the project was to evaluate global animal health priorities and the risk they could pose to the European Union. This understanding would assist in ensuring the most effective allocation of research funding. The project led to the development of a disease database containing a gap analysis and prioritisation model for 52 infectious diseases of animals. The objective of this paper is to describe the different steps in the development of the database (Section Construction and content), describe its utility (Section Utility) and discuss how it could assist policy makers in targeting research funding (Section Discussion). It should be noted that the focus of the database is on research needs with respect to control tools in the form of diagnostics, vaccines and pharmaceuticals. It does not necessarily consider disease control strategies or other aspects of disease control such as disease modelling, surveillance and regulatory support.

Methods

General approach

The DISCONTOOLS project was organised as shown in Fig. 1. All European and Global organisations with an interest in animal health research were invited to join the Stakeholder Forum. It included organisations ranging from farmers, veterinarians and the pharmaceutical industry to chief veterinary officers, research institutes and related projects funded by the European Commission. The Project Management Board (PMB) comprised 10 representatives from the Stakeholders selected to represent research, industry, users and public bodies. The membership is listed in Table 1.

Five work packages or working groups were established each reporting to the PMB. Of these two working groups one on disease prioritisation, the other on gap analysis were involved in developing the database (See Fig. 1). Membership of the two working groups consisted of approximately 15 people and was by invitation along with nominations from the stakeholders and interested parties. It was important that each of the groups was balanced with members with appropriate expertise from research, industry, users (including farming and veterinary profession) and regulators as well as the European Commission and international organisations.

The development of the database was preceded by a review of existing processes for prioritisation and gap analysis by the PMB in order to steer the methodology adopted. Subsequently, the disease list was selected and prioritisation methodology developed, followed by expert opinion elicitation to provide content to the database. The prioritisation methodology was subdivided in the development of Disease & Product analysis document (D&P), a prioritisation model and gap analysis model.

Review of existing prioritisation models

A worldwide review of existing models was carried out. In public health, a number of studies have methodically prioritised communicable diseases and pathogens [7–15]. In the field of animal health, most studies have focused on

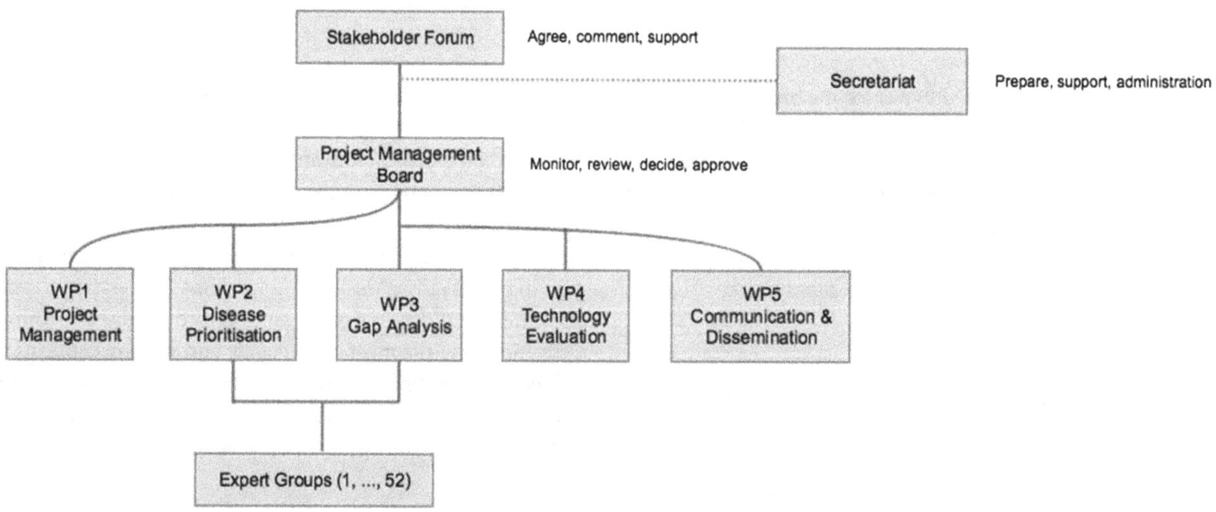

Fig. 1 Organisation of the DISCONTOOLS project

Table 1 Organisations represented in the Project Management Board of DISCONTOOLS

Organisation	Description
Copa-Cogeca	European union for agricultural organisations and cooperatives
CVO's	Chief Veterinary Officers
DG Research	Directorate-General for Research and Innovation of the European Commission
EAEVE	European Association of Establishments for Veterinary Education
EMIDA ERA-net	Coordination platform of research on emerging infectious diseases of animals
EMVD	European Manufacturers of Veterinary Diagnostics
EPIZONE	International network of veterinary research institutes working on epizootic animal diseases
FVE	Federation of Veterinarians of Europe
HMA	Heads of Medicines Agencies
IFAH-Europe	International Federation for Animal Health Europe
MEDVETNET	European Network of Excellence for Zoonoses Research
OIE	World organisation for animal health

prioritisation of food-borne and zoonotic pathogens [13, 16–20]. In addition, studies have also been conducted with the specific aims of prioritising surveillance of wildlife pathogens [21], disease control for poverty alleviation [22], non-regulatory animal health issues [23] and exotic diseases and emerging animal health threats [24, 25].

Although methodological approaches differ, priority-setting studies typically follow a series of steps: (i) selecting a group of diseases/pathogens for prioritization; (ii) identifying a list of appropriate and measurable criteria to assess diseases/pathogens; (iii) defining a range of levels for each criterion; (iv) determining the relative importance by means of a weight or score for each level and criterion; (v) aggregating to produce an overall score for each disease/pathogen; and (vi) ranking diseases/pathogens by their overall score to derive a recommended list for prioritization [26]. It was evident that risk-based priority-setting should be systematic, flexible, reproducible and informative to public policy. The criteria must be explicit, measurable, relevant and objective wherever possible. However, the methodology and criteria required will depend on the goal of prioritisation, so a clear definition of the aim is essential. The priority-setting process should be transparent and open to discussion and revision. In addition, it is considered preferable to define a disease as specifically as possible (e.g. brucellosis of cattle versus brucellosis in general) and to consider how the model can evolve over time in order to remain of value. On the basis of the review, and considering the goal of DISCONTOOLS, i.e. identifying research needs of infectious animal diseases in the EU, the main steps which have been followed include establishing a list of relevant infectious diseases and gathering relevant information on each disease. It was considered essential that the scoring system allows diseases to be ranked based on total scores and/or on scores for particular criteria (e.g. impact on public health).

Establishment of disease list

The working groups of the DISCONTOOLS project were created by inviting stakeholders to become involved in WP2, WP3 and/or WP4 with the PMB taking care of WP1 and WP5 (see Fig. 1). In parallel, the PMB invited an expert to Chair each of WP2, WP3 and WP4. The WPs then established a list of 52 priority diseases to be included in the prioritisation exercise. The starting point for the list of diseases was from the Action Plan of the ETPGAH which referred to 47 diseases. In addition, it was considered important not to lose sight of endemic diseases or disease syndromes (e.g. internal parasites, mastitis). Therefore, 3 groups of diseases were defined as follows:

(1) epizootic diseases: infectious diseases which pose a risk for introduction or spread in the EU and for which tools for optimum detection, surveillance and control would be beneficial;
(2) food producing animal complexes: major enzootic diseases of livestock in Europe;
(3) zoonotic diseases: infectious diseases of animals that are important for human health and for their socio-economic effects.

The geographic dimension of the project was primarily European. Naturally, where a disease was not present in Europe, a global perspective was taken into account. The expert groups were asked to highlight and take into account strains and species where the economic impact was the highest not only in Europe, but worldwide.

After discussions of the working groups of DISCONTOOLS a final list of 52 diseases was agreed. The list was not considered to be exhaustive, but representative of most disease scenarios. Infectious diseases of aquatic animals or companion animals without a zoonotic implication were not considered.

Results

Prioritisation methodology

Disease and product analysis document

A D&P was developed for each disease by the working groups of the DISCONTOOLS project in order to have key information available prior to scoring of the different criteria. The D&P is a reference document that provides the detailed and relevant information for each disease which is necessary to support the scoring for the prioritisation and gap analysis models. It contains 23 main sections with sub-headings covering a wide range of aspects such as description and characteristics of the disease, route of transmission, zoonotic potential, control tools available, and socio-economic impact. The full list of sections may be consulted at www.discontools.eu/diseases under the custom report section. For each section, an additional column headed "Gaps identified" was included in the D&P to gather further information on the gaps in knowledge and products of each disease. The document was completed by the expert groups who were asked to reach a consensus on the final text which was then reviewed by the PMB.

Prioritisation model

The criteria, levels within each of the criteria, scores and weighting coefficients that were used in the prioritisation model can be viewed in Table 2. Six criteria were considered:

Table 2 The prioritisation model: criteria considered, levels within the criteria, scores and applied weighting coefficients (Coef)

Criteria	Scores					Coef	Total (score*coef)
Disease knowledge	0	1	2	3	4	2.5	/100
1. Speed of spread							
2. Number of species involved							
3. Persistence of infectious agent in the environment							
4. Risk of spread to susceptible populations							
5. Potential for silent spread							
6. Wildlife reservoir and potential spread							
7. Vector reservoir and potential spread							
8. Variability of the agent							
9. Understanding of fundamental immunology							
10. Host pathogen interaction							
Impact on animal health and welfare	0	1	2	3	4	8.33	/100
1. Disease impact on production							
2. Duration of animal welfare impact							
3. Proportion of animals affected and suffering pain/injury/distress as a result of the disease							
Impact on public health – human health	0	1	2	3	4	4.16	/100
1. Impact of occurrence on human health							
2. Likelihood of occurrence							
3. Impact of occurrence on food safety							
4. Transmissibility (spread from animals to humans)							
5. Spread in humans							
6. Bioterrorism potential							
Impact on wider society	0	1	2	3	4	8.33	/100
1. Economic direct impact (including cumulative cost, e.g. enzootic vs. epizootic)							
2. Economic indirect impact (social, market)							
3. Agriterrorism potential							
Impact on trade	0	1	2	3	4	6.25	/100
1. Impact on international trade due to existing regulations							
2. Impact on EC trade due to existing regulations							
3. Potential for regionalisation							
4. Impact on security of food supply							
Control tools	+2	+1	0	−1	−2	16.66	/100
1. Appropriate diagnostics							
2. Appropriate vaccines							
3. Appropriate pharmaceuticals							
Total Score							

(1) disease knowledge
(2) impact on animal health and welfare
(3) impact on public health
(4) impact on wider society
(5) impact on trade
(6) control tools

An interpretation guide (http://www.discontools.eu/upl/1/default/doc/1233_PrioInterV3-1-20110303.pdf) was developed to help the expert groups decide on the appropriate scores to apply to each criterion. The expert groups were asked to reach a consensus for the scoring of each criterion. A 5 – tiered scoring system was chosen as this appeared to offer a greater flexibility across the various criteria. The scoring scale applied to the 5-tiered system is as follows: for the first five sections 0, +1; +2; +3; +4 are used; for the sixth section dealing with control tool scores of +2; +1; 0; −1; −2 are used. This scoring scale was selected to highlight the differences in control tools for each disease in the sense that if for a particular disease a vaccine exists that has a high level of efficacy, quality, safety and availability, then a negative score will be attributed to the final total score of the concerned disease to diminish its priority as an effective tool is available. On the contrary, if control tools are missing, then a positive score will be added to the total score meaning that the disease will be higher in the prioritised list of diseases.

The weighting coefficient for each level of a criterion was computed as follows:

$$W = \frac{100}{X * I}$$

where W = the weighting coefficient, X is the maximum score of a level within a criterion and I is the number of levels within a criterion. This ensured that the maximum score of each criterion was 100 and that the different criteria were attributed the same weight in the overall score.

As there are 6 criteria for each disease, the scores could be grouped, listed, ranked or presented in a wide range of ways using either the overall score or the individual scores for each criteria.

Gap analysis model of control tools

The criteria, levels within each of the criteria, scores and weighting coefficients that were used in the gap analysis model can be viewed in Table 3. Gap analysis considered 3 areas: diagnostic, vaccine and pharmaceutical gaps. The scoring system goes from +2 (important gap) to −2 (current tools are appropriate and no need to focus research in this area). As with the prioritisation model, an interpretation guide was developed to facilitate consistency in scoring (http://www.discontools.eu/upl/1/default/doc/1235_GapAna-Inter-V3-1.pdf).

Table 3 The gap analysis model: criteria considered, levels within the criteria, scores and applied weighting coefficients (Coef)

Criteria	Scores	Coef	Total (score*coef)
Diagnostic tools	2 1 0 −1 −2	4.17	/100
1. Availability[a]			
2. Prevention and control - Differentiation of infected from vaccinated (DIVA)			
3. Strategic reserve			
4. Capacity of production			
5. Market potential			
6. Affordable			
7. Quality/stability durability			
8. Sensitivity			
9. Specificity			
10. Reproducibility			
11. Simplicity/ease of use			
12. Speed			
Vaccination tools	2 1 0 −1 −2	4.55	/100
1. Commercial availability[a]			
2. Monitoring for infection in a vaccinated population			
3. Strategic reserve			
4. Capacity of production			
5. Market potential			
6. Affordable			
7. Quality/stability			
8. Safety of vaccines			
9. Efficacy			
10. Immunity			
11. Convenience of use			
Pharmaceutical tools	2 1 0 −1 −2	4.55	/100
1. Availability[a]			
2. Prevention and control			
3. Strategic reserve			
4. Capacity of production			
5. Market potential			
6. Cost			
7. Quality			
8. Safety animal			
9. Safety consumer/user concerns			
10. Safety environment			
11. Resistance			
Total Score:			

[a]A maximum score of 20 was given to the whole criterion when there isn't any product available (not even under development)

Expert opinion elicitation

An expert group leader was appointed for each disease and was asked to engage other experts. Where possible each group was asked to include experts with laboratory and diagnostic expertise, an epidemiologist, an industry representative and an individual with economic/trade expertise. The leader was expected to organise a physical or e-meeting in order to provide the information as described below. The names of the experts are published on the DISCONTOOLS website.

The average number of experts per group was 7. For 43 of the 52 included diseases (83%) the expert groups involved at least 4 members considered to cover the requested expertise (diagnostic, epidemiology, industry, economics). However for 9 diseases (17%), ≤3 experts were included (i.e. contagious bovine pleuropneumonia, swine influenza virus, peste des petits ruminants, rift valley fever, liver fluke, bovine herpes virus type 1, leptospirosis, salmonella, Crimean congo haemorrhagic fever).

Utility

DISCONTOOLS website

The DISCONTOOLS website contains two main sections: (i) work group pages and (ii) the disease database. The work group pages contain relevant minutes, documents and presentations related to meetings of the project management board.

The disease database contains the full D&P, along with a 2-page summary to make it easy to interpret the outcome. All the available information can be filtered for specific diseases or specific sections of the analysis and the customized reports can be downloaded in.pdf or.xls format. There is also a tool to enable web site users to provide comments on the D&P to the DISCONTOOLS secretariat. The prioritisation model and gap analysis model can be consulted for one or more diseases simultaneously and the specific scores for individual levels of criteria can be consulted or downloaded through custom reports.

Ranking of diseases by prioritisation model, disease category and gap analysis model

In Table 4, diseases are ranked based on the total score of the prioritisation model. The Table is very useful in terms of providing a 'Big Picture' view and shows that the top ranked diseases comprise mostly zoonotic diseases and epizootic (often exotic) diseases. This, in turn, helps to guide funders who are working in an international environment and with a broad remit in terms of priorities. In Table 5, the diseases were ranked within disease category. This provides an opportunity to identify priorities within different research domains. As such, funders with an interest in public health will look to the zoonoses ranking. In contrast, funders focusing on international trade will have a great interest in the epizootic diseases ranking and funders who are focusing on the efficiency of production, especially within individual countries, will have a great interest in the ranking of food producing animal complexes. The results of the gap analysis model can be used to obtain more details of the gaps in control tools. As an example, in Table 6 we provide the scores of the gap analysis model for diagnostics, vaccines and pharmaceuticals for the top 10 ranked diseases within each disease category. In general, this table highlights the major gap in pharmaceuticals for the epizootic diseases which is not surprising as the availability of antivirals for the majority of diseases is very limited or non-existent at present. In contrast, for the food producing animal complexes, the picture is more diverse with, dependent on the disease, remaining gaps in diagnostics and vaccines and less so in pharmaceutical development. For the zoonotic diseases, good diagnostics are generally available and the analysis highlights the need for research into vaccine development. It should be noted that, whilst the gap is identified, in many cases, it is unlikely that a pharmaceutical solution would be pursued, for example Bluetongue.

Discussion

The aim of the DISCONTOOLS project was to build a prioritisation model and gap analysis on control tools as a means of prioritising research on infectious animal diseases with the support of stakeholders via a very open consultation process in the animal health research community.

The major achievement of this project consists of the wide and standardized consultation of the animal health research community, involving a total of 342 animal health scientists from all over the world. The establishment of expert groups was an important step in itself because it brought together scientists from different backgrounds and expertise often leading to lively debate, the challenge of assumptions and the identification of research gaps within their field. Where expert groups could not reach consensus, this was recorded in the D&P under the "Gap" section because it represents a gap in knowledge that needs to be filled by research.

An example is the benefit of bees to pollination. At the outset of the discussion, it was suggested by some of the participants that crop yields could decline by 65% without bees. However, when it was pointed out that wild insects have a more important role in pollination than honey bees, major crop species such as cereals are self-pollinating and many others are wind pollinated [27], it was agreed that the impact would be considerably less and it was noted that work needs to be done in

Table 4 Ranking of 52 infectious diseases of animals by the overall score of the prioritisation model

Disease	Overall score
Nipah virus	464
Peste des petits ruminants	385
African swine fever	373
Rift valley fever	365
Bovine tuberculosis	359
Foot and mouth disease	310
Non tse-tse transmitted animal trypanosomiasis	296
African horse sickness	294
Cryptosporidiosis	291
Salmonellosis	282
Contagious bovine pleuropneumonia	269
Leishmaniosis	262
Brucellosis	254
Leptospirosis	250
Classical swine fever	247
Lumpy skin disease	244
Bluetongue	241
Orthopox	237
Hepatitis E virus	237
Poultry coccidiosis	226
Paratuberculosis	223
Anthrax	220
Campylobacter	219
Sheep and goat pox virus	218
Q-fever	214
Rabies	212
Avian Influenza	209
Verocytotoxigenic *Escherichia coli*	209
Liver fluke	202
Chlamydophila abortus	197
Nematodes	193
Porcine circo virus type 2	183
Bovine viral diarrhoea virus	183
Bovine spongiform encephalopathy	180
Small ruminant mastitis	179
Varroa mite	177
Staphylococcus aureus mastitis	175
Theileria	174
Mycoplasma bovis	173
Echinococcosis	167
Swine influenza virus	162
Congo crimean haemorrhagic fever	162
Swine *Actinobacillus pleuropneumonia*	159
Bovine respiratory syncytial virus	153
Parapox	152
Swine mycoplasma	143
Cysticercosis	130
Swine vesicular disease	118
West Nile Virus	118
Bovine herpes virus type 1	107
Porcine reproductive and respiratory syndrome virus	107
Environmental/Streptococcal mastitis	83

this area to determine the real impact. Having had this discussion, it was recognised that efforts should be made to control *Varroa* mite as the bee sector – with its various products – is valuable (roughly estimated in the consortium at €640 million per annum) and needs to be protected.

As was done in Table 3, it is possible to rank diseases by total scores of the prioritisation model. The total score is valuable in highlighting the overall importance of some diseases. Nipah virus obtained the highest score. This was an interesting outcome and its high ranking is confirmed in other recent studies to prioritize diseases of food-producing animals and zoonoses [25, 28]. In the case of FMD, it scores highly due to knowledge gaps along with its impact on animal health and welfare, society and trade even though we have good diagnostics and vaccines. Given the impact of the disease, we need heat stable multi-valent vaccines and need to focus research in this area.

It might be surprising that the overall total for FMD (310) in the prioritisation model is lower than that for ASF (373) but an examination of the score in each of the six separate categories (Table 2) which make up the prioritisation model it is apparent where the variation exists. In the case of ASF the score is higher for the impact on international trade, animal health and welfare and significantly higher for control tools where there is no vaccine and diagnostic tests need to be improved.

Despite the maximally standardized consultation rounds and the use of a validation system in the form of Work Packages 2 and 3 and the PMB, the final ranking of diseases should be interpreted with caution. The total scores also hide specific research needs within a disease. In the case of nematodes for example, the total score hides the pressing need to assign resources to the development of vaccines in this area [29]. To avoid the user missing key data, the "Interpretation of the Scores Guide" was developed as well as the two page summary for each disease.

Table 5 Ranking of 52 infectious diseases of animals by disease category based on the prioritisation model

1. Epizootic diseases	Score	2. Food producing animal complexes	Score	3. Zoonoses	Score
Peste des petits ruminants	385	Poultry coccidiosis	226	Nipah virus	464
African swine fever	373	Paratuberculosis	223	Bovine tuberculosis	359
Rift valley fever	365	Liver fluke	202	Non tse-tse transmitted animal trypanosomiasis	296
Foot and mouth disease	310	Nematodes	193	Cryptosporidiosis	291
African horse sickness	294	Porcine circo virus type 2	183	Salmonellosis	282
Contagious bovine pleuropneumonia	269	Bovine viral diarrhoea virus	183	Leishmaniosis	262
Classical swine fever	247	Small ruminant mastitis	179	Brucellosis	254
Lumpy skin disease	244	Varroa mite	177	Leptospirosis	250
Bluetongue	241	*Staphylococcus aureus* mastitis	175	Hepatitis E virus	237
Orthopox	237	Theileria	174	Anthrax	220
Sheep and goat pox virus	218	*Mycoplasma bovis*	173	Campylobacter	219
Avian Influenza	209	Swine influenza virus	162	Q-fever	214
Parapox	152	Swine *Actinobacillus pleuropneumonia*	159	Rabies	212
Swine vesicular disease	118	Bovine respiratory syncytial virus	153	Verocytotoxigenic *Escherichia coli*	209
West Nile Virus	118	Swine mycoplasma	143	*Chlamydophila abortus*	197
		Bovine herpes virus type 1	107	Bovine spongiform encephalopathy	180
		Porcine reproductive and respiratory syndrome virus	107	Echinococcosis	167
		Environmental/Streptococcal mastitis	83	Congo crimean haemorrhagic fever	162
				Cysticercosis	130

The latter is of particular assistance to the non-specialist user who wants an overview of the critical research needs. Depending on the aim of the research, it may be more informative to compare specific criteria only between diseases (e.g. disease knowledge, impact on wider society, etc.). Two critical factors that can affect the results are: (i) the choice of the weighting coefficients and (ii) the different composition of each expert group. The different criteria of the prioritisation model such as disease knowledge, impact on animal health and welfare, etc. received an equal weight. However, depending on the user, different weight attributions may be desirable. Recently, novel methods have been developed to identify criteria important to different stakeholders by using the nominal group technique and attribute relative weights to the criteria using a wide consultation of different stakeholders and conjoint analysis [26]. This can result in different rankings according to the criteria and weights defined by different stakeholders (e.g. the public vs. health professionals) and provide additional insights to the decision maker on the spending of research funds [19]. In contrast to other prioritisation studies where all diseases were scored by the same expert panel, e.g. [13, 28], in the DISCONTOOLS project, each disease was scored by a different expert panel. This may have introduced bias due to inter-personal differences in scoring, but was considered necessary in order to adequately capture the current status of knowledge and gaps for control tools for each disease.

The epidemiological situation of infectious animal diseases can change rapidly (e.g. the current epidemic of the new porcine epidemic diarrhoea virus [30]), and biotechnological developments constantly change the landscape of diagnostics, vaccines and pharmaceuticals. As a consequence, the prioritisation exercise should be repeated regularly [28]. To this end, the database has been placed on a public website with the possibility that the public and research community can provide comments. This was deliberately done to provide an environment where the information in the D&P and the scores could be challenged. The idea is to gather comments over time and then ask the expert group to consider comments made and adjust the information and scoring on the site as appropriate. It is foreseen that the diseases will be systematically reviewed by the expert groups over a 5-year cycle, taking on board the latest technical advances. In fact, this process has already commenced and updated information on the site is available for African swine fever, Foot and mouth disease, Nematodes and Verocytotoxigenic *E. coli*.

Conclusion

A database was established with the intention of identifying and prioritising research needs in the control of infectious

Table 6 Scores from the gap analysis model for the top-10 ranked diseases within each disease category[a]

Disease	Diagnostics	Vaccines	Pharmaceuticals
1. Epizootic diseases			
Peste des petits ruminants	−5	−10	**20**
African swine fever	−50	**40**	**40**
Rift valley fever	**29**	**18**	**40**
Foot and mouth disease	−32	−20	**40**
African horse sickness	−18	**20**	**10**
Contagious bovine pleuro pneumonia	**9**	**30**	**25**
Classical swine fever	−23	−50	**40**
Lumpy skin disease	**27**	−5	**40**
Bluetongue	−27	−15	**40**
Orthopox	**18**	**40**	**15**
2. Food producing animal complexes			
Coccidiosis	**9**	**5**	−35
Paratuberculosis	0	0	**40**
Liver fluke	−9	**40**	−25
Nematodes	−5	**40**	−65
Bovine viral diarrhoea virus	−27	−10	**40**
Porcine circo virus type 2	**20**	−40	**40**
Small ruminant mastitis	−23	−5	−50
Varroa mite	**40**	**40**	−10
Staphylococcus aureus mastitis	**14**	0	−30
Theileria	**27**	**40**	−30
3. Zoonotic diseases			
Nipah virus	0	0	0
Bovine tuberculosis	−18	**10**	**40**
Non tse-tse transmitted trypanosomiasis	**32**	**40**	**15**
Cryptosporidiosis	0	**40**	−45
Salmonellosis	−23	−30	−35
Leishmaniosis	−14	**35**	−20
Brucellosis	−5	**20**	**40**
Leptospirosis	−5	**5**	−60
Hepatitis E virus	−32	**40**	**40**
Anthrax	**36**	**5**	−45

Positive scores (indicating a gap) were highlighted in bold
[a]Decimals were rounded to the first integer. This may cause apparent deviations between the sum of the individual and the total score

animal diseases in the EU. If the focus of research is now placed on the priorities identified, it will hasten the development of diagnostics, vaccines and pharmaceuticals and reduce the 20% loss in production potential, valued at €28 billion per year in the EU. Funders of research including the European Commission, member states, foundations, trusts along with private industry should use the database to prioritise and focus future research. This will deliver benefits in terms of animal health and welfare but also public health, societal benefits and a safe and secure food supply. The employed method and results should not be considered fixed, but by refining the scoring methodology, challenging and updating the available information on a regular basis and incorporating new diseases, the DISCONTOOLS database has the potential to become a reference point used by stakeholders when prioritising research.

Abbreviations
D&P: Disease and Product analysis document; ETPGAH: European Technology Platform for Global Animal Health; EU: European Union; OIE: World Organisation for Animal Health; PMB: Project Management Board

Acknowledgements
We wish to thank all Expert Group leaders and members of Expert Groups and stakeholders for their invaluable contribution to the success of the DISCONTOOLS Project.

Funding
This project was funded by the 7th framework programme of the EU (grant agreement number 211316) and currently receives funding from different research funding bodies from EU member states.

Authors' contributions
DOB conceived the study, coordinated the project and supervised the manuscript. JS assisted in project management, wrote the manuscript and the disease summaries. JC wrote the manuscript and manages the database from 2014. MD managed the project and maintained the database from 2008 to 2013. All authors read and approved the final manuscript.

Authors' information
DOB was the coordinator of the project under the 7th framework programme on behalf of IFAH-Europe but is currently no longer employed by this organisation. JC is the current project manager commissioned by IFAH-Europe.

Competing interests
Being a stakeholder driven project, all those involved in the chain from research to commercialisation of products including universities, regulators, farming and veterinary representative organisations along with the pharmaceutical industry contributed to the outcome of this study. The authors declare that they have no financial or personal relationships with other people or organisations that could have inappropriately influenced the present study and manuscript.

Consent for publication
Name of disease experts are published below the disease information where written consent has been given. Experts retain the right to access, change or remove their personal data.

Author details
[1]International Federation for Animal Health Europe, Avenue de Tervueren 168, box 81150 Brussels, Belgium. [2]Institute of Infection and Global Health, University of Liverpool, Liverpool, UK. [3]Avia-GIS, Risschotlei 33, 2980 Zoersel, Belgium.

References

1. Vallat B. One World, One Health. In: Editorials from the Director-General. Publisher: World Organisation for Animal Health (oie). 2009. http://www.oie.int/en/for-the-media/editorials/detail/article/one-world-one-health/. Accessed 20 Aug 2014.
2. Benmansour A. Animal Health and Welfare ERA-net (anihwa). 2012. https://www.anihwa.eu/About-Anihwa/Project-description. Accessed 20 Aug 2014.
3. Anonymous. Common financial framework for the food chain. 2014. http://ec.europa.eu/food/animal/diseases/index_en.htm. Accessed 20 Aug 2014.
4. IFAH. Annual Report 2013 International Federation for Animal Health-Europe. 2014. p. 12.
5. EUROSTAT. Key figures on Europe, 2013 digest of the online Eurostat yearbook. Luxembourg: Piirto Jukka; 2013. p. 184.
6. European Technology Platform for Global Animal Health. Action plan. 2007. http://www.etpgah.eu/action-plan.html. Accessed 20 Aug 2014, 52 pp.
7. Rushdy A, O'Mahony M. PHLS overview of communicable diseases 1997: results of a priority setting exercise. Commun Dis Rep CDR Wkly. 1998;8:S1–S12.
8. Weinberg J, Grimaud O, Newton L. Establishing priorities for European collaboration in communicable disease surveillance. Eur J Public Health. 1999;9:236–40.
9. Doherty JA. Establishing priorities for national communicable disease surveillance. Can J Infect Dis. 2000;11:21–4.
10. Horby P, Rushdy A, Graham C, O'Mahony M. PHLS overview of communicable diseases 1999. Comm Dis Publ Health. 2001;4:8–17.
11. WHO. Setting priorities in communicable disease surveillance. Global Alert and Response publications. 2006; 32 pp.
12. Krause G, Working Group on Prioritisation at the Robert Koch Institute. Prioritisation of infectious diseases in public health–call for comments. Euro Surveill. 2008;13(40):18996.
13. Cardoen S, Van Huffel X, Berkvens D, Quoilin S, Ducoffre G, Saegerman C, Speybroeck N, Imberechts H, Herman L, Ducatelle R, Dierick K. Evidence-based semiquantitative methodology for prioritization of foodborne zoonoses. Foodborne Pathog Dis. 2009;6:1083–96.
14. Balabanova Y, Gilsdorf A, Buda S, Burger R, Eckmanns T, Gartner B, Gross U, Haas W, Hamouda O, Hubner J, Janisch T, Kist M, Kramer MH, Ledig T, Mielke M, Pulz M, Stark K, Suttorp N, Ulbrich U, Wichmann O, Krause G. Communicable diseases prioritized for surveillance and epidemiological research: results of a standardized prioritization procedure in Germany, 2011. Plos One. 2011;6:e25691.
15. Cox R, Sanchez J, Revie CW. Multi-criteria decision analysis tools for prioritising emerging or re-emerging infectious diseases associated with climate change in Canada. Plos One. 2013;8:e68338.
16. Havelaar AH, van Rosse F, Bucura C, Toetenel MA, Haagsma JA, Kurowicka D, Heesterbeek JH, Speybroeck N, Langelaar MF, van der Giessen JW, Cooke RM, Braks MA. Prioritizing emerging zoonoses in the Netherlands. Plos One. 2010;5:e13965.
17. Ng V, Sargeant J. An empirical and quantitative approach to the prioritization of zoonotic diseases of public health importance in Canada. Ecohealth. 2011;7:S114.
18. Sargeant J, Ng V. The current state of knowledge of zoonoses and the implications for research outcomes in disease prioritization in Canada. Ecohealth. 2011;7:S34.
19. Ng V, Sargeant JM. A quantitative approach to the prioritization of zoonotic diseases in north America: a health professionals' perspective. Plos One. 2013;8:e72172.
20. FAO/WHO. Multicriteria-based ranking of risk management of food-borne parasites. Microbiological Risk Assessment Series. 2014;23:302.
21. McKenzie J, Simpson H, Langstaff I. Development of methodology to prioritise wildlife pathogens for surveillance. Prev Vet Med. 2007;81:194–210.
22. Heffernan C. Panzootics and the poor: devising a global livestock disease prioritisation framework for poverty alleviation. Rev Sci Tech – OIE. 2009;28:897–907.
23. More SJ, McKenzie K, O'Flaherty J, Doherty ML, Cromie AR, Magan MJ. Setting priorities for non-regulatory animal health in Ireland: Results from an expert Policy Delphi study and a farmer priority identification survey. Prev Vet Med. 2010;95.198–207.
24. Vilas VJD, Voller F, Montibeller G, Franco LA, Sribhashyam S, Watson E, Hartley M, Gibbens JC. An integrated process and management tools for ranking multiple emerging threats to animal health. Prev Vet Med. 2013;108:94–102.
25. Brookes VJ, Hernandez-Jover M, Cowled B, Holyoake PK, Ward MP. Building a picture: prioritisation of exotic diseases for the pig industry in Australia using multi-criteria decision analysis. Prev Vet Med. 2014;113:103–17.
26. Ng V, Sargeant JM. A stakeholder-informed approach to the identification of criteria for the prioritization of zoonoses in Canada. Plos One. 2012;7:e29752.
27. Garibaldi LA, Steffan-Dewenter I, Winfree R, Aizen MA, Bommarco R, Cunningham SA, Kremen C, Carvalheiro LG, Harder LD, Afik O, Bartomeus I, Benjamin F, Boreux V, Cariveau D, Chacoff NP, Dudenhoffer JH, Freitas BM, Ghazoul J, Greenleaf S, Hipolito J, Holzschuh A, Howlett B, Isaacs R, Javorek SK, Kennedy CM, Krewenka KM, Krishnan S, Mandelik Y, Mayfield MM, Motzke I, Munyuli T, Nault BA, Otieno M, Petersen J, Pisanty G, Potts SG, Rader R, Ricketts TH, Rundlof M, Seymour CL, Schuepp C, Szentgyorgyi H, Taki H, Tscharntke T, Vergara CH, Viana BF, Wanger TC, Westphal C, Williams N, Klein AM. Wild pollinators enhance fruit set of crops regardless of honey bee abundance. Science. 2013;339:1608–11.
28. Humblet MF, Vandeputte S, Albert A, Gosset C, Kirschvink N, Haubruge E, Fecher-Bourgeois F, Pastoret P-P, Saegerman C. Multidisciplinary and evidence-based method for prioritizing diseases of food-producing animals and zoonoses. Emerg Infect Dis. 2012;18. doi: 10.3201/eid1804.111151
29. Vercruysse J, Schetters TPM, Knox DP, Willadsen P, Claerebout E. Control of parasitic diseases using vaccines: an answer to drug resistance? Rev Sci Tech – OIE. 2007;26:105–15.
30. Chen Q, Li G, Stasko J, Thomas JT, Stensland WR, Pillatzki AE, Gauger PC, Schwartz KJ, Madson D, Yoon KJ, Stevenson GW, Burrough ER, Harmon KM, Main RG, Zhang J. Isolation and characterization of porcine epidemic diarrhea viruses associated with the 2013 disease outbreak among swine in the United States. J Clin Microbiol. 2014;52:234–43.

4

Clinical, serological and echocardiographic examination of healthy field dogs before and after vaccination with a commercial tetravalent leptospirosis vaccine

Andrea M. Spiri[1,2], Sabrina Rodriguez-Campos[4], José M. Matos[3], Tony M. Glaus[3], Barbara Riond[1], Claudia E. Reusch[3], Regina Hofmann-Lehmann[1,2] and Barbara Willi[1,3*]

Abstract

Background: Leptospirosis is a re-emerging bacterial zoonosis caused by spirochetes of the genus *Leptospira*. Severe disease has been reported in dogs in Europe despite vaccination with bivalent *Leptospira* vaccines. Recently, a tetravalent canine *Leptospira* vaccine (Nobivac® L4) was licenced in Europe. The goal of this study was to investigate clinical signs, microscopic agglutination test (MAT) titres, haematology, blood biochemistry, cardiac (c) Troponin I levels and echocardiography before and after vaccination with this tetravalent vaccine. Forty-eight healthy dogs were prospectively enrolled and vaccinated twice, 3–4 weeks apart (T0 and T1). Before vaccination (T0) and 16–31 days after the second vaccination (T2), MAT (n = 48), haematology (n = 48), blood biochemistry (n = 36) and cTroponin I measurements (n = 29) were performed, and MAT was repeated 347–413 days after the second vaccination (T3, n = 44). Echocardiography was performed before the first and second vaccination (T0 and T1, n = 24).

Results: Mild and transient clinical signs within 5 days following the first and second vaccination occurred in 23% and 10% of the dogs, respectively. Before the first vaccination (T0), all dogs showed negative MAT titres for the tested serovars except for Canicola (50% with titres 100–400). At T2, positive MAT titres to the serovars Canicola (100%), Australis (89%), Grippotyphosa (86%), Bratislava (60%), Autumnalis (58%), Copenhageni (42%), Pomona (12%), Pyrogenes (8%) and Icterohaemorrhagiae (2%) were found. Median to high titres (≥ 400) were most common to the serovar Canicola (92%) and less common to the serovars Australis (41%), Grippotyphosa (21%), Bratislava (12%), Autumnalis (4%), Pyrogenes (4%) and Pomona (2%). At T3, positive MAT titres (titre range: 100–400) were found in 2–18% of the dogs to serovars of the vaccine serogroups and in 2–18% of the dogs to the non-vaccine serovars Pomona, Autumnalis, Pyrogenes and Ballum. Haematology, blood biochemistry, cTroponin I levels and echocardiography results did not change significantly following vaccination.

Conclusions: Clinical signs following vaccination with Nobivac® L4 were transient and mild in all cases. Seroconversion differed considerably among individual dogs and among the vaccine serogroups.

Keywords: Nobivac® Lepto 6, *Leptospira*, Tetravalent vaccine, Vaccination, Seroconversion, Microscopic agglutination test, Adverse events

* Correspondence: bwilli@vetclinics.uzh.ch
[1]Clinical Laboratory, Vetsuisse Faculty, University of Zurich, Winterthurerstr. 260, 8057 Zurich, Switzerland
[3]Clinic for Small Animal Internal Medicine, Vetsuisse Faculty, University of Zurich, Winterthurerstr. 260, 8057 Zurich, Switzerland
Full list of author information is available at the end of the article

Background

Leptospirosis is a re-emerging bacterial zoonosis of global importance caused by spirochetes of the genus *Leptospira* [1]. Dogs can be infected with a wide range of pathogenic *Leptospira* serovars and shed the leptospires in their urine during acute infection [2]. Leptospires can survive for months in water and moist soil [3], and indirect transmission through contact with contaminated soil or water is thought to play an important role in the epidemiology of leptospirosis.

In Europe, canine leptospirosis in dogs has gained increasing attention in the last several years [4]. Following infection with pathogenic leptospires, dogs can develop a severe, multi-systemic disease associated with high mortality [2]. Besides this severe course of infection, mild clinical signs and asymptomatic infections have been documented. Acute leptospirosis in dogs is mainly associated with acute kidney or liver injury and respiratory signs associated with pulmonary haemorrhage [5]. Furthermore, myocarditis has been documented in humans with leptospirosis and has also been suspected in infected dogs [6, 7]. The clinical manifestation of leptospirosis depends not only on the causative serovar but also on host-specific factors such as age and the immune status of the dog [8].

The most commonly used diagnostic test for leptospirosis in dogs is the demonstration of antibodies in the microscopic agglutination test (MAT). Serial dilutions of patient sera are thereby incubated with a selection of pathogenic *Leptospira* serovars, and agglutination of the organisms is assessed by darkfield microscopy. Cross-reactivity among serovars only allows for a serogroup-specific diagnosis, and positive titres following vaccination, previous exposure and during chronic asymptomatic infection complicate the interpretation of the results [2]. Generally, the serovar that gives the highest titre is regarded as the infecting serogroup or serovar, although this diagnosis is, at best, presumptive [9]. Post-vaccination titres have been assessed in small groups of dogs following vaccination with bivalent and tetravalent vaccines [10–12]. These studies revealed that titres usually decline by 4 months after vaccination, although persistently high titres have been documented which have been explained by natural exposure to *Leptospira* field serovars [10]. PCR can be used as an alternative diagnostic method to detect leptospiral DNA in biological samples such as blood, urine or tissue. However, leptospires can only transiently be detected in the blood and urine of infected animals [13], and antibiotic therapy is thought to clear bacteraemia and leptospiruria [14]. The detection of the agents in biological samples by bacterial culture is a definitive proof of infection [2], but leptospires are fastidious organisms requiring special culture media, and they grow very slowly after 2 to up to 24 weeks in culture, making this diagnostic procedure impractical in a clinical setting.

Despite the introduction of efficient bivalent *Leptospira* bacterin vaccines some decades ago [15], clinical leptospirosis has recently been documented among numerous vaccinated dogs in Europe [16]. The currently licenced bivalent *Leptospira* vaccines in Europe contain serovars belonging to the serogroups Canicola and Icterohaemorrhagiae. These vaccines have been shown to prevent leptospirosis caused by serovars belonging to these two serogroups, but the vaccines induce only partial or no immunity to heterologous serogroups [17–19]. Canicola and Icterohaemorrhagiae were previously thought to be the main serogroups causing clinical leptospirosis in dogs. Recent seroepidemiological studies revealed, however, that dogs are susceptible to a broad range of serovars. In Europe, antibodies against the serogroups Icterohaemorrhagiae, Canicola, Grippotyphosa, Pomona, Australis and Sejroe have most commonly been documented in clinically healthy and diseased dogs [4].

In 2012, a new canine tetravalent inactivated *Leptospira* vaccine (Nobivac® L4, in Switzerland licenced as Nobivac® Lepto 6, MSD Animal Health GmbH, Luzern, Switzerland) that contains antigens from serovars from four different serogroups, including Canicola, Icterohaemorrhagiae, Australis and Grippotyphosa was licenced in Europe [20, 21]. Because serology represents the mainstay in the diagnosis of leptospirosis in dogs, the serological response following vaccination can interfere with the interpretation of MAT results in suspect clinical cases [22]. So far, no data on the serological response following vaccination with this novel tetravalent vaccine have been published. Furthermore, recent pharmacovigilance reports from Germany and Switzerland suggest that adverse events after vaccination with *Leptospira* vaccines have significantly increased since 2013 and 2014, respectively, following the introduction of novel, multivalent *Leptospira* vaccines in these countries [23, 24]. The authors of the reports speculated that the increasing number of *Leptospira* serovars included in these vaccines could result in higher antigenicity of the vaccines. However, studies investigating the incidence of adverse events following the vaccination of dogs did not reveal a significant increase in hypersensitivity reactions following *Leptospira* vaccination when compared with other vaccines [25, 26]. Finally, there have been recent anecdotal reports describing cardiac abnormalities suspicious of acute myocarditis after vaccination (S. Jenni, personal communication). Specifically, at the second vaccination, new heart murmurs had been auscultated that had not been present at the first vaccination. Subsequent echocardiographic examinations reportedly had revealed left ventricular dilation and hypocontractility with mitral annulus dilation and associated mitral insufficiency as the explanation for the murmur.

The goal of the present study was to evaluate the serological response of dogs after vaccination with a commercially available, inactivated, tetravalent *Leptospira* vaccine and to investigate whether the dogs showed clinical signs and alterations in haematology, blood biochemistry and echocardiography following vaccination.

Methods

Study design, sample and data collection and sample processing

This monocentric, longitudinal, prospective study was performed at the Clinic for Small Animal Internal Medicine, University of Zurich, between August 2013 and May 2015. Dogs were prospectively enrolled within the study when they met the following inclusion criteria: older than 8 weeks of age, judged clinically healthy by the owner, in good general health according to clinical examination, no vaccination within 4 weeks and no medical therapy within 2 months prior to study enrolment, with the exception of antiparasitic treatment. The study design and number of dogs that received each procedure are shown in Table 1. The day of the first vaccination was defined as T0. All dogs were vaccinated twice with a commercial tetravalent leptospirosis vaccine (Nobivac® L4, in Switzerland licenced as Nobivac® Lepto 6, MSD Animal Health GmbH) 3–4 weeks apart (T0 and T1). Additional vaccine components licenced for concurrent administration were applied as required (Table 1). Blood samples were collected by venipuncture before the first (T0) and second vaccination (T1) and 41–54 days (T2) and 368–434 days after the first vaccination (T3). Blood samples were processed or frozen at −80 °C within 4 h of collection. A medical history and clinical examination were performed at each presentation by a veterinary surgeon (AS) or a board-certified internal medicine specialist (BW). Echocardiography was performed before the first (T0) and second vaccination (T1) by board-certified cardiologists (JM, TG) at the division of cardiology, Vetsuisse Faculty, University of Zurich. Adverse vaccine events were suspected when clinical signs occurred within 5 days of vaccination and belonged to one of the following groups: lethargy or inappetence, local reaction at the injection site (signs of tenderness or pain, cutaneous swelling or mass, lameness in a limb close to the injection site), non-specific signs (periuria, diarrhoea, vomiting) or a hypersensitivity reaction (swelling of the face, hives or bumps on the face or body, hypersalivation, tachypnoea, or respiratory distress). Data on adverse vaccine events were collected from the medical history and clinical examination performed at each presentation.

Haematology, blood biochemistry and cTroponin I

Haematology and blood biochemistry tests and measurements of cTroponin I were performed at the Clinical Laboratory, Vetsuisse Faculty, University of Zurich. Haematology was performed from EDTA anticoagulated whole blood within 4 h of sample collection. Blood biochemistry was determined batch-wise from serum samples stored at −80 °C. Haematology and blood biochemistry were run on a Sysmex XT-2000iV (Sysmex Corporation, Kobe, Japan) [27] and Cobas Integra 800 instrument (Roche Diagnostics AG, Rotkreuz, Switzerland), respectively. The clinical chemistry parameters included: albumin, total protein, alanine aminotransferase (ALAT), alkaline phosphatase (AP), bilirubin, urea, creatinine and lipase. The laboratory's device-specific reference intervals were applied. cTroponin I was measured on an Immulite 1000 (Siemens Healthcare Diagnostics GmbH, Zurich, Switzerland). The serum cTroponin I concentration was measured using a commercially available assay that had been validated for the dog [28]. The test's lower limit of detection was 0.2 ng/mL, and cTroponin I values exceeding 0.2 ng/mL were considered increased.

Table 1 Study design and number of dogs that received each procedure

Time point	T0	T1	T2	T3
Days after first presentation	0	20–28	41–54	368–434
Procedure/number of dogs				
Vaccination	48	48	-	44
Clinical examination	48	48	48	44
Echocardiography	24	24	-	-
MAT	48	-	48	44
Haematology	48	-	48	-
Blood biochemistry	36	-	36	-
cTroponin I	29	-	29	-
Number of dogs receiving other vaccine components				
Nobivac® DHPPi	16	3	-	-
Nobivac® Pi	10	1	-	-

Microscopic agglutination test

The MAT was performed at the National Reference Laboratory for animal leptospirosis at the Institute of Veterinary Bacteriology, Vetsuisse Faculty, University of Bern, Switzerland. The MAT was performed batch-wise from serum samples stored at −80 °C that were sent by priority mail at room temperature to the laboratory. Samples were examined for the presence of antibodies against a standard panel of 14 pathogenic *Leptospira* strains commonly used in Switzerland (Table 2) by MAT according to Office International des Epizooties (OIE) standards [29]. To prevent inter-observer variability, all samples were tested by the same person. The end-point titre refers to the reciprocal of the highest serum dilution at which at least 50% agglutination occurs. In this study, sera with a titre of 100, indicating past exposure to *Leptospira* [8], were considered seropositive.

Echocardiography

Echocardiographic examinations were performed with continuous ECG monitoring on laterally recumbent unsedated dogs using a GE Vivid 7 ultrasound unit (Vivid 7, GE Medical Systems, Munich, Germany). Standard two-dimensional, M-mode and colour Doppler echocardiographic views were obtained from standard right parasternal views using a 7 MHz transducer. The primary focus was qualitative left ventricular size and function as well as valvular integrity and function. Quantitated parameters were left ventricular diameter in diastole and systole (LVDd and LVDs, respectively), the shortening fraction (%FS) from M-Mode images, and the left atrial to aortic ratio (LA/Ao) in short axis [30, 31].

Statistical analyses

Statistical analyses were performed using Analyse-it® for Microsoft Excel version 1.0.5.0 (Analyse-it Software, Ltd., Leeds, United Kingdom) and GraphPad Prism 5.03 (GraphPad Software, Inc., CA, USA). The Wilcoxon signed rank test (p_w) was used to compare the results from the same dog at two different time points. Correlation between MAT titres and time elapsed since the last *Leptospira* vaccination was assessed using the Spearman rank correlation test (correlation coefficient: r_{sp}). Proportions between groups were analysed with the Fisher's exact test (p_F). *P*-values <0.05 were considered significant.

Results

Characteristics of the study population

A total of 48 dogs were included in the study. The characteristics of the study population are shown in Table 3. All but one dog had previously received a *Leptospira* vaccine; all vaccine products were inactivated bivalent *Leptospira* vaccines containing serovars from the serogroups Canicola and Icterohaemorrhagiae. The vaccines belonged to several different brands (Canigen® L (*n* = 28), Canigen® 7 (*n* = 1), Virbac, Glattbrugg, Switzerland; Canimed® L (*n* = 1), Eurican® L (*n* = 1), Merial, Lyon, France; Nobivac® Lepto (*n* = 8), Vetamun® Lepto (*n* = 6), MSD Animal Health GmbH; Vanguard® 7 (*n* = 2), Zoetis Schweiz GmbH, Zurich, Switzerland). All 48 dogs completed the primary vaccination schedule, and 44 dogs were sampled after 1 year (T3, Table 1); the remaining four dogs died within 1 year after vaccination for unrelated reasons (*n* = 2), moved to another country (*n* = 1) or did not keep the appointment after

Table 2 The 14 *Leptospira spp.* strains used as live antigens in the microscopic agglutination test[a]

Genomospecies	Serogroup	Serovar	Strain
Leptospira interrogans	Australis	Australis	Ballico
	Australis	Bratislava	Jez-Bratislava
	Autumnalis	Autumnalis	Akiyami
	Bataviae	Bataviae	Swart
	Canicola	Canicola	Hond Utrecht IV
	Icterohaemorrhagiae	Icterohaemorrhagiae	RGA
	Icterohaemorrhagiae	Copenhageni	M20
	Pomona	Pomona	Pomona
	Pyrogenes	Pyrogenes	Salinem
	Sejroe	Hardjo	Hardjoprajitno
Leptospira borgpetersenii	Ballum	Ballum	Mus127
	Tarassovi	Tarassovi	Perepelitsin
	Sejroe	Sejroe	M84
Leptospira kirschneri	Grippotyphosa	Grippotyphosa	Moskva V

[a]All reference strains were obtained from the Royal Tropical Institute (KIT), Amsterdam, The Netherlands

Table 3 Characteristics of the 48 dogs of this study

Parameter	Number of dogs	Range	Median	95% CI[a]
Age (years)	48	0.4–14	5	4.2–6.3
Body weight (kg)	48	5.5–51.2	21	18.0–25.1
Days to prior leptospirosis vaccination	47	31–1745	379	386.5–640.5
Parameter	Number of dogs (%)			
Gender				
Female intact	16 (33)			
Female castrated	16 (33)			
Male intact	14 (29)			
Male castrated	2 (4)			
Pedigree				
Yes	39 (81)			
No	9 (19)			
Breed				
Barzoi	8 (17)			
Beagle	4 (8)			
Labrador Retriever	5 (10)			
Jack Russel Terrier	2 (4)			
Rhodesian Ridgeback	2 (4)			
Shetland Sheepdog	6 (13)			
Malinois	2 (4)			
Whippet	2 (4)			
Other breeds[b]	8 (17)			

[a]CI, confidence interval
[b]Other breeds comprised: Old German Shepherd Dog, Australian Kelpie, Bavarian Mountain Hound, Golden Retriever, German Wirehaired Pointer, Small Munsterlander, Poitevin, Schipperke (each n = 1)

1 year (n = 1). The two dogs that died were 11 and 14 years old and were euthanized because of histiocytic sarcoma or acute monoparesis that occurred 137 and 340 days after the second vaccination, respectively.

Clinical examination

Clinical examination was unremarkable in 75–90% of the dogs at each presentation (Additional file 1). Clinical findings included vaginal discharge due to juvenile vaginitis or heat, conjunctivitis, faint heart murmurs, splenomegaly, focal pyoderma, inflammation or fistula in the anal region, red and scaly ears, fluid-filled bowel loops, enlarged prostate and depigmentation of the nose.

Following the first and second vaccination, adverse vaccine events were reported by the owners of 11 (23%) and 5 (10%) dogs, respectively (Additional file 1). The clinical signs occurred within 5 days of vaccination and were transient and mild in all cases. The clinical signs mainly included local reactions at the injection site, lethargy or inappetence. Three dogs showed a single episode of vomiting or periuria. A total of 6 out of 11 dogs with adverse events after the first vaccination had received additional vaccine components (Nobivac® DHPPi, n = 3, Nobivac® Pi, n = 3). None of the five dogs with adverse events after the second vaccination had received additional vaccine components. The proportion of animals that showed adverse vaccine events was not significantly different between dogs that had or had not received additional vaccine components (p_F = 1.0). Other anamnestic abnormalities that occurred after 5 days of vaccination were reported in 5 (10%) and 4 (8%) dogs after the first (T0) and second vaccination (T1), respectively. They included a single episode of vomiting or diarrhoea 10–14 days after vaccination, a depigmentation of the planum nasale that started 7 days after vaccination, acute trembling and a focal epileptic seizure 3 and 4 weeks after vaccination, respectively, coughing 3 weeks after vaccination, a reduced general condition 10 days after vaccination and tenesmus due to prostate enlargement 3 weeks after vaccination. At the time of the 1-year booster vaccination (T3), two dogs had died (see above), one dog had developed laryngeal paralysis, one dog suffered from idiopathic epilepsy and one dog had developed and recovered from an acute encephalitis.

Microscopic agglutination test

MAT results for the 14 tested serovars are shown in Table 4 for the serogroups included in the vaccine and in Table 5 for the serogroups that are not included in the vaccine. At first presentation and before the first vaccination (T0), all dogs had negative MAT titres (< 100) for all tested serovars, except for the serovar Canicola, for which 50% of the dogs showed titres ≥100 at T0 (Table 4). All of the seropositive dogs had been previously vaccinated with a vaccine that contained a serovar of the serogroup Canicola. In the 20 dogs with titres of 100, the previous *Leptospira* vaccine had been given 101–1745 days prior to study enrolment. In the three dogs with titres of 200, the leptospirosis vaccine had been given 176–554 days prior to study enrolment, and in the one dog with a titre of 400, the vaccine had been given 129 days before enrolment. There was no significant correlation between the MAT titres to the serovar Canicola and the time elapsed since the last vaccination ($r_{sp} = -0.006$).

Positive MAT titres (≥ 100) measured after the second vaccination (T2) were most common for the serovar Canicola (100%), followed by the serovars Australis (89%), Grippotyphosa (86%), Bratislava (60%), Autumnalis (58%), Copenhageni (42%), Pomona (12%), Pyrogenes (8%) and Icterohaemorrhagiae (2%, Tables 4 and 5). Median to high titres (≥ 400) were most commonly found for the serovar Canicola (92%), followed by the serovars Australis (41%), Grippotyphosa (21%), Bratislava (12%), Autumnalis (4%), Pyrogenes (4%) and Pomona (2%); none of the dogs developed titres ≥400 for the serovars Copenhageni or Icterohaemorrhagiae. Maximal MAT titres measured at T2 for the serovars were as follows: Canicola (3200), Australis (3200), Grippotyphosa (800), Bratislava (800), Autumnalis (3200), Copenhageni (200), Pomona (400), Pyrogenes (800) and Icterohaemorrhagiae (100).

At the 1-year booster appointment (T3), 2–18% of the dogs showed positive MAT titres to serovars of the vaccine serogroups, and the titres were generally low (< 400, Table 4). A total of 2–18% of the dogs showed positive MAT titres to the non-vaccine serovars Pomona, Autumnalis, Pyrogenes and Ballum (Table 5). The seven dogs with an MAT titre of 400 against the serovar Pyrogenes at T3 had negative titres against the other tested serovars at this time point and had also been seronegative for the serovar Pyrogenes following the second vaccination (T2). Positive MAT titres were not detected at any time point during the study for *L. interrogans* serovar Bataviae or for *L. borgpetersenii* serovars Tarassovi, Hardjo and Sejroe (data not shown).

Haematology, blood biochemistry and cTroponin I

The haematological parameters determined before (T0) and after the second vaccination (T2) revealed no significant differences, with the exception of a slight but significant increase in haematocrit ($p_W = 0.02$) and a decrease in total monocyte count at T2 compared to T0 ($p_W = 0.04$; Additional file 2). For the blood biochemistry results, significant differences between T0 and T2 were only evident for the AP activity (decrease; $p_W = 0.04$) and the urea concentration (increase; $p_W = 0.03$; Additional file 3). These differences were small, and the median AP activity and urea concentration remained within the reference range at both time points. The cTroponin I concentrations were obtained in 29 dogs. At T0, cTroponin I concentrations were below the detection limit in 27 dogs; two dogs (both Barzois) had measurable cTroponin I levels of 0.39 and 0.50 ng/mL. At T2, cTroponin I concentrations were below the detection limit in 27 dogs; two dogs (both Barzois) had measurable cTroponin I levels of 0.23 and 0.29 ng/mL; both dogs had had undetectable values at T0. There was no significant difference between the cTroponin I levels at T0 and T2.

Table 4 Microscopic agglutination test results for the vaccine serogroups before and after vaccination

Species	*L. interrogans*			*L. interrogans*			*L. interrogans*			*L. interrogans*			*L. interrogans*			*L. kirschneri*		
Serogroup	Canicola			Icterohaemorrhagiae			Icterohaemorrhagiae			Australis			Australis			Grippotyphosa		
Serovar	Canicola			Copenhageni			Icterohaemorrhagiae			Bratislava			Australis			Grippotyphosa		
Time point	T0	T2	T3	T0	T2	T3	T0	T2	T3	T0	T2	T3	T0	T2	T3	T0	T2	T3
Percentage of dogs with titre																		
< 100	50	0	91	100	58	95	100	98	98	100	40	98	100	11	82	100	14	95
100	**42**	**2**	**9**	0	**33**	**5**	0	**2**	**2**	0	**19**	0	0	**27**	**11**	0	**42**	**5**
200	**6**	**6**	0	0	**9**	0	0	0	0	0	**29**	**2**	0	**21**	**7**	0	**23**	0
400	**2**	**34**	0	0	0	0	0	0	0	0	**10**	0	0	**25**	0	0	**19**	0
800	0	**29**	0	0	0	0	0	0	0	0	**2**	0	0	**8**	0	0	**2**	0
1600	0	**27**	0	0	0	0	0	0	0	0	0	0	0	**6**	0	0	0	0
3200	0	**2**	0	0	0	0	0	0	0	0	0	0	0	**2**	0	0	0	0
Total number of dogs	48	48	44	48	48	44	48	48	44	48	48	44	48	48	44	48	48	44

Positive titres are shown in bold

Table 5 Microscopic agglutination test results for selected non-vaccine serogroups before and after vaccination

Species	*L. interrogans*			*L. interrogans*			*L. interrogans*			*L. borgpetersenii*		
Serogroup	Pomona			Autumnalis			Pyrogenes			Ballum		
Serovar	Pomona			Autumnalis			Pyrogenes			Ballum		
Time point	T0	T2	T3	T0	T2	T3	T0	T2	T3	T0	T2	T3
Percentage of dogs with titre												
< 100	100	88	87	100	42	95	100	92	82	100	100	98
100	0	**8**	**9**	0	**50**	**5**	0	**4**	**2**	0	0	**2**
200	0	**2**	**2**	0	**4**	0	0	0	0	0	0	0
400	0	**2**	**2**	0	**2**	0	0	**2**	**16**	0	0	0
800	0	0	0	0	0	0	0	**2**	0	0	0	0
1600	0	0	0	0	0	0	0	0	0	0	0	0
3200	0	0	0	0	**2**	0	0	0	0	0	0	0
Total number of dogs	48	48	44	48	48	44	48	48	44	48	48	44

Positive titres are shown in bold

Echocardiography

Left ventricular (LVDd) and left atrial (LA/Ao) size did not significantly change between the first (T0) and the second (T1) vaccination, and mitral insufficiency could not be documented in any dog. Additionally, systolic function, as assessed by LVDs and %FS, did not change significantly between T0 and T1. Looking at individual dogs, there was not any dog that showed a notable increase in LVDd or LVDs. In none of the dogs could any arrhythmia be recognized at any time point during the study.

Discussion

This is the first independent study evaluating the serological and clinical response in field dogs following vaccination with a novel tetravalent *Leptospira* vaccine. Our results suggest that the vaccine was generally well tolerated and that there was marked variation among individual dogs and among different vaccine serovars regarding the extent of seroconversion following vaccination.

Up to 23% of the dogs in this study showed clinical signs following vaccination, but they were mild and transient in all cases and did not include anaphylactoid reactions. *Leptospira* vaccines have been said to carry an increased risk of adverse events in puppies younger than 12 weeks of age and in small-breed dogs [32], but a recent study evaluating the incidence rate of owner-reported post-vaccination adverse events found no significant increase in hypersensitivity reactions in dogs vaccinated against *Leptospira* compared with other vaccines [25]. In the present study, most of the adverse vaccine events included discomfort at the injection site and transient lethargy and inappetence. These are common clinical signs induced by vaccination and have also been reported for other vaccine products [33]. Because additional vaccine components were administered in six of the eleven dogs that showed clinical signs after the first vaccination, the clinical signs could also have been attributable to other vaccine components. However, there was no significant difference in the frequency of adverse events between dogs that did or did not receive other vaccine components at the first or second vaccination. In this study, we decided to administer additional vaccine components as indicated to mimic the situation in the field, where *Leptospira* vaccines are usually administered together with other vaccine components registered for concurrent application. In light of the high incidence and mortality rate of clinical leptospirosis in dogs in Europe [4, 5, 16], the benefit of vaccinating dogs with this novel tetravalent vaccine highly outweighs the risk of adverse events following vaccination.

The highest MAT titres after vaccination for the tested serovars were observed for the serovars Canicola, Australis, Grippotyphosa, Bratislava and Autumnalis; the MAT titres were generally low (up to 200) for the vaccine serovar Copenhageni (serogroup Icterohaemorrhagiae), with only 42% of the study population showing positive titres after the second vaccination. One recent study evaluated vaccine-associated *Leptospira* antibodies in client-owned dogs following vaccination with four different tetravalent *Leptospira* vaccines (all containing the serovars Canicola, Grippotyphosa, Icterohaemorrhagiae and Pomona) [10]. The authors found a comparable percentage of dogs with positive titres for the serovars Canicola (100%), Grippotyphosa (72%) and Bratislava (44%) after vaccination as in the present study, but in contrast to our results, 94% of the dogs developed positive titres to the serovar Icterohaemorrhagiae. The four vaccines tested in the previous study were different from the vaccine used in the present study; different vaccines could vary in their potential to induce seroconversion to vaccine serovars depending on the strains used in the vaccines. Alternatively, natural exposure or differences in immune status could have affected the vaccine responses of individual dogs in our study. Accordingly, we observed highly variable vaccine responses among individual dogs, as also reported in previous studies [10]. It could be argued that we missed the maximal MAT titres against the Icterohaemorrhagiae serogroup, because we sampled the dogs only once 16–31 days after the second immunization, whereas a previous study followed the MAT titres for several weeks following immunization [10]. However, Martin et al. found the highest MAT titres for the vaccine serovars at weeks 4 and 7 after the start of immunization, which is similar to the time point used in the present study to evaluate seroconversion following vaccination. Importantly, a lack of seroconversion does not imply lack of immune protection against the vaccine serovar Copenhageni. Evaluating the protective potential of *Leptospira* vaccines by use of MAT titres does not provide the entire picture, because previous studies have shown that post-vaccination titres may not correlate with protection [11, 34].

Seroconversion following vaccination was also observed for some non-vaccine serovars, including Autumnalis, Pomona and Pyrogenes. This finding is not unexpected and can be explained by cross-reactivity in MAT among different *Leptospira* serovars. MAT titres are not serovar-specific, and also in recent studies, dogs developed positive titres against non-vaccine serovars following vaccination with bi- and tetravalent *Leptospira* vaccines [10–12]. In one study, dogs showed even highest titres to non-vaccine serovars [12]. In the present study, one dog showed maximal seroconversion for the non-vaccine serovar Autumnalis following vaccination, with a titre of 3200 in MAT, although the titres for all of the vaccine serovars were negative at that time except for the serovar Canicola (800). Besides vaccination, natural exposure to the serovar Autumnalis coinciding with vaccination could have accounted for seroconversion in this animal. However, the dog showed no clinical signs or abnormalities in haematology and blood biochemistry compatible with leptospirosis at that time. Our results indicate that even high titres (≥ 800) against non-vaccine serovars should be interpreted with caution in vaccinated dogs exhibiting signs consistent with leptospirosis.

Half of the dogs showed positive MAT titres at study enrolment for the serovar Canicola, although vaccines containing this serovar had been administered to the dogs up to 1745 days prior to sampling. The dog is assumed to be a natural reservoir host of *L. interrogans* serovar Canicola, and before the introduction of efficient vaccines, clinical leptospirosis in dogs has commonly been associated with this serovar. Because the present study was performed in privately owned dogs with outdoor access, natural exposure to leptospires in addition to vaccination could have resulted in antigenic stimulation in these dogs. Our results are in contrast to an earlier study that evaluated *Leptospira* antibodies in privately owned dogs in Switzerland between 1991 and 1996 [35]. In that study, 34% of the dogs showed positive *Leptospira* antibody titres, with seroconversion to other serovars, e.g., Bratislava, Australis, Icterohaemorrhagiae, Pomona and Grippotyphosa, being common. Moreover, in a survey of 259 dogs from Switzerland over a 10-year-period before the introduction of the tetravalent vaccine, only 12.3% of the dogs showed seropositivity to serovar Canicola [5]. We cannot conclude from the present data whether the positive MAT titres to Canicola were due to previous vaccination or natural exposure to this serovar. However, in light of the large time span elapsed since the last vaccination in some of the seropositive dogs, natural exposure seems likely, and vaccination against this serovar can still be advocated.

In the present study, dogs were specifically examined for evidence of myocarditis due to anecdotal reports of cardiac changes after vaccination with this new vaccine. There is some credibility to such a potential association, because natural infection with leptospirosis may, indeed, cause myocarditis. Even though clinically important myocarditis is rare in dogs and people after natural infection [6, 36], subclinical myocarditis may be quite commonly present in both species based on biochemical abnormalities, specifically the elevation of cTroponin I [6], and histopathological findings [7]. Furthermore, myocarditis has been documented as an adverse event following vaccination in humans, such as after smallpox vaccination [37]. The present study found no echocardiographic, electrocardiographic or biochemical evidence of subclinical vaccine-induced myocarditis. Based on the limited number of dogs included in the present study, myocarditis as a rare complication of leptospirosis vaccination cannot, however, completely be ruled out.

The present study has some limitations. Due to the prospective study design, the number of dogs included in the study was too small to evaluate rare adverse events induced by the vaccine. This could be assessed by large retrospective studies and pharmacovigilance data. The present study also did not follow the course of the MAT titres after vaccination and therefore cannot evaluate the time point of maximal MAT titres and the duration of seropositivity induced by the vaccine. Third, the inclusion of other vaccine components could have influenced the clinical and serological response of the dogs. However, we chose this setting to most accurately mimic the situation in the field, where *Leptospira* vaccines are commonly administered together with other vaccine components licenced for concurrent administration. Finally, measurements of cTroponin I were only obtained before the first and 16–31 days after the second vaccination. It can be argued that an elevation might have been present earlier after vaccination. However, the complete absence of any evidence of morphological, functional and electrical cardiac abnormalities makes clinically important myocardial damage very unlikely.

Conclusions

The present study indicates that the novel tetravalent *Leptospira* vaccine Nobivac® L4 is generally well-tolerated and that clinical signs following vaccination were mild and transient. Seroconversion following vaccination differed considerably among individual dogs and among the vaccine serovars. High titres to non-vaccine serovars were present in some dogs following vaccination, which hampers the interpretation of single MAT titres in vaccinated dogs with clinical signs consistent with leptospirosis. In the light of the high incidence and mortality rate associated with clinical leptospirosis in dogs in Europe, vaccination with this tetravalent vaccine can be advocated for every dog with potential exposure to leptospires.

Additional files

Additional file 1: Medical history and clinical examination findings at different time points before and after vaccination. (DOCX 37 kb)

Additional file 2: Selected haematology results of the dogs before and after vaccination. Values outside the reference range are shown in bold, significant differences between T0 and T2 are shown in italics. (DOCX 35 kb)

Additional file 3: Selected blood biochemistry results before and after vaccination. Values outside the reference range are shown in bold, significant differences between T0 and T2 are shown in italics. (DOCX 35 kb)

Abbreviations

ALAT: Alanine aminotransferase; AP: Alkaline phosphatase; CI: Confidence interval; cTroponin I: Cardiac Troponin I; %FS: Fractional shortening (%); MAT: Microscopic agglutination test; LA/Ao: Left atrial to aortic ratio; LVDd: Left ventricular diameter in diastole; LVDs: Left ventricular diameter in systole; OIE: Office International des Epizooties; p_F: *p*-value of Fisher's exact test; p_W: *p*-value of Wilcoxon signed rank test; r_{sp}: Correlation coefficient of Spearman rank correlation test; T0: Before first vaccination; T1: Second vaccination 20–28 days after the first vaccination; T2: 41–54 days after the first and 16–31 days after the second vaccination; T3: 368–434 days after the first vaccination and 347–413 days after the second vaccination (1 year booster)

Acknowledgements

The authors thank the technicians of the Clinical Laboratory for their excellent laboratory assistance and Stefanie Müller from the Institute of Veterinary Bacteriology for excellent technical assistance.

Funding

AS was supported by a research grant (Forschungskredit, FK-53210-01-01) from the University of Zurich. The funding body played no role in the design of the study and collection, analysis, and interpretation of data and in writing the manuscript.

Authors' contributions

BW, RHL and CR conceived the study. BW and AS were responsible for the study coordination and the data and sample collection. SRC was responsible for the serological analyses by MAT. BR was responsible for the haematology and blood biochemistry tests. JM and TG performed the echocardiography examinations. BW drafted the manuscript. BW, AS, CR and RHL edited the manuscript. All of the authors read and approved the final manuscript.

Competing interests

The authors declare that they have no competing interests.

Author details

[1]Clinical Laboratory, Vetsuisse Faculty, University of Zurich, Winterthurerstr. 260, 8057 Zurich, Switzerland. [2]Center for Clinical Studies, Vetsuisse Faculty, University of Zurich, Winterthurerstr. 260, 8057 Zurich, Switzerland. [3]Clinic for Small Animal Internal Medicine, Vetsuisse Faculty, University of Zurich, Winterthurerstr. 260, 8057 Zurich, Switzerland. [4]Institute of Veterinary Bacteriology, Vetsuisse Faculty, University of Bern, Länggassstr. 122, 3001 Bern, Switzerland.

References

1. Sykes JE, Hartmann K, Lunn KF, Moore GE, Stoddard RA, Goldstein RE. 2010 ACVIM small animal consensus statement on leptospirosis: diagnosis, epidemiology, treatment, and prevention. J Vet Intern Med. 2011;25(1):1–13. doi:10.1111/j.1939-1676.2010.0654.x.
2. Schuller S, Francey T, Hartmann K, Hugonnard M, Kohn B, Nally JE, et al. European consensus statement on leptospirosis in dogs and cats. J Small Anim Pract. 2015;56(3):159–79. doi:10.1111/jsap.12328.
3. Alexander AD, Evans LB, Baker MF, Baker HJ, Ellison D, Marriapan M. Pathogenic leptospiras isolated from Malaysian surface waters. Appl Microbiol. 1975;29(1):30–3.
4. Ellis WA. Control of canine leptospirosis in Europe: time for a change? Vet Rec. 2010;167(16):602–5. doi:10.1136/vr.c4965.
5. Major A, Schweighauser A, Francey T. Increasing incidence of canine leptospirosis in Switzerland. Int J Environ Res Public Health. 2014;11(7):7242–60. doi:10.3390/ijerph110707242.
6. Mastrorilli C, Dondi F, Agnoli C, Turba ME, Vezzali E, Gentilini F. Clinicopathologic features and outcome predictors of *Leptospira interrogans* Australis serogroup infection in dogs: a retrospective study of 20 cases (2001-2004). J Vet Intern Med. 2007;21(1):3–10.
7. Shah K, Amonkar GP, Kamat RN, Deshpande JR. Cardiac findings in leptospirosis. J Clin Pathol. 2010;63(2):119–23. doi:10.1136/jcp.2009.069575.
8. Levett PN. Leptospirosis. Clin Microbiol Rev. 2001;14(2):296–326. doi:10.1128/CMR.14.2.296-326.2001.
9. Goris MG, Hartskeerl RA. Leptospirosis serodiagnosis by the microscopic agglutination test. Curr Protoc Microbiol. 2014;32:Unit 12E 5. doi:10.1002/9780471729259.mc12e05s32.
10. Martin LE, Wiggans KT, Wennogle SA, Curtis K, Chandrashekar R, Lappin MR. Vaccine-associated Leptospira antibodies in client-owned dogs. J Vet Intern Med. 2014;28(3):789–92. doi:10.1111/jvim.12337.
11. Barr SC, McDonough PL, Scipioni-Ball RL, Starr JK. Serologic responses of dogs given a commercial vaccine against *Leptospira interrogans* serovar pomona and Leptospira kirschneri serovar grippotyphosa. Am J Vet Res. 2005;66(10):1780–4.
12. Midence JN, Leutenegger CM, Chandler AM, Goldstein RE. Effects of recent Leptospira vaccination on whole blood real-time PCR testing in healthy client-owned dogs. J Vet Intern Med. 2012;26(1):149–52. doi:10.1111/j.1939-1676.2011.00852.x.
13. Greenlee JJ, Alt DP, Bolin CA, Zuerner RL, Andreasen CB. Experimental canine leptospirosis caused by *Leptospira interrogans* serovars pomona and bratislava. Am J Vet Res. 2005;66(10):1816–22.
14. Fraune CK, Schweighauser A, Francey T. Evaluation of the diagnostic value of serologic microagglutination testing and a polymerase chain reaction assay for diagnosis of acute leptospirosis in dogs in a referral center. J Am Vet Med Assoc. 2013;242(10):1373–80. doi:10.2460/javma.242.10.1373.

15. Jull DJ, Heath KR. The evaluation of a combined *L. canicola* and *L. icterohaemorrhagiae* vaccine on hamsters and dogs. J Small Anim Pract. 1961;1:245–58.

16. Kohn B, Steinicke K, Arndt G, Gruber AD, Guerra B, Jansen A, et al. Pulmonary abnormalities in dogs with leptospirosis. J Vet Intern Med. 2010;24(6):1277–82. doi:10.1111/j.1939-1676.2010.0585.x.

17. Sonrier C, Branger C, Michel V, Ruvoen-Clouet N, Ganiere JP, Andre-Fontaine G. Evidence of cross-protection within *Leptospira interrogans* in an experimental model. Vaccine. 2000;19(1):86–94.

18. Plesko I, Lataste-Dorolle C. Intertype immunity relations of leptospira strains belonging to the 'Australia' serogroup. Biologia. 1970;25:403–11.

19. Adler B, Faine S. The antibodies involved in the human immune response to leptospiral infection. J Med Microbiol. 1978;11(4):387–400. doi:10.1099/00222615-11-4-387.

20. Klaasen HL, van der Veen M, Molkenboer MJ, Sutton D. A novel tetravalent Leptospira bacterin protects against infection and shedding following challenge in dogs. Vet Rec. 2013;172(7):181. doi:10.1136/vr.101100.

21. Klaasen HL, van der Veen M, Sutton D, Molkenboer MJ. A new tetravalent canine leptospirosis vaccine provides at least 12 months immunity against infection. Vet Immunol Immunopathol. 2014;158(1–2):26–9. doi:10.1016/j.vetimm.2013.08.002.

22. Andre-Fontaine G. Diagnosis algorithm for leptospirosis in dogs: disease and vaccination effects on the serological results. Vet Rec. 2013;172(19):502. doi:10.1136/vr.101333.

23. Hoffmann A, Schwedinger E, Werner G, Cussler K. Pharmakovigilanzreport Tierimpfstoffe. Deutsches Tierärzteblatt. 2016;8:1176–8.

24. Müntener CR, Bruckner L, Kupper J, Althaus FR, Schäublin M. Vigilance der Tierarzneimittel: Gemeldete unerwünschte Wirkungen im Jahr 2013. Schweiz Arch Tierheilkd. 2014;156(11):519–25.

25. Yao PJ, Stephenson N, Foley JE, Toussieng CR, Farver TB, Sykes JE, et al. Incidence rates and risk factors for owner-reported adverse events following vaccination of dogs that did or did not receive a Leptospira vaccine. J Am Vet Med Assoc. 2015;247(10):1139–45. doi:10.2460/javma.247.10.1139.

26. Moore GE, Guptill LF, Ward MP, Glickman NW, Faunt KK, Lewis HB, et al. Adverse events diagnosed within three days of vaccine administration in dogs. J Am Vet Med Assoc. 2005;227(7):1102–8.

27. Weissenbacher S, Riond B, Hofmann-Lehmann R, Lutz H. Evaluation of a novel haematology analyser for use with feline blood. Vet J. 2011;187(3):381–7. doi:10.1016/j.tvjl.2010.01.005.

28. Gallay-Lepoutre J, Belanger MC, Nadeau ME. Prospective evaluation of Doppler echocardiography, tissue Doppler imaging and biomarkers measurement for the detection of doxorubicin-induced cardiotoxicity in dogs: a pilot study. Res Vet Sci. 2016;105:153–9. doi:10.1016/j.rvsc.2016.02.001.

29. Office International des Epizooties (OIE). Chapter 2.1.9. Leptospirosis. In: Terrestrial Manual. 7th ed; 2012. p. 251–64.

30. Thomas WP, Gaber CE, Jacobs GJ, Kaplan PM, Lombard CW, Moise NS, et al. Recommendations for standards in transthoracic two-dimensional echocardiography in the dog and cat. Echocardiography Committee of the Specialty of cardiology, American College of Veterinary Internal Medicine. J Vet Intern Med. 1993;7(4):247–52.

31. Rishniw M, Erb HN. Evaluation of four 2-dimensional echocardiographic methods of assessing left atrial size in dogs. J Vet Intern Med. 2000;14(4):429–35.

32. Paul MA, Appel M, Barrett R, Carmichael LE, Childers H, Cotter S, et al. Report of the American animal hospital association (AAHA) canine vaccine task force: executive summary and 2003 canine vaccine guidelines and recommendations. J Am Anim Hosp Assoc. 2003;39(2):119–31.

33. Day MJ. Vaccine side effects: fact and fiction. Vet Microbiol. 2006;117:51–8.

34. Minke JM, Bey R, Tronel JP, Latour S, Colombet G, Yvorel J, et al. Onset and duration of protective immunity against clinical disease and renal carriage in dogs provided by a bi-valent inactivated leptospirosis vaccine. Vet Microbiol. 2009;137(1–2):137–45. doi:10.1016/j.vetmic.2008.12.021.

35. Steger-Lieb A, Gerber B, Nicolet J, Gaschen F. An old disease with a new face: canine leptospirosis does not lose its relevance. Schweiz Arch Tierheilkd. 1999;141(11):499–507.

36. Abgueguen P, Delbos V, Blanvillain J, Chennebault JM, Cottin J, Fanello S, et al. Clinical aspects and prognostic factors of leptospirosis in adults. Retrospective study in France. J Inf Secur. 2008;57(3):171–8. doi:10.1016/j.jinf.2008.06.010.

37. Engler RJ, Nelson MR, Collins LC Jr, Spooner C, Hemann BA, Gibbs BT, et al. A prospective study of the incidence of myocarditis/pericarditis and new onset cardiac symptoms following smallpox and influenza vaccination. PLoS One. 2015;10(3):e0118283. doi:10.1371/journal.pone.0118283.

5

Immunization against GnRF in adult cattle: a prospective field study

Gaby Hirsbrunner[1*], Sarah Rigert[2], Fredi Janett[3], Jürg Hüsler[4], Philipp Schnydrig[5], Ester Lopez[6], Sue Amatayakul-Chantler[6] and Adrian Steiner[1]

Abstract

Background: Suppression of cyclic activity in cattle is often desired in alpine farming and for feedlot cattle, not intended for breeding. A cattle specific anti-GnRF vaccine (Bopriva™) is registered for use in heifers and bulls in different countries. In adult cows vaccinated with Bopriva™, the median period until recurrence of class III follicles was 78 days from the day of the 2nd vaccination and reversibility could be proven, as out of 11 experimental cows 10 cows became pregnant at first, and one cow at second insemination. In the present study, 76 healthy, cyclic Eringer heifers and cows were vaccinated twice with Bopriva™ 3-7 weeks apart, to prevent estrus during alpine pasturing. Blood samples were taken for progesterone and GnRF antibody titer analysis on the day of inclusion (7–9 d before the first vaccination) and at the first vaccination. At the same time, gynaecological examinations were performed. When estrus occurred in the course of the alpine pasturing season, a gynaecological examination was done including analysis of a blood sample (progesterone, anti-GnRF antibody titer). Cows were followed for fertility out to 26 months post second vaccination.

Results: Median duration of estrus suppression was 191 days after the second vaccination (when the 2 vaccinations were given 28–35 days apart). From $n = 13$ cows showing signs of estrus on the alpine pasture, $n = 7$ could not be confirmed in estrus (serum progesterone value >2 ng/ml, no class III follicles seen using ultrasonography). Median duration between second vaccination and next calving was 496 days (25%/75% quartiles: 478/532 days).

Conclusion: Bopriva™ induced a reliable and reversible suppression of estrus for more than 3 months in over 90% of the cows.

Keywords: Cattle, Anti-GnRF, GnRH, Immunization, Estrus, Antibody titer, Eringer breed

Background

Estrus suppression is desired by cattle owners for feedlot animals not intended for breeding and for animals in seasonal breeding management (e.g. summer pasturing in the Alps). Young heifers and older beef cows are often unintentionally pregnant at slaughter (Federal Food Safety and Veterinary Office: Projekt Schlachtung von trächtigen Rindern – Prävalenz und Gründe der Schlachtung). Immunization against GnRF has been used to reduce sexual behavior and to prevent the development of secondary sexual characteristics in males [1–8], and for suppression of estrous cycles [9] and prevention of unwanted pregnancies in females [10, 11]. GnRF antibody titers, ovarian function, progesterone concentration and uterine weight differed significantly between immunized and non-immunized heifers [9]. In adult cows vaccinated with Bopriva™ (Zoetis Australia Limited, 38–42 Wharf Road, West Ryde, NSW 2114, Australia), the median period until recurrence of class III follicles (> 9 mm in diameter and less than 2 cm; [12]) was 78 days from the day of the 2nd vaccination [13]. It was also shown that the absence of class III follicles was the best clinical indicator of anestrus.

Estrous behavior of the cows, though, was inhibited for 30 weeks (180 days after second vaccination). Reversibility could be proven, as 10 out of 11 cows fell pregnant soon after first, and 1 cow after the second insemination [13]. In pastures with commingling of cows from different farms of origin, non-pregnant cows may cause agitation and accidents in the herd because of recurring estrous behavior. This is especially accentuated

* Correspondence: gaby.hirsbrunner@vetsuisse.unibe.ch
[1]Clinic for Ruminants, Vetsuisse Faculty, University of Berne, Bremgartenstrasse 109a, CH-3012 Berne, Switzerland
Full list of author information is available at the end of the article

in the Swiss Eringer breed, raised for fighting and selected for dominance abilities [14]. Estrus suppression during pasture commingling is highly valued, but currently, with the exception of intravaginal progesterone devices, no pharmaceuticals are approved in Switzerland for suppression of cycling activity in food-producing animals. Immunization against GnRF is a likely animal-friendly alternative. Therefore, the aim of this prospective study was to evaluate the duration and efficiency of an active immunization against GnRF using Bopriva™ for estrus suppression in free range adult Eringer cattle during mountain pasturing in the Swiss Alps. Their fertility variables in the subsequent breeding season were described. We hypothesized that the vaccination induced estrus suppression would last longer than 80 days after the 2nd vaccination and that it would be reversible.

Methods

Animals, inclusion and exclusion criteria

From April to May 2014, n = 76 heifers and cows of the Eringer breed (confirmed non-pregnant) spending the summer free ranging on the Alps with daily supervision were included in the study. Animals suffering from purulent vaginal discharge, inseminated less than 30 days before and with a history of recurring ovarian cysts were excluded from the study. The history of the cows and the structure of the farms were investigated by a questionnaire for the owners. Calving dates and number of inseminations in the preceding and subsequent season were additionally sourced from the Swiss animal movement data base (www.agate.ch) and the Eringer breeding association.

Gynaecological examination

The cows were examined twice (at inclusion and first vaccination) within 7–9 days including a vaginoscopy, a rectal palpation of the genital tract and an ultrasonographical examination. Uterine symmetry and tone, cervical opening and properties, and amount of vaginal discharge were recorded [15]. Using ultrasonography (Magic 500, Eickemeyer, Eickemeyer Medizintechnik, Appenzell, Schweiz), the number of follicles was recorded and assigned to 1 of 3 categories, according to the classification of Moreira et al. [16]: class I follicles (≤5 mm in diameter), class II follicles (6–9 mm in diameter), and class III follicles (>9 mm and <2 cm in diameter) [12]. The presence of a corpus luteum (CL) was also noted.

Blood sampling, GnRF antibody titer and progesterone

In all animals, blood was sampled at inclusion, at first and second vaccination and at the time of the first heat after estrus suppression. The blood samples were collected by venipuncture from the coccygeal vein into heparinized tubes, centrifuged (4000 x g, 10 min), and plasma was then stored at −18 °C for later analysis.

GnRF antibody titers were determined by dissociation enhanced lanthanide fluorescence immunoassay (DELFIA) (PerkinElmer Pty Ltd., Glen Waverly, Australia), and results were expressed as relative light units (RLU). Briefly, 384-well streptavidin coated plates (PerkinElmer Pty Ltd., Glen Waverly, Australia) were coated for 1 h at room temperature with 1 μg/mL biotinylated modified GnRH peptide in DELFIA buffer (50 mM Tris-HCl, 0.9% NaCl, 0.05% Tween 20, 20 μM EDTA, 0.2% ovalbumin). Plates were washed and then incubated for 1 h at RT with 50 μL aliquots of cattle samples serially diluted to 1/800 in DELFIA buffer. Unbound plasma and antibodies were removed by washing, and bound antibody was detected by incubating plates for a further 1 h with 50 μL of europium labeled protein G (PerkinElmer Pty Ltd., Glen Waverly, Australia). After washing off excess europium labeled protein G, DELFIA Enhancement Solution (PerkinElmer Pty Ltd., Glen Waverly, Australia) was added to all wells to dissociate bound lanthanide from the antigen forming a highly fluorescent chelate. After 10 min, the intensity of fluorescence was measured by excitation at 340 nm and emission readings at 615 nm using a time resolved fluorometer (Envision 2102 Multireader, Perkin Elmer). Pooled non-vaccinated cattle samples served as a negative control. Unknown samples were compared to serial dilutions of a standard positive reference immune cattle sample. Calculation of a standard curve and reading of unknown samples were performed using the WorkOut 2.5 software (Dazdaq Solutions Ltd., East Sussex, England). Intra- and inter-assay CV were 6.7% and 8.5%, respectively. Serology titers showed a 120 fold range from 3850 RLU titers units for negative samples to 495,000 titers units for immune samples, with 11,500 RLU being taken as the lower cut-off differentiating positive from negative samples. Lowest detection level of GnRF antibody titer was 3850 units [13].

Progesterone concentration was measured using radioimmunoassay (Immunotech, Beckman Coulter, Sinsheim, Germany). The intra-assay coefficient of variation (CV)% was 5.3% and the inter-assay CV% 7.7% determined by using a bovine pool serum, measured 30 times within a test routine and between 25 assay runs. The analytical sensitivity was 0.05 ng/mL and the measurement range was 0.05–50 ng/mL. The assay was performed according to the manufacturer's instructions.

Treatment; GnRF vaccine

The treatment consisted of two vaccinations with the anti-GnRF vaccine Bopriva™ (Bopriva, Zoetis Australia Limited, 38–42 Wharf Road, West Ryde, NSW 2114, Australia) 4 weeks apart whenever applicable. Bopriva™ contains an analogue of GnRF linked to a carrier protein accompanied by a synthetic aqueous adjuvant (400 μg GnRF-protein-conjugate per mL) and is registered with claims to suppress testosterone blood levels in post-pubertal bulls as well as to suppress estrous behavior in post-pubertal heifers. The dosage used for both the initial and the booster vaccination was 400 µg GnRF-protein-conjugate (1 mL Bopriva™). All injections were administered subcutaneously on the right side of the neck.

All animal experimentation was performed with permission and in accordance to Swiss law (https://www.blv.admin.ch/blv/en/home/tiere/tierversuche.html; Nr. G54/3616).

Clinical evaluation, side effects

Behaviour and food intake was carefully observed by the owners. If activity and / or food intake was judged to be reduced for more than 25%, a veterinarian was consulted. The injection site was palpated for signs of heat, swelling and sensitivity daily for 1 week. Estrous behavior observation was conducted daily during alpine pasturing by the responsible herdsmen.

Follow-up

Owners were instructed to immediately report if animals showed estrous behavior. When estrous behavior was observed, a gynaecological examination was performed and another blood sample was taken for analysis of GnRF-antibody titer and serum progesterone concentration. In the cows' first heat after the alpine season, blood samples were planned to be taken and examined.

All owners completed a second questionnaire concerning the first heat of the cows, number of inseminations until next pregnancy and reasons for leaving the farm. Data of subsequent calving was taken from the Swiss animal transportation internet portal (www.agate.ch).

Statistical analysis

The continuous variables are described as mean, sd, median and quartiles, the categorical with absolute and relative frequencies. The primary endpoint "period from 2nd vaccination to estrus" was analyzed with the non-parametric Kaplan-Meier survival function, since some of the cows were slaughtered before coming in heat which is considered as censored time periods. The different periods of the different groups were compared with the log rank test. Several explanatory factors were investigated with the Cox regression. A *p*-value <0.05 indicated a significant result.

Results

Animals, inclusion and exclusion criteria

Ten cows and heifers were excluded because of a missing second vaccination, culling due to other reasons than fertility problems during the alpine pasturing season. Seventy-six animals (13 heifers and 63 cows) were included. Before the alpine pasturing season 90% of the owners took care of their animals themselves, whereas 10% of the owners used a communal cattle shed. All owners preferred seasonal calving from September to December. Concerning the use of the cows, 58.3% of the owners indicated to milk them for a mean of 180 days, 37.5% used them as beef (suckling) cows for a mean of 120 days, and 4.2% of the owners neither milked them nor let the calf suckle. Mean herd size was 10 cows and 4 heifers, 96% of these animals spent the summer on the Alps.

Cows' histories

Median age of the cows and heifers was 5.3 yr. (range: 1.8–10.9 yr). First calving age of the cows was 3.1 yr. (median; range 1.8–4.8 yr). Preceding intercalving period was 445.9 days (mean; range: 311–779 days). Conception index for the preceding pregnancy was 1.5 (median), conception rate at first insemination was 50% and at second insemination was 51.7%. Signs of heat were considered "good" in 67.6%, "moderate" in 26.5% and "not observed" in 5.9% according to the owner's judgment.

Culling rate due to fertility problems was 9.4%.

Gynaecological examination at inclusion / first vaccination

On the day of inclusion, 10 animals suffered from an urovagina. At the time of inclusion and time of first vaccination 67 and 70 animals, respectively had a small uterus that was retractable onto the floor of the pelvis. None of the animals had proliferations of the most caudal cervical ring. A functional CL was present in 46 and 47 of cattle at the time of inclusion and the time of the first vaccination, respectively. Median number of class I-II-III follicles was 2–1-0 at inclusion and 2–1-1 at first vaccination (Additional file 1).

GnRF vaccine; side effects

The 2 vaccinations were performed 20–49 days apart (median 32 days). None of the owners identified any serious adverse side effects in their cows. Most of the cows treated with Bopriva™ showed a slight swelling at the injection site, varying in severity, and moderate local pain for 2–9 days after vaccinations.

GnRF antibody titer and progesterone

The GnRF antibody titer at the inclusion of the study and on the day of the first vaccination was below the detection limit (3800 units). At the second vaccination, the titers ranged between 3850 and 236,998 units (median: 17,870 units) in 62 cows, while in 12 cows, the titer was still below the detection limit (2 results missing). Median titers in heifers at second vaccination and at first signs of heat were higher compared to median values in cows (Table 1). Median antibody titer of animals seen with signs of heat was 3850 (range 3850–16,623).

Table 1 Anti-GnRF antibody titer (DELFIA) in heifers and pluriparous cows at first and second vaccination and at first signs of estrus on the Alp and after the alpine season

	heifers	pluriparous cows
First vaccination		
Median	3850	3850
25% quartile	3.850	3850
75% quartile	3850	3850
Second vaccination		
Median	28,919	15,520
25% quartile	19,501	10,939
75% quartile	41,899	22,494
Estrus signs on the Alp pasture (n = 1 heifer, n = 12 pluriparous cows)		
Median	3850	3850
25% quartile		3850
75% quartile		10,231
First signs of estrus after the alpine season		
Median	17,772	3850
25% quartile	13,885	3850
75% quartile	35,420	10,775

Serum progesterone values ranged from 0.3 to 40 ng/ml (median: 4.7 ng/ml) at first examination. At first vaccination, the serum progesterone levels ranged from 0.3–40 ng/ml (median: 6 ng/ml), with 15 cows ≤2 ng/ml. At the second vaccination, the serum progesterone levels ranged from 0.2–32.1 ng/ml (median: 2.8 ng/ml) with 33 cows ≤2 ng/ml.

Vaccination induced anestrus

One heifer and twelve cows showed signs of estrus while on pasture and 30 animals were detected after return to the farm of origin (alpine season 100–150 days depending on climate). Median duration of estrus suppression after the second vaccination was 113 days (<28 days between the 2 vaccinations), 191 days (28–35 days between the 2 vaccinations) and 229 days (>35 days between the 2 vaccinations). The cox regression was started with the period "2nd vaccination to heat" in days and the explanatory factors "cow", "serum progesterone value at 1st and 2nd vaccination" and the categorized variable "period between the 2 vaccinations". The latter was grouped in group 1 (< 28 days), group 2 (28–35 days), and group 3 (> 35 days). The backward selection revealed only group 1 as a significant factor with $p < 0.0001$. Figure 1 shows the percentages of days between the second vaccination and heat in the three groups. Plasma progesterone at the time of the first and second vaccination did not affect duration of estrus suppression.

Follow-up

Follow-up data were included until 26 months after the second vaccination. Out of the 76 cows, 35 cows were culled within a median of 134 days after the second vaccination. From these 35 cows, 23 were culled without being inseminated (planned to be culled after alpine pasturing), 7 were culled for fertility reasons and 5 for reasons other than fertility problems. Median duration between second vaccination and subsequent calving in 37 cows was 496 d. Calving data of four cows was not available, but they were pregnant in the 2015/2016 season.

Discussion

Our hypothesis was confirmed: the cows' estrus was suppressed for more than 80 d. The alpine pasturing season lasts for a minimum of 100 d, depending on the weather. Therefore, the length of cycle suppression for cows vaccinated with Bopriva™ was satisfactory, and depended on the length of the period between the 2 vaccinations (medians ranged from 113 to 229 days). To our knowledge, this variability in response in females has not been described yet, whereas in bulls it is known, that the duration of testosterone suppression is dependent on the type of adjuvant used, and the number of and the interval between the vaccinations (3–4 weeks versus 6–8 weeks) [17]. GnRF antibody titers at second vaccination and at first signs of heat were increased in heifers as compared to pluriparous cows. As only 17% of the animals included were heifers, a statistical difference could not be determined between the 2 groups. Only twelve cows and one heifer were observed with signs of estrus during alpine pasturing. However, seven of these animals had serum progesterone values >2 ng/ml, no class III follicles when examined on the alpine pasture, but median antibody titers were below the detection limit. In mares vaccinated against GnRF, estrous behavior occurred in anovulatory mares, as only small amounts of estradiol are needed for induction of estrous signs [18]. The characteristics of the old breed "Eringer" are known to be dominant and hot-tempered [14] and might be intensified in the alpine pasturing systems. In older bulls "learnt behaviors" may contribute to sexual behaviors that persist following vaccination with Bopriva™ (personal communication Sue Amatayakul-Chantler). It is possible that the behavioral signs of estrus in cattle may not always be related to findings on the ovaries and serum progesterone concentrations.

The GnRF antibody titer increases 2–3 weeks after the first vaccination and peaks 2 weeks after the second vaccination. Due to alpine pasturing logistics, it was not feasible to measure the anti GnRF antibody titer during the alpine season, except for those cows observed in heat in which serum samples could be taken on the Alps. Median duration between second vaccination and subsequent calving was 496 days. This period consists of 280 days pregnancy and 150 days of alpine pasturing and a voluntary waiting

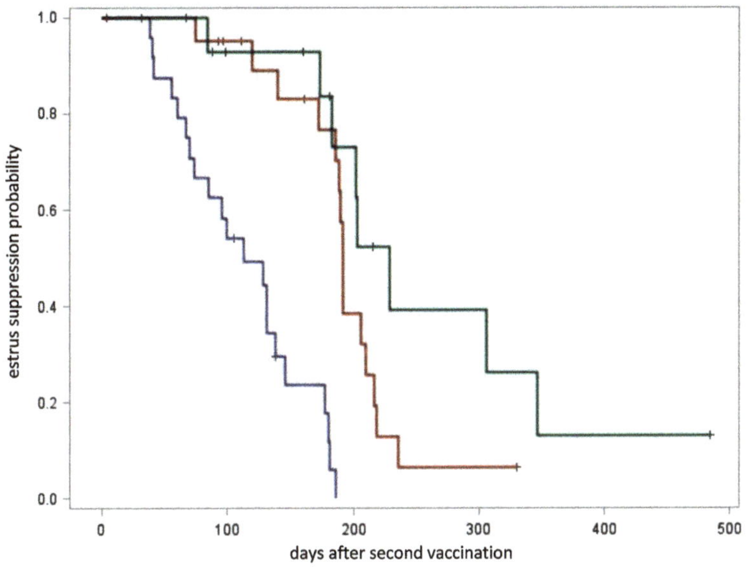

Fig. 1 Kaplan Meyer graph representing the percentage of cattle within group 1–3, versus the duration of the period between second vaccination and estrus. The median times are 113, 191 and 229 days in the three groups. Group 1 (*blue*) = < 28 days, group 2 (*brown*) = 28–35 days, and group 3 (*green*) = > 35 days between the vaccinations. † mean censored data

period of 50–70 days, as alpine pasturing and cow fight rules demand a seasonal calving, with 80% of the calvings occuring between October and December [19]. The calving month and seasonal calving were the most important reasons for a prolonged calving to conception interval in this breed [19]. Therefore, the evaluation of classic fertility variables is difficult in the Eringer cows and vaccinated with Bopriva™, as their preceding calving was between October 2012 and March 2014. Owners prefer to let the cows open instead of allowing them to calve during the wrong season of the year.

Unfortunately, 29% (23/76) of the cows were culled within 6 months after the alpine season e.g. before the end of the subsequent breeding season. For the owners of those cows, it was important that the estrous cycle of the cows be suppressed during the alpine season, so cows could be slaughtered in the fall or winter, when meat prices are higher. In the remaining cows, the culling rate due to fertility problems was 9.2% similar to 9.4% from the preceding season. Our results support those from a previous study that Bopriva™ does not negatively impact bovine fertility [13].

Conclusion

We can highly recommend anti-GnRF vaccination (Bopriva™) for reversible suppression of estrus in Eringer cattle spending the summer on alpine pasture. For a period of 28–35 days between the two vaccinations anestrus is lasting up to 216 days with a median of 191 days. If a longer period of cycle suppression is desired, the period between the two vaccinations should be >35 days. Seventy percent of the cows calved in the subsequent calving seasons.

Abbreviations

CL: Corpus luteum; DELFIA: Dissociation enhanced lanthanide fluorescence immunoassay; GnRF: Gonadotropin Releasing Factor; GnRH: Gonadotropin Releasing Hormone; RLU: Relative light units

Acknowledgements

We thank Zoetis Animal Health for their support and the Eringer owners for providing the data of their cows.

Funding

The study was not funded. Zoetis only guaranteed analysis of GnRF antibody titers for free.

Authors' contributions

GH: planned and coordinated the study, organized the shipping of the samples to Zoetis, was responsible for the animal experimentation application, wrote the manuscript. SR: was responsible for the questionnaire, performed the gynaecological examinations and vaccinations and the blood samplings. FJ: helped with the planning of the study and his experience with Bopriva™ in male animals. JH: calculated all statistical analyses. PS: did his master thesis on the history of the cows and heifers included, and analyzed the questionnaires The thesis is available from the corresponding author on request. EL: helped with the planning of the study concerning the vaccination and the interpretation of the antibody titers. SA: helped with the planning of the study based on her experience with Bopriva™. AS: helped with the coordination of the study and the manuscript. All authors read and approved the final manuscript.

Consent for publication

Not applicable.

Competing interests
The study was not funded; SA had no influence on the analysis of the results and will not profit from this study.

Author details
[1]Clinic for Ruminants, Vetsuisse Faculty, University of Berne, Bremgartenstrasse 109a, CH-3012 Berne, Switzerland. [2]Tierarztpraxis Arche, CH-3952 Susten, Switzerland. [3]Department of Farm Animals, Vetsuisse-Faculty, University of Zurich, Winterthurerstrasse 260, CH-8057 Zurich, Switzerland. [4]Institute of Mathematical Statistics and Actuarial Science, Sidlerstrasse 5, CH-3012 Berne, Switzerland. [5]Institut for Veterinary Bacteriology, Länggassstrasse 122, CH-3012 Berne, Switzerland. [6]Zoetis Research and Manufacturing, 45 Poplar Road, Parkville, VIC A-3052, Australia.

References

1. Cook RB, Popp JD, Kastelic JP, Robbins S, Harland R. The effects of active immunization against GnRHon testicular development, feeedlot performance, and carcass characteristics of beef bulls. J Anim Sci. 2000; doi:10.2527/2000.78112778x.
2. D'Occhio MJ, Aspden WJ, Trigg TE. Sustained testicular atrophy in bulls actively immunized against GnRH: potential to control carcase characteristics. Anim reprod sci. 2001; http://doi.org/10.1016/S0378-4320(01)00091-4.
3. Finnerty M, Enright WJ, Roche JF. Testosterone, LH and FSH episodic secretory patterns in GnRH-immunized bulls. J Reprod Fertil. 1998;114(1):85.
4. Janett F, Gerig T, Tschuor AC, Amatayakul-Chantler S, Walker J, Howard R, Piechotta M, Bollwein H, Hartnack S, Thun R. Effect of vaccination against gonadotropin-releasing factor (GnRF) with Bopriva(R) in the prepubertal bull calf. Anim reprod sci. 2012; http://doi.org/10.1016/j.anireprosci.2012.02.012.
5. Janett F, Lanker U, Jörg H, Hässig M, Thun R. Die Kastration männlicher Lämmer mittels Immunisierung gegen GnRH. Schweiz. Archiv Tierheilk. 2003; doi:10.1024/0036-7281.145.6.291.
6. Janett F, Lanker U, Jörg H, Meijerink E, Thun R. Unterdrückung der Fortpflanzungsaktivität durch aktive Immunisierung gegen GnRH beim adulten weiblichen Schaf. Schweiz. Archiv Tierheilk. 2009; doi:10.1024/0036-7281.151.2.53.
7. Theubet G, Thun R, Hilbe M, Janett F. Effect of vaccination against GnRH (Bopriva(R)) in the male pubertal calf. Schweizer Archiv Tierheilk. 2010; doi:10.1024/0036-7281/a000106.
8. Thompson DL. Immunization against GnRH in male species (comparative aspects). Anim reprod sci. 2000; http://doi.org/10.1016/S0378-4320(00)00116-0.
9. Geary TW, Grings EE, MD MN, de Avila DM, Reeves JJ. Use of recombinant gonadotropin-releasing hormone antigens for immunosterilization of beef heifers. J Anim Sci. 2006;84:343.
10. Prendiville DJ, Enright WJ, Crowe MA, Finnerty M, Hynes N, Roche JF. Immunization of heifers against gonadotropin-releasing hormone: antibody titers, ovarian function, body growth, and carcass characteristics. J Anim Sci. 1995; doi:10.2527/1995.7382382x.
11. Bell M, Daley CA, Berry SL, Adams TE. Pregnancy status and feedlot performance of beef heifers actively immunized against gonadotropin-releasing hormone. J Anim Sci. 1997; doi:10.2527/1997.7551185x.
12. Vanholder T, Opsomer G, deKruif A. Aetiology and pathogenesis of cystic ovarian follicles in dairy cattle: a review. Reprod Nutr Dev. 2006; doi:10.1051/rnd:2006003.
13. Balet L, Janett F, Husler J, Piechotta M, Howard R, Amatayakul-Chantler S, Steiner A, Hirsbrunner G. Immunization against gonadotropin-releasing hormone in dairy cattle: antibody titers, ovarian function, hormonal levels, and reversibility. J Dairy Sci. 2014; doi:10.3168/jds.2013-7602.
14. Plusquellec P, Bouissou M. Behavioural characteristics of two dairy breeds of cows selected (Hérens) or not (Brune des Alpes) for fighting and dominance ability. Appl Anim Behav Sci. 2001;72:1.
15. Sheldon IM. The postpartum uterus. Vet Clin North Am (Food Animals). 2004; doi:10.1016/j.cvfa.2004.06.008.
16. Moreira F, de la Sota RL, Diaz T, Thatcher WW. Effect of day of the estrous cycle at the initiation of a timed artificial insemination protocol on reproductive responses in dairy heifers. J Anim Sci. 2000; doi:10.2527/2000.7861568x.
17. Amatayakul-Chantler S, Hoe F, Jackson JA, Roca RO, Stegner JE, King V, Howard R, Lopez E, Walker J. Effects on performance and carcass and meat quality attributes following immunocastration with the gonadotropin releasing factor vaccine Bopriva or surgical castration of *Bos indicus* bulls raised on pasture in Brazil. Meat Sci. 2013; doi:10.1016/j.meatsci.2013.04.008.
18. Imboden I, Janett F, Burger D, Crowe MA, Hässig M, Thun R. Influence of immunization against GnRH on reproductive cyclicity and estrous behavior in the mare. Theriogenology. 2006; doi:10.1016/j.theriogenology.2006.04.038.
19. Pfister P. Studie über die Fruchtbarkeit der Eringerrasse von 2003–2007. Berne: Vetsuisse Faculty of Berne; Thesis; 2009.

6

Feed-based vaccination regime against streptococcosis in red tilapia, *Oreochromis niloticus* x *Oreochromis mossambicus*

M. S. Ismail[1], A. Siti-Zahrah[2], M. R. M. Syafiq[2], M. N. A. Amal[3], M. Firdaus-Nawi[1] and M. Zamri-Saad[1,4*]

Abstract

Background: Streptococcosis is an important disease of tilapia throughout the world. In Malaysia, streptococcosis outbreak was commonly reported during the 3-month period of high water temperature between April and July. This study describes the duration of protection following single and double booster dose regimes against streptococcosis in tilapia using a feed-based vaccine containing formalin-killed *Streptococcus agalactiae*. A total of 510 tilapias of 120 ± 10 g were selected and divided into 3 groups. Fish of Group 1 were vaccinated at weeks 0 and 2 (single booster group) while fish of Group 2 were vaccinated at weeks 0, 2 and 6 (double booster group) with a feed-based vaccine against streptococcosis. Fish of Group 3 was not vaccinated. Serum samples were collected weekly to determine the antibody level while samples of eye, brain and kidney were collected for bacterial isolation. At week 10, all fish were challenged with live *S. agalactiae* and the survival rate was determined.

Results: Both vaccinated groups showed significant ($p < 0.05$) increase in the antibody levels following the first booster dose, which lasted until week 6. Group 2 showed consistent high level of antibody following the second booster dose at week 6 and remained high until week 12. Challenge trial at week 10 resulted in 45 %, 70 % and 0 % rate of survival for Groups 1, 2 and 3, respectively.

Conclusion: Double booster regime is most suitable to be applied for feed-based vaccination against streptococcosis prior to the start of the hot season.

Keywords: Vaccination regime, Streptococcosis, Red tilapia, Feed-based vaccine

Background

Tilapia is one of the most cultured fish species in the world with China, Egypt and Philippines as major producers [1]. However, with extensive aquaculture activity, farmed fish are affected by environmental fluctuations and husbandry management, which cause stress to the fish and contribute to infections by a wide variety of pathogens [2].

Streptococcosis is one of the major diseases of fish that leads to staggering losses. It is caused by two main species; *Streptococcus agalactiae* and *S. iniae*, affecting a wide range of both freshwater and marine fish species. In Malaysia, most outbreaks of streptococcosis in tilapia are caused by *S. agalactiae* that are influenced by the high water temperature above 31 °C during the hot months of April to July [3].

Vaccination is the most viable option to control streptococcosis in fish [2]. Injection is the most potent route of vaccination as it produces a stronger immune response compared to other routes of vaccination such as spray and immersion [4, 5]. However, the injection method requires a certain level of manpower, technical prowess and proper equipment. Therefore, a more practical route of vaccination is the oral route as there is no direct contact between handler and fish [6]. Furthermore, no specific technical skill is needed to apply the vaccine to the fish. However, oral vaccination results in lower efficacy and shorter period of protection [2]. This paper determines the duration of systemic IgM response and efficacy of the newly developed

* Correspondence: mzamri@upm.edu.my
[1]Department of Veterinary Laboratory Diagnosis, Faculty of Veterinary Medicine, Universiti Putra Malaysia, 43400 Serdang, Malaysia
[4]Present address: Institute of Bioscience, Universiti Putra Malaysia, 43400 Serdang, Malaysia
Full list of author information is available at the end of the article

feed-based vaccine against challenge by field strain of *S. agalactiae*.

Methods

The fish

Red tilapia (*Oreochromis mossambicus* x *O. niloticus*) fingerlings of approximately 2 in. in length were acquired from a hatchery in Tapah, Perak. Upon arrival at the experimental station, the fish were kept in 2 thousand litres capacity fibreglass tanks at 27 °C with running water and aerators. The fish were fed *ad-libitum* twice daily until they reached approximately 100 g bodyweight. Prior to the start of the experiment, the fish were screened for bacterial colonization and antibody level to ensure that they were free from infection by *S. agalactiae* [7].

Bacterial culture

Streptococcus agalactiae strain TP 749B was used in this study. The strain was isolated from an outbreak of streptococcosis in cage-cultured red tilapia in 2007 at Sungai Pahang, Malaysia [8]. The stock that was kept in glycerol at −20 °C was thawed to room temperature overnight prior to use.

Formalin-killed bacteria

The formalin-killed bacteria for vaccine preparation were prepared according to the method of Firdaus-Nawi et al. [6]. Briefly, stock culture of *S. agalactiae* (TP 749B) was streaked onto 5 % blood agar and incubated at 30 °C for 24 h. Propagation of *S. agalactiae* was done by inoculating 10 colonies from the blood agar into Brain Heart Infusion Broth (BHIB) and incubated in a shaker incubator at 150RPM, 30 °C for 24 h. Following incubation, the bacterial concentration was determined using the standard plate count technique [9]. The *S. agalactiae* cells were then harvested by centrifugation (6000 × g, 10 min) and washed with phosphate-buffered saline (PBS) followed by centrifugation (6000 × g, 10 min) for 3 times to remove the medium residue. Afterwards, 10 % buffered formalin was added into the washed pellet to reach a final concentration of 0.5 % formalin before the mixture was kept overnight at 4 °C to kill the bacteria. Then, the bacteria cells were washed again with PBS with centrifugation (6000 × g, 10 min) for 3 times to remove the formalin residue from the culture. The formalin-killed bacteria were re-suspended in sterile PBS solution to obtain the final bacteria concentration of 6.7×10^7 CFU/mL. The suspension was streaked onto blood agar and incubated for 24 h at 37 °C to ensure that all *S. agalactiae* were killed. To improve the vaccine antigenicity, Freund's incomplete adjuvant (FIA) was added to a final concentration of 10 % before it was thoroughly mixed with pelletted feed to give a final concentration of 10^6 cells/kg of feed [6].

Experimental design

A total of 510 red tilapia hybrid (*Oreochromis mossambicus* x *O. niloticus*) fish with an average weight of 120 ± 10 g were selected and equally divided into 3 groups; the single booster, double booster and control groups. Ten fish were placed into each of the 51 glass aquaria containing 100 L water at an average water temperature of 29 °C, provided with aeration and running water with 12-h light and dark periods. The fish were fed with commercial feed (Cargill, Malaysia).

At the start of the experiment, the vaccine was orally administered on day 0 by feeding the fish with feed containing the vaccine at 4 % body weight twice; at 8 am and 3 pm. To ensure that all treated fish received the feed-based vaccine, they were deprived of feed for 24 h and while feeding, the feed-based vaccine was distributed slowly and evenly in each glass aquaria. For single booster group, vaccination was repeated on day 14, while the double booster group received the feed-based vaccine on days 14 and 42. The unvaccinated control group was given regular commercial feed without the vaccine. On other days, all fish were fed with normal commercial pellet throughout the 14-week study period.

Serum samples to determine the antibody level were collected from 10 fish of each group at weekly intervals beginning from day 0 until day 98 when the experiment was terminated. The same procedure was replicated and data from both experiments were pooled and analysed.

Challenge trial

The challenge trial was carried out at week 10 of the experiment. Twenty fish from each of the three groups were transferred into 6 glass aquaria without running water. These 20 selected fish from each group were kept in 2 aquaria at the rate of 10 fish per aquarium as duplicate. A fresh inoculum containing live virulent cells of *S. agalactiae* strain NF958 at a concentration of 1.0×10^9 CFU/ml was prepared before 0.5 ml of the inoculum was injected intraperitoneal (i.p.) into each fish. The fish were anaesthetized with *Tricaine methanesulfonate* (MS-222) prior to the i.p. injection [6]. After challenged, all fish were closely observed at hourly intervals for behavioural and physical changes. Fish that died within the first 6 h were excluded from the experiment while fish that showed advanced clinical signs of the infection were euthanized. At the end of day 7 post-challenge, all surviving fish were killed by an overdose of MS-222. They were subjected to post-mortem examination before samples of brain, eye and kidneys were collected for bacterial isolation. The level of protection or relative percentage survival (RPS) value was then determined [10].

$$RPS = 1 - (\%\ \text{immunized group mortality}/\ \%\ \text{control group mortality}) \times 100$$

Bacterial isolation

Organ samples were streaked onto blood agar and were incubated at 37 °C for 18 to 24 h. Following incubation dominant colonies were sub-cultured to obtain pure colonies before they were subjected to Gram staining, oxidase and catalase tests. Isolates that were Gram-positive, cocci shaped and catalase negative were subjected to API 20 STREP bacteria identification kit (BioMerieux, France). The Gram-positive cocci but catalase positive were subjected to API STAPH (BioMerieux, France). Similarly, Gram-negative isolates, which were oxidase negative, were subjected to API 20E while those that were oxidase positive were subjected to API 20NE (BioMerieux, France). The API colour codes were referred to the APILAB PLUS program (BioMerieux, France) for species and genus determination of the isolates. Cultures that were identified as *S. agalactiae* by API20 STREP were further confirmed by API 20STREP and BLAST analysis of 16S rRNA sequence of PCR product [11].

Enzyme-linked immunosorbent assay

All serum samples were subjected to indirect ELISA [12, 13] that detected the IgM. Coating antigen was prepared by culturing *S. agalactiae* into brain-heart infusion broth and incubated for 24 h in shaker incubator at 30 °C, 150 rpm. Bacterial concentration was determined using standard plate count technique before harvested by centrifugation and washed with phosphate buffer saline (PBS). The bacterial pellet was then resuspended in carbonate-bicarbonate buffer (pH 9.6) to a final concentration of 2.5×10^5 CFU/ml. The suspension was boiled in water bath at 97 °C for 20 min to kill the bacteria and cooled to room temperature prior to use as coating antigen.

Flat-bottomed microtitre plates were coated with 100 μL coating antigen and were left overnight at 4 °C before washed twice with PBS + 0.05 % Tween 20 (PBST). Then, 200 μL of 1 % bovine serum albumin (BSA) was added to block unspecific binding sites and incubated in 37 °C for 1 h. This was followed by adding 100 μL of serum (1:1000) into the reaction and similarly incubated. After that, 100 μL of goat anti-tilapia hyperimmune serum, diluted 1:10,000 was added and incubated again. Next, 100 μL of conjugated rabbit anti-goat IgM-horseradish peroxidase (Nordic, Netherland) diluted to 1:10,000 was added into the reaction and incubated. After washed for three times with PBST, bound conjugates were detected by adding 100 μL of TMB One substrate solution (Promega, USA) before the reaction was stopped with 0.2 mol/L sulphuric acid. The absorbance was determined at 450 nm wavelength (Bio-Rad, USA).

The cut-off value is the highest possible true-positive rate [14] that is used as an indication of protection. It was determined by performing ELISA on 100 serum samples collected from non-immunized tilapia obtained from farms that had no history of streptococcosis infection and did not practice vaccination against the target organism. After subtracting the blank wells, the average OD value was times 2 to get the cut-off value of 0.2 OD.

Statistical analysis

The significance value of the results was calculated by using one way analysis of variance (ANOVA) employed by Tukey HSD in Statistix 9 software (Analytical software, USA). The results were considered as significant at $p < 0.05$.

Results

Serum antibody response

The serum IgM antibody levels of all groups prior to vaccination showed insignificant ($p > 0.05$) differences. Following vaccination, both vaccinated groups showed significantly ($p < 0.05$) higher IgM levels compared to the control group. Following the first booster dose at week 2, the increasing pattern continued for both vaccinated groups and reached peak at week 3. The level, however, started to decrease insignificantly ($p > 0.05$) in the following week but significantly ($p < 0.05$) thereafter to reach the non-protective cut-off value ($p > 0.05$) at weeks 5 and 6 (Fig. 1). In the first 6 weeks post-vaccination, both vaccinated groups showed insignificantly ($p > 0.05$) high IgM value. However, following second booster in week 6, the antibody level significantly ($p < 0.05$) increased again to reach peak at week 8 before declining thereafter until week 12 (Fig. 1). The vaccinated group that received a single booster showed gradual decline in IgM levels to reach the same level ($p > 0.05$) as the cut-off value by week 7 and below the cut-off value thereafter until the end of the experimental period. At time of challenge in week 10, the IgM level of the double booster group was significantly ($p < 0.05$) higher while the single booster and control groups were significantly ($p < 0.05$) lower than the protective cut-off value (Fig. 1).

Challenge trial

Following intraperitoneal challenge, fish mortality was observed among the control group as early as 24 h post-challenge. Clinical symptoms were apparent in the control group, which included lethargy, exophthalmia, erratic

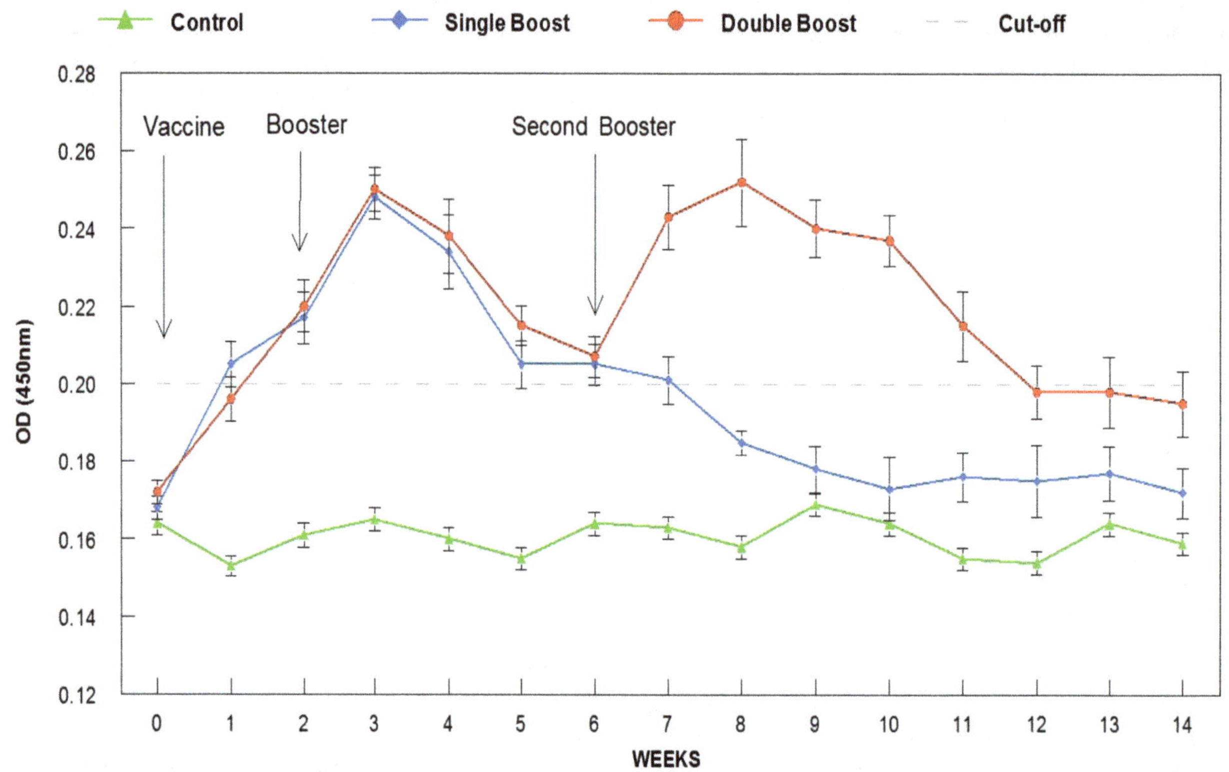

Fig. 1 Serum antibody (IgM) response following oral vaccination with a feed-based vaccine. Double booster at weeks 2 and 6 prolonged the high antibody levels for up to 12 weeks compared to the single booster at week 2 that lasted 6 weeks

swimming, inflammation at injection area and loss of appetite while few vaccinated fish showed signs of lethargy and loss of appetite. At the end of day 7 post-challenge, none of the unvaccinated control fish had survived compared to 45 % and 70 % survival rates of single and double booster vaccinated fish, respectively (Table 1).

Post-mortem examinations revealed congested kidney, enlarged spleen, pale liver and soft, watery brain. Haemorrhages were also registered in various organs including liver, gastrointestinal organs and brain.

Bacterial isolation

Streptococcus agalactiae was successfully re-isolated from the brain, eye and kidney of all dead fish. The presence of clear zone around cultured colonies was suggestive of β-haemolytic *S. agalactiae* that was confirmed by BLAST analysis of 16S rRNA sequence of PCR product.

Discussion

As development in aquaculture industry continues to expand, many vaccines against many diseases are made available with the purpose of controlling disease outbreaks. Commercial vaccines for tilapia against streptococcosis are currently available in many countries and are widely used. The most common type of vaccine for streptococcosis is the injectable vaccine, administered via intraperitoneal route as it provides the best protection against streptococcosis. Immersion vaccines such as AQUAVAX™ and GARVETIL™ (Intervet Pty. Ltd.) are

Table 1 Comparative fish mortality, survival and relative percentage survival (RPS) between controls unvaccinated fish, fish vaccinated with single booster, and fish vaccinated with double booster regimes followed by intraperitoneal challenge with 0.5 mL of 1.0×10^9 CFU/mL of live *Streptococcus agalactiae*

Group	Number of Fish	Mortality (n) Post-challenge							Survival	RPS
		D1	D2	D3	D4	D5	D6	D7	Rate (%)	
Single Booster	20	6	3	0	1	1	0	0	45	45^b
Double Booster	20	3	2	0	1	0	0	0	70	70^c
Control	20	7	5	3	3	2	0	0	0	0^a

^{a,b,c}Different superscripts indicate significant difference ($p < 0.05$)

available and are claimed to be more practical for administration but lower in efficacy [5]. The focus of these commercial vaccines, however, was mainly for large farms that can afford high manpower, technicality and facilities for carrying out such vaccinations. Small-scale private farmers in Southeast Asia such as Vietnam, Malaysia, Indonesia and Thailand, however, are unlikely to be able to afford labor-intensive vaccine protocols requiring special equipment. They, therefore, require an easier, cost effective, user friendly and less stressful method of vaccination, which is what oral vaccination can provide [14]. Furthermore, large scale fish producers can also benefit from oral vaccination since an effective, feed-based vaccine could greatly reduce stress in the production fish by avoiding handling during vaccination and lower the cost associated with manpower and equipment.

It is well documented that different routes of vaccination give different intensity of immune response and thus, different vaccine efficacy [13]. Vaccination via intraperitoneal and intramuscular injections triggers a systemic immune response with high antibody levels in a short period of time. This provides longer protection compared to immersion and oral exposure that triggers local mucosal immunity [15, 16]. Nevertheless, if sufficient amount of antigen is managed to be transported and reach the end gut segment of fish such as carp, both local and systemic immune responses are induced [17]. The second gut segment of fish especially grouper plays an important role in oral vaccination as it participates in the transportation and presentation of antigen from intestinal lumen to intraepithelial macrophages [7]. These macrophages ingest the antigen presented by this route and remigrate from the intestine to lymphoid organs mainly the spleen and kidney before initiating systemic immune response [17]. Similar mechanisms are believed to occur in tilapia.

Our earlier study revealed that feed-based bacterin without adjuvant was able to stimulate IgM response for a brief period of 3 weeks [6]. Addition of incomplete Freund's adjuvant was able to prolong the response to 6 weeks but was not long enough to cover the 3-month critical period. Therefore, in this study, different oral vaccination regimes were tested in trying to maintain immune response and protective efficacy to cover the 3-month critical period. Administration of second booster at week 6 resulted in a significant increase in the level of serum IgM for up to week 12, covering the 3-month period required for protection of tilapia during the hot months of April to July. This was further clarified following challenge at week 10 when 45 % and 70 % of the single booster and double booster groups survived, respectively. Therefore, double booster provided longer period of high antibody titre that protected at least 70 % of the fish. This is in agreement with earlier studies that show that a repetition of vaccine dosage or booster dose provides better immune responses and lasting protection [18, 19].

A vaccine that provides 70 % protection is considered a good vaccine, but an excellent vaccine provides >80 % protection [20]. Furthermore, oral vaccination stimulates both mucosal and systemic immune responses, which is an advantage since natural streptococcosis involves entrance of the pathogen through mucosal organs of mouth and skin before entering the blood stream [21]. Naturally, the pathogens initially encounter the mucosal barrier of skin and gut lining before reaching the blood stream. Many studies have highlighted on the presence of some key components of mucosal immunity, particularly the IgT or IgZ antibody that are associated with mucosal immunity in fish. Furthermore, the role of intestinal T cells and their functions, particularly in antigen uptake mechanisms at mucosal surfaces has been highlighted, which is important in mucosal vaccination strategies [22]. Similarly, a study in grouper revealed that oral administrations of antigen stimulate the gut-associated lymphoid tissue of the intestine leading to higher level of IgM [7].

Conclusion

In conclusion, oral vaccination using feed-based vaccine containing formalin-killed bacteria is a viable option in tilapia vaccination against streptococcosis as it can provide systemic immune response against *S. agalactiae*. Administration of second booster dose provides longer period of protection that last for at least 12 weeks at a rate of 70 % protection.

Acknowledgements
Technical assistance from Mr. Shahidan, Mr. Fahmi and Mrs Nur Nazifah is gratefully appreciated.

Funding
The study was partially funded by the AgroBiotechnology Institute, the Ministry of Science, Technology and Innovation Malaysia.

Authors' contribution
MSI collected and analysed data, and drafting of manuscript. SZA designed the experiment and revised manuscript. MRMS collected and processes the samples and analysed data. MNAA designed the experiment, analysed data and revised the manuscript. MFN collected and analysed data. MZS designed experiment, analysed data and revised manuscript. All authors read and approved the final manuscript.

Competing interests
The authors declare that they have no competing interests.

Consent for publication
Not applicable.

Author details
[1]Department of Veterinary Laboratory Diagnosis, Faculty of Veterinary Medicine, Universiti Putra Malaysia, 43400 Serdang, Malaysia. [2]National Fish Research and Disease Diagnosis, Fisheries Research Institute, 11960 Batu Maung, Penang, Malaysia. [3]Department of Biology, Faculty of Science, Universiti Putra Malaysia, 43400 Serdang, Malaysia. [4]Present address: Institute of Bioscience, Universiti Putra Malaysia, 43400 Serdang, Malaysia.

References

1. FAO. Cultured aquatic species information programme, *Oreochromis niloticus* (Linnaeus, 1758). FAO Fisheries and Aquaculture Department; http://www.fao.org/fishery/culturedspecies/Oreochromis_niloticus/en. 2015; Accessed 25 Sept 2015.
2. Zamri-Saad M, Amal MNA, Siti-Zahrah A, Zulkafli AR. Control and prevention of streptococcosis in cultured tilapia in Malaysia: a review. Pertanika J Trop Agric Sci. 2014;37:389–410.
3. Amal AMN, Zamri-Saad M. Streptococcosis in tilapia *(Oreochromis niloticus):* a review. Pertanika J Trop Agric Sci. 2011;34:195–206.
4. Klesius PH, Shoemaker CA, Evans JJ. Efficacy of single and combined *Streptococcus iniae* vaccine administered by intraperitoneal and intramuscular routes in tilapia (*Oreochromis niloticus).* Aquaculture. 2000;188:237–46.
5. Silva BC, Martins ML, Jatoba A, Neto CCB, Vieira FN, Pereira GV, Jeronimo GT, Seiffert WQ, Mourino JLP. Hematological and immunological responses of Nile tilapia after polyvalent vaccine administration by different routes. Pesq Vet Brasil. 2009;29:874–80.
6. Firdaus-Nawi M, Sabri MY, Hanan Y, Siti-Zahrah A, Zamri-Saad M. Efficacy of feed-based adjuvant vaccine against *Streptococcus agalactiae* in *Oreochromis* spp. in Malaysia. Aquacul Res. 2013a;45:87–96.
7. Firdaus-Nawi M, Zamri-Saad M, Nik-Haiha NY, Zuki ABS, Effendy AWM. Histological assessment of intestinal immuno-morphology of tiger grouper juvenile, *Epinephelus fuscoguttatus.* SpringerPlus. 2013b;2:611–23.
8. Amal MNA, Zamri-Saad M, Siti-Zahrah A, Zulkafli AR. Water quality influences the presence of *Streptococcus agalactiae* in cage cultured red hybrid tilapia, *Oreochromis niloticus* x *Oreochromis mossambicus.* Aquacul Res. 2013;46:313–23.
9. Wohlsen T, Bates J, Vesey G, Robinson WA, Katouli M. Evaluation of the methods for enumerating coliform bacteria from water samples using precise reference standards. Lett Appl Microbil. 2006;42:350–6.
10. Amend DF. Potency testing of fish vaccines. Dev Biol Standard. 1981;49:447–54.
11. Abuseliana A, Daud H, Saleha AA, Khairani-Bejo S, Alsaid M. *Streptococcus agalactiae* the aetiological agent of mass mortality in farmed red tilapia *(Oreochromis* spp.). J Anim Vet Adv. 2013;9:2640–6.
12. Shelby RA, Shoemaker CA, Evans JJ, Klesius PH. Development of an indirect ELISA to detect humoral responses to *Streptococcus iniae* infections of Nile tilapia, Oreochromis niloticus. J Appl Aquacul. 2001;11:35–44.
13. Grabowski LD, LaPatra SE, Cain KD. Systemic and mucosal antibody response in tilapia, *Oreochromis niloticus* (L.) following immunization with *Flavobacterium columnare.* J Fish Dis. 2004;27:573–81.
14. Holten-Andersen L, Dalsgaard I, Nylen J, Lorenzen N, Buchmann K. Determining Vaccination Frequency in Farmed Rainbow Trout Using Vibrio anguillarum O1 Specific Serum Antibody Measurements. PLoS One. 2012; 7(11):e49672. doi:10.1371/journal.pone.0049672.
15. Rombout JHWM, Kiron V. Mucosal Vaccination of Fish. In: Guddings R, Lillehaug D, Evensen O, editors. Fish Vaccination. Chichester: John Wiley & Sons, Ltd; 2014. doi:10.1002/9781118806913.ch6.
16. Thune RL, Collins LA, Penta MP. A comparison of immersion, immersion/oral combination and injection methods for the vaccination of channel catfish, *Ictalurus punctatus* against *Edwardsiella ictaluri.* J World Aquacul Soc. 1997; 28:193–201.
17. Pereira GV, da Silva BC, Vieira FN, Seiffert WQ, Ushizima TT, Mourino JLP, Martins ML. Vaccination strategies with oral booster for surubim hybrid *(Pseudoplatystoma corruscans x P. reticulatum)* against haemorrhagic septicaemia. Aquacul Res. 2013;46:1831–41.
18. Rombout JHWM, van den Berg AA. Immunological importance of the second gut segment of carp. I. Uptake and processing of antigens by epithelial cells and macrophages. J Fish Biol. 1989;35:13–22.
19. Chettri JK, Deshmukh S, Holten-Anderssen L, Jaafar RM, Dalsgaard I, Buchman K. Comparative evaluation of administration methods for a vaccine protecting rainbow trout against *Yersinia ruckeri* O1 biotype 2 infection. Vet Immun Immunopath. 2013;154:42–7.
20. Chettri JK, Jaafar RM, Skov J, Kania PW, Dalsgaard I, Buchman K. Booster immersion vaccination using diluted *Yersinia ruckeri* bacterin confers protection against ERM in rainbow trout. Aquacult. 2015;440:1–5.
21. Jarp J, Tverdal A. Statistical aspects of fish vaccination trials. Dev Biol Standard. 1997;90:311–20.
22. Iregui CA, Comas J, Vasquez GM, Verjan N. Experimental early pathogenesis of *Streptococcus agalactiae* infection in red tilapia *Oreochromic* spp. J Fish Dis. 2016;39:205–15.

7

Immunogenic potential of a *Salmonella* Typhimurium live vaccine for pigs against monophasic *Salmonella* Typhimurium DT 193

Tobias Theuß[1*], Elke Ueberham[2], Jörg Lehmann[2], Thomas Lindner[1] and Sven Springer[1]

Abstract

Background: Monophasic *Salmonella* Typhimurium (mSTM) strains account for up to 8.6% of all human Salmonellosis cases. They have an increasing prevalence during recent years and several human cases with hospitalisation were reported. These strains are often isolated from pigs and pork - one primary source of human infection. A *Salmonella* Typhimurium (STM) live vaccine has been proven successful in controlling of STM infections in pigs for many years. The aim of this study was to test the immunogenicity of the vaccine in weaners during oral challenge with a virulent mSTM strain and to examine the kinetics of STM-specific IgA, IgM and IgG antibodies induced by vaccination and infection.

Results: Despite clinical signs being present in both groups, the vaccination led to a significant reduction of diarrhoea, overall clinical symptoms and a milder elevation of the body temperature. Necropsy revealed fewer pathological lesions in the gastrointestinal tract of vaccinated compared to control animals. Moreover, in the ileal and caecal mucosa and in the ileocaecal lymph nodes the challenge strain burden was significantly reduced by vaccination. Significant differences in the antibody responses of both groups were present during the vaccination period and after infection. In vaccinated animals *Salmonella*-specific IgA and IgG antibody levels increased significantly after vaccination and were even more pronounced in response to challenge. In contrast, similarly low levels of IgM antibodies were detected during the vaccination period in both vaccinated and non-vaccinated animals. However, after challenge IgM antibody levels increased significantly in control pigs while neither IgA nor IgG antibodies were detectable.

Conclusion: The data demonstrate that mSTM can evoke clinical signs in weaners. Due to the vaccination their incidence and magnitude were significantly milder. Vaccination also led to a significantly reduced challenge strain burden in the intestine and the lymph nodes which is comparable to previous studies using the same vaccine in a challenge with biphasic STM. Therefore, it is concluded that this vaccine induces immunity against monophasic and biphasic STM strains. Furthermore, the results of antibody profiles in response to vaccination and infection provide additional evidence for humoral immune mechanisms triggered during *Salmonella* infection or vaccination.

Keywords: Salmonella Typhimurium, Vaccination, Infection, Salmoporc, IgM, IgA, IgG, Serology, ELISA, Antibody response

* Correspondence: tobias.theuss@idt-biologika.de
[1]IDT Biologika GmbH, Business Unit Animal Health, Research and Development, Am Pharmapark, 06861 Dessau-Rosslau, Germany
Full list of author information is available at the end of the article

Background

Salmonella Enteritidis (SE), *Salmonella* Typhimurium (STM) and monophasic *Salmonella* Typhimurium strains (mSTM) were the most common reported serovars detected in human foodborne salmonellosis in the EU during recent years [1]. While confirmed infections with SE showed a decreasing incidence within the last years, those with STM and mSTM are progressively taking their place. In 2014 and 2015, 25.2% or 28.8% of all diagnosed cases of human Salmonellosis were attributed to these strains, respectively [1].

Monophasic *Salmonella* Typhimurium are often isolated from pigs and pork [1, 2]. Normally, they are multidrug-resistant and belong to phage type DT 120 and DT 193 (Anderson) [2]. In contrast to biphasic STM (seroformula 4,[5],12:i:1,2) their monophasic variants are lacking the H-antigen (seroformula 4,[5],12:i:-) according to the Kauffmann-White-LeMinor-Scheme [2]. Several diffuse outbreaks involving human cases with requirement of hospitalization have been reported [3–5].

Besides hygienic procedures at the barn level a STM live vaccine (Salmoporc®/Salmoporc STM®, IDT Biologika) based on an attenuated STM strain has been proven successful in controlling of STM infections in pigs for many years as shown in several laboratory [6–9] and field trials [10]. However, all of the mentioned laboratory studies have shown protection against STM. Protection against mSTM has not been confirmed in laboratory studies so far but is very likely upon consideration of the results of a large field study in the UK [10].

Although both humoral and cell-mediated immune mechanisms play an important role in the control of *Salmonella* infections [11], the detection of antibodies in blood serum or meat juice is of special interest as serology was and still is used in several governmental surveillance programs (e.g. Denmark, Belgium, Germany, Ireland, Sweden, The Netherlands).

Several commercial ELISA kits were developed but two different approaches dominated. Either an ELISA, based on a mix of LPS-antigen that is directed against *Salmonella*-specific IgG (Salmotype® PigScreen, Labor Diagnostik Leipzig, Leipzig, Germany; Swine Salmonella Ab Test, IDEXX, Hoofddorp, The Netherlands) or a test based on a whole-cell lysate of purified STM (Salmotype® Pig STM-WCE ELISA, Labor Diagnostik Leipzig) [12]. The latter test also allowed discrimination between *Salmonella*-specific IgM, IgA, and IgG [12]. Although this ELISA kit is no longer commercially available, it can be applied as an in-house format in our laboratory.

Numerous studies aimed to analyse the antibody response after STM infection [13–15] or vaccination [16]. However, to the best of our knowledge no approaches have been conducted to study the serological response of vaccination and subsequent challenge infection with STM in pigs.

Therefore, the aim of this study was to test the immunogenic potential of the vaccine against mSTM and to investigate the kinetic of antibody response to immunization and infection induced by the vaccine or the challenge strain, respectively.

Methods

Weaners at the age of 4 weeks ($n = 16$, dam: German Landrace x German Large White, sire: Pietrain) were randomly selected from 4 sows and included in this study. All animals derived from the livestock of IDT Biologika GmbH and were owned by the company. The weaners were serologically negative for *Salmonella* spp. (< 10 OD %) and were tested bacteriologically negative for *Salmonella* spp. (individual faecal samples) prior to the beginning of the trial. All weaners were randomly selected to either the vaccination or the control group ($n = 8$ per group), which were housed separately in air-conditioned high-security rooms (BSL 2). The weaners were allocated in groups of 4 animals. Food and water were provided ad libitum and a commercial diet without anti-*Salmonella* ingredients (e.g. probiotics, prebiotics) was fed. The animal trial was conducted according to the German law of animal welfare (Reference no. 42502–3-753 IDT, Landesverwaltungsamt Sachsen-Anhalt). The study was performed as a randomized and blinded trial.

The vaccination group received 1.0 ml of the live attenuated *Salmonella* Typhimurium vaccine (Salmoporc®/Salmoporc STM®, IDT Biologika, Dessau-Rosslau, Germany) adjusted with physiologic saline solution at the minimal dose of 5×10^8 CFU/ml. The vaccine strain was attenuated by chemical induced mutagenesis followed by phenotypical selection and is adenine/histidine auxotrophic. The control group received physiologic saline solution as placebo. The animals were vaccinated twice orally at an interval of 3 weeks using an oral drencher kit (IDT Biologika, Dessau-Rosslau, Germany) (study days 0 and 21). For drenching a second person fixed the animal in a slight upright position prior administration of the vaccine/placebo in the buccal cavity.

Three weeks after the 2nd administration of the vaccine (study day 42), both groups were orally infected with 5×10^9 CFU/ml of a virulent *S. enterica* 4,[5],12:i: (DT 193) wild-type strain (kindly provided by Dr. W. Rabsch, National Reference Centre for *Salmonella* and other Enteric Bacterial Pathogens, Robert Koch Institute, Wernigerode, Germany) resistant to ampicillin (A), streptomycin (S), sulfamerazine (Su) and oxytetracycline (T). The challenge strain was administered to each pig in 5.0 ml sugar solution using an oral drench as described above.

Clinical scores were recorded daily during the challenge period according to the following scheme:

(i) diarrhoea (0 = none, 1 = yes, pulpy consistency, 2 = yes, liquid consistency)
(ii) depression (0 = none, 1 = reduced alertness, 2 = animal apathetic)
(iii) food intake (0 = normal, 1 = reduced, 2 = no food intake)
(iv) body temperature (in °C)

Summative 'diarrhoea scores' and 'clinical scores' (all scores added, including diarrhoea) were estimated daily for every group.

All animals were euthanized 6 or 7 days post challenge (p.chall.; study days 48 or 49, respectively; 4 animals of each group per day) by intravenous pentobarbital administration (Release® 500, WDT, Garbsen, Germany) during ketamine and azaperone anesthesia (Ursotamin®, Serumwerk Bernburg, Bernburg, Germany; Stresnil®, Elanco, Bad Homburg, Germany).

The quantitative determination of the number of challenge strain organisms ($\log_{10}$ CFU/g) of the ileal or caecal mucosa, and the ileocaecal lymph nodes was carried out using the Koch spread-plate method as previously described [6]. In brief, after weight assessment the tissue samples were homogenized (Ultra-Turrax T25, Janke & Kunkel, IKA®-Labortechnik Staufen, Germany) and a 10-fold dilution series was prepared. The number of bacteria was then estimated by plating out the homogenate on desoxycholate citrate agar supplemented with antibiotics ('ASSuT,' see above). The incubation was performed at 37 ± 1 °C for 24 h under aerobic conditions. Samples which failed to grow when plated out directly were examined according to DIN ISO 6579:2002/A1:21,007 Annex D. Blood samples for serology were taken before the 1st (B0) and 2nd (B1) vaccination, before (B2) as well as 6/7 days p.chall. (B3) in the course of the necropsy. After coagulation of the fibrin clot at 20 °C for 4 h, all samples were centrifuged for 10 min at 3500 x g. The sera were then collected and stored at −20 °C until analysis.

All serum samples were tested using a commercially available ELISA kit (Swine Salmonella Ab Test, IDEXX, Hoofddorp, The Netherlands) that detects IgG antibodies against *Salmonella*-specific LPS. This analysis was performed at IVD Diagnostik (Hannover, Germany) according to the manufacturer's instruction (cut-off < 10 OD%).

Furthermore, all samples were analysed with an optimized in-house WCE ELISA for determining the *Salmonella*-specific IgM, IgA, and IgG immunoreactivity according to the following instruction. The Salmoporc®/Salmoporc STM® vaccine strain was grown overnight for seeding a fresh logarithmic culture which was harvested at an optical density of 0.3 (wavelength = 600 nm; Saphire 2, Microplate reader, Tecan Group Ltd., Männedorf, Switzerland). The bacteria were lysed in 8 M urea at 60 °C for 5 min and centrifuged at 12,000 x g for 10 min. Protein content of supernatant was determined by Bradford assay (SIGMA Aldrich, Deisenhofen, Germany) and 10 µg/ml protein was immobilized onto a 96-well flat-bottomed microplate (Medisorp™, Nunc, Wiesbaden, Germany) at 4 °C overnight. Plates were washed three times with phosphate-buffered saline, 154 mM NaCl, 0.05% Tween (3× PBS-T) and blocked with Superblock™ blocking buffer (Thermo Fisher Scientific, Schwerte, Germany). Swine sera were diluted 12.5-fold for IgM and IgA or 200-fold for IgG determination. After preincubation with soluble *E. coli* proteins, which were prepared from logarithmic culture by lysis with 8 M urea at 60 °C for 5 min and spinning down at 12,000 x g for 10 min, for 1 h at room temperature in order to quench cross-reactivity. Preadsorbed sera were incubated with plate-immobilized STM antigen for 1 h at room temperature in duplicate. Afterwards, antigen-bound IgM, IgG, and IgA antibodies were detected by isotype-specific secondary antibodies against swine IgM, swine IgG or swine IgA (goat anti-swine, all from Bethyl Labs., Montgomery, TX, USA) conjugated to horse radish peroxidase (HRP) and visualized after another washing step by incubating the plates with TMB-E (3,3′,5,5′-tetramethybenzidine) substrate (Moss, Pasadena, MD, USA). Enzymatic reaction was stopped by adding 0.5 M sulphuric acid.

Finally, the optical density (OD) was measured at a wavelength of 450 nm. Colour intensity, which was proportional to the amount of bound antibodies, was calculated into OD% by setting the intensity of a hyper-immune serum ('hyper-immune serum 97.4') to 100%. This hyper-immune serum was derived from a pig which was three-fold vaccinated with Salmoporc®/Salmoporc STM® [7] and served as positive control on each plate. The ELISA result is given as OD% relative to the hyper-immune serum.

Statistical analyses were done using a two-tailed Mann-Whitney U test with a level of significance of $p < 0.05$ (SPSS Version 15.0, IBM). The null hypothesis was defined as equal results in the vaccinated and in the control group with respect to the outcome variables. The alternative hypothesis was that the treatment groups will differ. Efficacy of the vaccine (bacteriology) was then assumed if the differences were significant in favour of the vaccination group.

Results

Rectal body temperatures

The rectal temperatures increased after challenge in both groups. However, vaccinated animals showed a lower increase of the rectal temperature and an earlier decline to physiological values compared to controls (Fig. 1). The differences between the groups were statistically significant at days 3, 4 and 5 p.chall. At the end of the observation period (day 6 p.chall.) both groups had nearly equivalent rectal temperatures.

Clinical examination

Clinical signs during the challenge period were predominantly recorded on days 3, 4, 5 and 6 post infection (p.i.). The vaccinated animals showed significantly lower 'diarrhoea score' and 'clinical score' on those days, when compared with the control group. Detailed information is given in Table 1.

At the end of the trial (day 6 p.chall.), 5 out of 8 control animals suffered from diarrhoea and all of the controls had at least one elevated value in the 'clinical score'. None of the vaccinated pigs showed persistent clinical signs at this day.

Gross pathological examination

Differences between the groups were also detected during the necropsy. Gross pathological findings were confined to the gastrointestinal tract. Catarrhal enteritis of the small intestine was seen in 37.5% of the vaccinated and 87.5% of the control pigs. The latter were additionally suffering from a focal to multifocal diphtheric enteritis in the caecum or colon. None of the vaccinated animals showed diphtheric lesions in the large intestine. Further lesions were not observed.

Bacteriology

All animals of both groups were found to be infected with the STM challenge strain after challenge. The challenge strain contents in the ileal and caecal mucosa and the ileocaecal lymph nodes were significantly reduced in vaccinated pigs ($p < 0.05$) (Table 2) compared to the non-vaccinated control group.

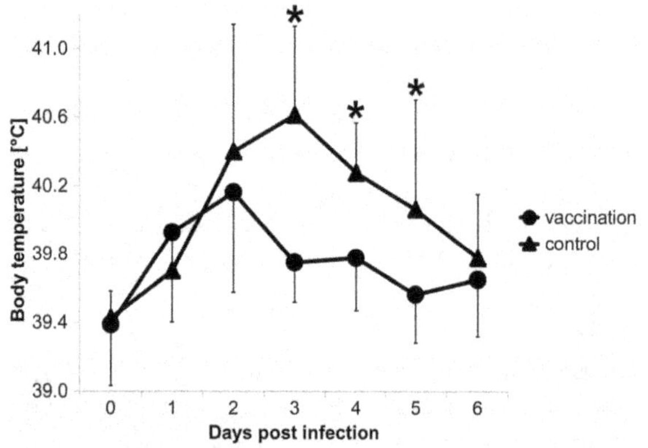

Fig. 1 Rectal temperatures during the challenge infection (mean ± standard deviation of each group per day post challenge). Asterisks point to significant differences between the groups ($p < 0.05$)

Table 1 Sums of diarrhoea and clinical score per group for each day post challenge

	Day 1	Day 2	Day 3	Day 4	Day 5	Day 6
Diarrhoea score						
Vaccination group	0	0	1	1	0	0
Control group	0	3	4	8	8	8
p value	1	0.233	0.233	0.031	0.013	0.013
Clinical score						
Vaccination group	3	4	4	4	0	0
Control group	0	9	11	20	19	19
p value	0.1	0.255	0.255	0.003	< 0.001	< 0.001

Serology I (Swine Salmonella Ab test)

Prior to the first vaccination (B0) all weaners were shown to be serologically negative for *Salmonella* sp. (< 2.25 OD%). At B1 (3 weeks after the 1st vaccination) no antibody response was detectable (Fig. 2). However, 3 weeks after the 2nd vaccination (B2, immediately before the challenge) the vaccinated animals had significant higher antibody levels than the control group. At slaughter (B3) a further remarkable increase of the antibody amounts was detected, but reached similar levels in vaccinated and non-vaccinated animals.

Serology II (STM-specific IgM, IgA, IgG)

Salmonella-specific IgM, IgA and IgG antibody isotypes showed different profiles during the vaccination and the subsequent challenge period. The results are shown in Fig. 2b–d and are specified as proportional constant of the OD%-values at two consecutive times. STM-specific IgM amounts were slightly increasing with the ageing of the piglets during the trial but without any appreciable differences between vaccinated and control pigs. The vaccination had no impact towards the IgM OD% values whereas in response to infection a 3.8-fold increase was detected, as a result of the acute infection. STM-specific IgA values were continuously increasing within the vaccination group starting after the first vaccination (4.4-fold increase from B1 to B2, 1.7-fold increase from B2 to B3). The differences between the groups were shown to be statistically significant from B1 until the end of the trial. In the control group a 5-fold increase of the OD% values was found at days 6/7 p.chall. STM-specific IgG amounts were nearly equivalent in vaccinated and control pigs until B1. Prior to the challenge (B2) the average amount of IgG significantly raised in vaccinated pigs, while the controls showed constantly low OD% levels. After the challenge a further 3-fold increase of the OD% values was detected in the vaccination group when compared with the values at B1. No increase of STM-specific IgG antibodies was observed in non-vaccinated animals.

Table 2 STM challenge strain contents in the ileal and caecal mucosa and ileocaecal lymph nodes (in CFU/g tissue: mean ± standard deviation)

Group	Number	Challenge strain content in lg CFU/g		
		Ileum	Caecum	Ileocaecal lymph nodes
Vaccinated	8	4.25 ± 1.25[a]	2.51 ± 2.06[a]	3.57 ± 0.20[a]
Control	8	5.72 ± 0.82	5.85 ± 1.27	4.43 ± 0.37

[a] $p < 0.05$ (Mann-Whitney U test)

Discussion

In this report we describe the immunogenicity of the vaccine Salmoporc®/Salmoporc STM® after challenge with a virulent mSTM DT193 strain including the results of the clinical, gross-pathological and bacteriological examination. Special emphasis was placed on the kinetics of the *Salmonella*-specific antibodies and a differentiated view on the isotypes IgM, IgA and IgG during the vaccination period and the subsequent infection.

Natural infections with STM are often asymptomatic [17–19] but they can also go along with enterocolitis, fever and inanition [20]. In this trial we used a high number of bacteria for inoculation in order to reliably trigger clinical signs. Following challenge infection, clinical signs were observed in both groups, including increased body temperatures, diarrhoea, loss of appetite or reduced general condition. It was clearly shown that the body temperature increased in both groups. However, the vaccinated animals returned significantly earlier to physiological body temperatures than animals of the control group did. The same could also be observed regarding the other clinical signs. Comparable results have previously been reported after challenge with a biphasic STM strain by Selke and colleagues [7].

Differences between both groups were also noted during post-mortem examination, as demonstrated by a significantly reduced prevalence of catarrhal enteritis and the absence of additional diphtheric enteritis in the large intestine of vaccinated animals. Especially the latter lesion is a typical morphological alteration associated

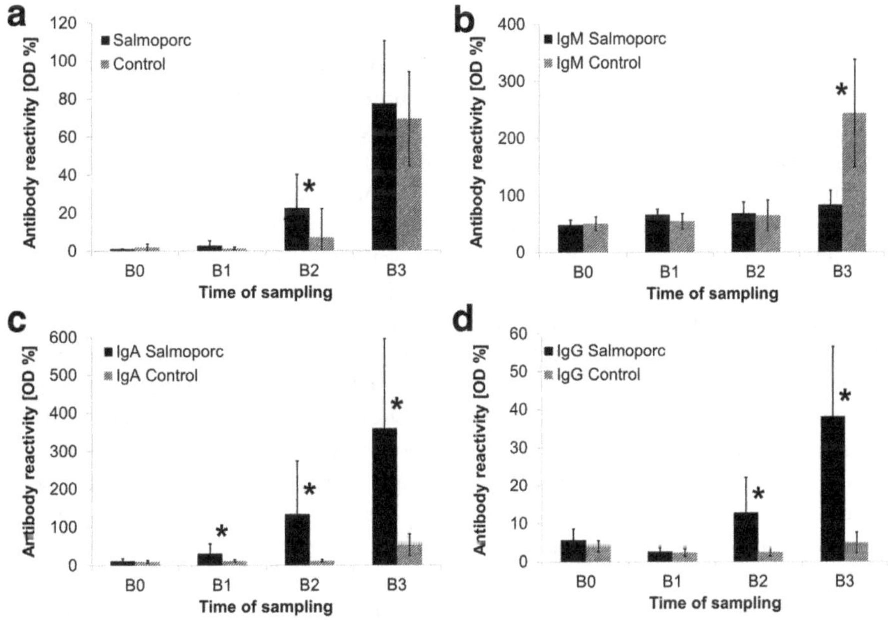

Fig. 2 Kinetics of the antibody response after oral vaccination and challenge (OD%, mean ± standard deviation). Asterisks point to significant differences between the groups ($p \leq 0.05$). B0 = study day 0, B1 = study day 21, B2 = study day 42, B3 = study day 48/49. **a** Following immunization (B2) significant differences between vaccinated and control animals became apparent. At the end of the challenge period both groups exhibit similar values (Swine Salmonella Ab Test). **b** The amount of IgM antibodies was nearly equivalent in both groups until challenge (B0 to B2). At B3 (day 6 post challenge), the IgM OD% values in the control group were found to be significantly increased to both, the IgM level of the control group at B2 and the IgM level at B3 of the vaccinated animals, which showed only a slight increase of STM-specific IgM due to the challenge infection (Ig-isotype specific in-house ELISA). **c** STM-specific IgA showed markedly increasing values in the vaccinated pigs during the vaccination period with a further increase during the challenge. In contrast, the control animals revealed only slightly increasing values during the whole animal trial (Ig-isotype specific in-house ELISA). **d** At the sampling point B0 and B1 statistical differences in terms of STM-specific IgG were neither detectable in the vaccinated nor in the control animals. Prior to and post challenge the vaccinated pigs showed significant higher values compared to the control group (Ig-isotype specific in-house ELISA)

with STM infections [20]. Comparable morphological findings were not described by Selke and colleagues [7]. They could only find subtle differences between the groups in terms of a reactive hyperaemia of the intestine. The absence of definite morphological changes could potentially be due to the lower infectious dose in their study (1×10^9 CFU/animal) or differences in the susceptibility of the weaners used in both studies.

During quantitative bacteriological examination we could demonstrate that the bacterial load of the challenge strain was significantly reduced in vaccinated animals. To the best of our knowledge, this is the first report of this particular vaccine that demonstrates efficacy against mSTM in a laboratory trial, as the protective potential against these strains was recently suggested by Davies and colleagues during a large-scale field study [10]. Despite this fact, the protective potential of the vaccine against STM has already been demonstrated in the past [6, 7].

When comparing our results to those reported in the literature with STM [6, 7] it can be concluded that the protective potential of the vaccine is nearly equivalent for both STM and mSTM. However, when considering the efficacy data of previous studies in more detail, it is striking that the bacterial loads in all of the three quantitatively examined tissues in the present report are higher [6, 7]. This might be attributed to the challenge strain. While in the two previous studies biphasic STM DT 104 have been used [6, 7], a virulent DT 193 was used in the present study, which was isolated during a serious human outbreak. This strain might have better colonization capability than the biphasic variants. However, despite the different values of the bacterial load in the mentioned studies and the present report, the reduction of the bacterial load (representing the vaccine's efficacy) is comparable.

Previoulsly, Methner demonstrated a direct correlation of the bacterial load in the caecum and the shedding of *Salmonella* through faeces in chickens [21]. This relationship has not been proven in pigs so far but is quite conceivable. Therefore, a reduction of the challenge strain content in the ileal and caecal mucosa, which are to be considered as the reservoir for *Salmonella* in pigs, should consequently lead to a reduction of STM shedding.

Vaccination against *Salmonella* induces both humoral and cell-mediated immune mechanism, as shown by Lehmann et al. [11] after vaccination of BALB/c mice with an attenuated *Salmonella* Enteritidis vaccine strain. And both immune mechanisms are crucial during *Salmonella* infections in chickens [22]. In our study, we confined on the humoral immune mechanisms but the cell-mediated immune response during vaccination and infection should likewise be studied in pigs in the future. The strong increase of the base line STM-specific IgG response following vaccination might be the result of T-cell-mediated class-switch recombination from IgM/IgG3 to downstream IgG subclasses (IgG2–6) in *Salmonella*-antigen activated B cells, which would imply the induction of cell-mediated immune mechanisms in the present vaccination model.

We could demonstrate an increase of the OD% values after vaccination using the LPS ELISA (Swine Salmonella Ab test). Nevertheless, the mean OD% values were still below current threshold values, for example the German threshold of 40 OD% [23]. This is in accordance with previous studies using the same vaccine [24, 25].

Within 1 week after infection a further increase of *Salmonella*-LPS specific antibody values was detected in both groups leading to almost the same OD% levels which has also been seen in previous studies [6]. The mean values of the animals were markedly above the threshold and would have been equally judged to be positive for *Salmonella*, independently from the trial group.

By the use of an Ig isotype-specific in-house ELISA we were able to study the kinetics of the relative amounts of IgM, IgA and IgG in pigs after oral vaccination and subsequent challenge. Antibody profiles have been shown by Trepnau and colleagues but without challenge [16]. Furthermore, the authors used a different vaccination scheme as well as an administration of the vaccine via the feeder (possibly reduced dose per animal). This and the fact that the ELISA applied for the differentiation of the immunoglobulin (Ig) isotypes in the previous study (Salmotype® Pig STM-WCE ELISA, Labor Diagnostik Leipzig) is no longer commercially available makes it difficult to compare the published results with those of the present study. Nevertheless, the overall kinetics of IgM, IgA and IgG in the previous report and in our study appear to be very similar.

STM-specific IgA and IgG antibody levels were elevated in response to vaccination with Salmoporc® and showed a further increase during the challenge whereas the OD% levels of the controls did not rise significantly 1 week after challenge. In contrast, STM-specific IgM levels were not elevated by vaccination whereas the challenge, which simulates a field infection, caused a significant increase in non-vaccinated animals within 1 week.

Mucosal pathogens are attacked in the first instance by a local immune response in terms of the secretion of IgA antibodies. This Ig isotype is mainly produced by gut associated lymphoid tissues and transported via luminal epithelial cells into the mucus [26]. Therefore, an activation of this first-line defence by vaccination is a crucial factor for protection against intestinal pathogens. IgA inhibits bacterial motility, circumvents adhesion to epithelial cells and neutralizes bacterial toxins. The first contact of the pathogen with the host proceeds via mucosa and thus bacteria which were neutralized by IgA, were finally hindered from entering host and colonizing organs [27].

Invasive pathogens are adequately combatted by IgG antibodies, which were found to be induced to a lesser degree in our study. Instead, a strong rise of IgA antibodies was detected after vaccination and infection. It has already been shown that innate IgA contributes in a significant manner to defence and recently, a long-lasting IgA memory response was reported to be developed especially after oral immunization [28, 29].

In the present study, a 12-fold increase of *Salmonella*-specific serum IgA in vaccinated animals (compared to controls) was detected. Given that about 30% of serum IgA originates from intestinal production [30] the content of IgA in mucus must be several fold higher than serum levels. A positive correlation between mucosal and systemic IgA levels has been shown [31].

The increase in serum levels of *Salmonella*-specific IgA might assist in eliminating *Salmonella* that evaded the first line mucosal defence and take part in defence of the gut across the hepato-biliary route as secretory IgA [26]. ELISA data show, that despite of the facultative intracellular pathogenic nature of *Salmonella* and the subsequent requirement of cell-mediated immunity to survive infection, humoral immunity mainly due to IgA antibody production decisively contributes to control of infection as previously shown by other authors [32]. Besides the gain of IgA an increase of IgG was present in the vaccinated animals after challenge, as well, which further confirms the immunogenic capacity of the vaccine.

Conclusion

An oral vaccination with a registered STM live vaccine makes clinical signs induced during a laboratory challenge infection of weaners with virulent mSTM milder. Furthermore, the vaccine is effective in reducing the bacterial count of the challenge strain in the gut and lymph nodes which consecutively would lead to a reduced persistence and shedding of STM/mSTM.

The kinetics of IgM, IgA and IgG were different in vaccinated and control animals. This reveals further information regarding the immune mechanisms being associated with STM infections and vaccination.

Abbreviations

ASSuT: Ampicillin, streptomycin, sulfamerazine, oxytetracycline; B0-B3: Blood sampling 0 – blood sampling 3; CFU: Colony forming unit; DT: Defined type; ELISA: Enzyme linked immunosorbent assay; HRP: Horse radish peroxidase; IgA: Immunoglobuline A; IgG: Immunoglobuline G; IgM: Immunoglobuline M; LPS: Lipopolysaccharide; mSTM: Monophasic *Salmonella* Typhimurium; OD: Optical density; p.chall.: Post challenge; SE: *Salmonella* Enteritidis; STM: *Salmonella* Typhimurium; TMB: 3,3′,5,5′-tetramethybenzidine; WCE: Whole cell extract

Acknowledgements

We are grateful to Dr. W. Rabsch (National Reference Centre for Salmonella and other Enteric Bacterial Pathogens, Robert Koch Institute, Wernigerode Branch, Burgstr. 37, 38855 Wernigerode, Germany) for kindly providing the challenge strain. We gratefully acknowledge Ulrike Scholz and the laboratory staff of IDT Biologika GmbH for excellent technical assistance.

Funding

This work was carried out without funding.

Authors' contributions

TT, SS and TL designed and performed the animal trial including vaccination, blood sampling, infection and necropsy as well as all laboratory work concerning the bacteriological analysis. EU and JL performed the ELISAs including all laboratory work for ELISA development. TT, EU and SS performed the statistical analysis. TT, EU, JL and SS wrote the manuscript. TL co-authored the draft of the manuscript. All authors contributed to data analysis. All the authors have read and approved the final manuscript.

Consent for publication

Not applicable

Competing interests

Three of the authors (TT, TL and SS) are employed by the manufacturer of the vaccine. The authors declare that they have no competing interests.

Author details

[1]IDT Biologika GmbH, Business Unit Animal Health, Research and Development, Am Pharmapark, 06861 Dessau-Rosslau, Germany. [2]Fraunhofer Institute for Cell Therapy and Immunology, Perlickstraße 1, 04103 Leipzig, Germany.

References

1. EFSA (European Food Safety Authority) and ECDC (European Centre for Disease Prevention and Control). The European Union summary report on trends and sources of zoonoses, zoonotic agents and food-borne outbreaks in 2014. EFSA J. 2015; doi:10.2903/j.efsa.2015.4329.
2. Hauser E, Tietze E, Helmuth R, Junker E, Blank K, Prager R, Rabsch W, Appel B, Fruth A, Malorny B. Pork contaminated with Salmonella enterica Serovar 4,[5],12:i:-, an emerging health risk for humans. Appl Environ Microbiol. 2010;14:4601–10.
3. Bone A, Noel H, Le Hello S, Pihier N, Danan C, Raguenaud ME, Salah S, Bellali H, Vaillant V, Weill FX, Jourdan-da Silva N. Nationwide outbreak of Salmonella enterica serotype 4,12:i:- infections in France, linked to dried pork sausage, march-may 2010. Euro Surveill. 2010;15:24.
4. Mossong J, Marques P, Ragimbeau C, Huberty-Krau P, Losch S, Meyer G, Moris G, Strottner C, Rabsch W, Schneider F. Outbreaks of monophasic Salmonella enterica serovar 4,5,12:i:- in Luxembourg, 2006. Euro Surveill. 2007;12:6.
5. Trüpschuch S, Laverde Gomez JA, Ediberidze I, Flieger A, Rabsch W. Characterisation of multidrug-resistant Salmonella Typhimurium 4, [5],12:i:- DT193 strains carrying a novel genomic island adjacent to the thrW tRNA locus. Int J Med Microbiol. 2010; doi:10.1016/j.ijmm.2010.02.001.
6. Springer S, Lindner T, Steinbach G, Selbitz HJ. Investigation of the efficacy of a genetically-stabile live Salmonella Typhimurium vaccine for use in swine. Berl Munch Tierarztl Wochenschr. 2001;114:9–10.
7. Selke M, Meens J, Springer S, Frank R, Gerlach G. Immunization of pigs to prevent disease in humans: construction and protective efficacy of a Salmonella enterica Serovar Typhimurium live negative-marker vaccine. Infect Immun. 2007; doi:10.1128/IAI.01908-06.
8. Leyman B, Boyen F, Verbrugghe E, van Parys A, Haesebrouck F, Pasmans F. Vaccination of pigs reduces Salmonella Typhimurium numbers in a model mimicking pre-slaughter stress. Vet J. 2012; doi:10.1016/j.tvjl.2012.04.011.
9. de RL, Maes D, Dewulf J, Butaye P, Pasmans F, Boyen F, Haesebrouck F, van der Stede Y. Use of a live attenuated Salmonella enterica serovar Typhimurium vaccine on farrow-to-finish pig farms. Vet J. 2014; doi:10.1016/j.tvjl.2014.09.012.

10. Davies R, Gosling R, Wales A, Smith R. Use of an attenuated live Salmonella Typhimurium vaccine on three breeding pig units: a longitudinal observational field study. Comp Immunol Microbiol Infect Dis. 2016; doi:10.1016/j.cimid.2016.03.005.
11. Lehmann J, Springer S, Werner C, Lindner T, Bellmann S, Straubinger R, Selbitz H, Alber G. Immunity induced with a Salmonella enterica serovar Enteritidis live vaccine is regulated by Th1-cell-dependent cellular and humoral effector mechanisms in susceptible BALB/c mice. Vaccine. 2006; doi:10.1016/j.vaccine.2006.03.024.
12. Roesler U, Szabo I, Matthies C, Albrecht K, Leffler M, Scherer K, Nöckler K, Lehmann J, Methner U, Hensel A, Truyen U. Comparing validation of four ELISA-systems for detection of Salmonella Derby- and Salmonella infantis-infected pigs. Berl Münch Tierärztl Wochenschr. 2011; doi:10.2376/0005-9366-124-265.
13. Brumme S, Arnold T, Sigmarsson H, Lehmann J, Scholz HC, Hardt W, Hensel A, Truyen U, Roesler U. Impact of Salmonella Typhimurium DT104 virulence factors invC and sseD on the onset, clinical course, colonization patterns and immune response of porcine salmonellosis. Vet Microbiol. 2007; doi:10.1016/j.vetmic.2007.04.032.
14. Szabó I, Scherer K, Roesler U, Appel B, Nöckler K, Hensel A. Comparative examination and validation of ELISA test systems for Salmonella typhimurium diagnosis of slaughtering pigs. Int J Food Microbiol. 2008; doi:10.1016/j.ijfoodmicro.2008.02.022.
15. Matiasovic J, Stepanova H, Kudlackova H, Havlickova H, Sisak F, Rychlik I, Chlebova K, Leva L, Osvaldova A, Gebauer J, Faldyna M. Immune response of pigs to Salmonella enterica serovar Derby and Typhimurium infections. Vet Microbiol. 2014; doi:10.1016/j.vetmic.2014.02.003.
16. Trepnau D, Ulrich E, Uhlig R, Lindner T, Selbitz H, Rosler U, Gabert J, Bergfeld U, Fehlhaber K, Brabetz W, Lehmann J. Antibody response after immunization with a Salmonella Typhimurium live vaccine in dependence on the way of application. Berl Munch Tierarztl Wochenschr. 2008; doi:10.2376/0005-9366-121-334.
17. Wood RL, Pospischil A, Rose R. Distribution of persistent Salmonella Typhimurium infection in internal organs of swine. Am J Vet Res. 1989;50:7.
18. Volf J, Stepanova H, Matiasovic J, Kyrova K, Sisak F, Havlickova H, Leva L, Faldyna M, Rychlik I. Salmonella enterica serovar Typhimurium and Enteritidis infection of pigs and cytokine signalling in palatine tonsils. Vet Microbiol. 2012; doi: 10.1016/j.vetmic.2011.10.004.
19. Boyen F, Haesebrouck F, Maes D, van Immerseel F, Ducatelle R, Pasmans F. Non-typhoidal Salmonella infections in pigs: a closer look at epidemiology, pathogenesis and control. Vet Microbiol. 2008; doi:10.1016/j.vetmic.2007.12.017.
20. Uzal FA, Plattner BL, Hostetter JM. Alimentary system. In: Maxie MG, editor. Pathology of domestic animals. St. Louis: Elsevier; 2016. p. 1–257.
21. Methner U. Erarbeitung eines Modells zur experimentellen oralen Infektion des Geflügels mit epidemiologisch bedeutsamen Salmonella-Serovaren. Leipzig: Diss. Univ; 1992.
22. Varmuzova K, Faldynova M, Elsheimer-Matulova M, Sebkova A, Polansky O, Havlickova H, Sisak F, Rychlik I. Immune protection of chickens conferred by a vaccine consisting of attenuated strains of Salmonella Enteritidis, Typhimurium and Infantis. Vet Res. 2016; doi:10.1186/s13567-016-0371-8.
23. Anon. Leitfaden Salmonellenmonitoring- und -reduzierungsprogramm für die Schweinefleischerzeugung. QS Qualität und Sicherheit GmbH. 2016. https://www.q-s.de/services/files/downloadcenter/4_leitfaeden/monitoringprogramme/salmonellenmonitoring_schwein/lf_salmo_sw_frei_01012017_d.pdf. Accessed 6 Nov 2017.
24. Lindner T, Springer S, Selbitz HJ: The use of a Salmonella Typhimurium live vaccine to control Salmonella Typhimurium in fattening pigs in field and effects on serological surveillance. 2007. http://lib.dr.iastate.edu/cgi/viewcontent.cgi?article=1097&context=safepork. Accessed 31 Jan 2017.
25. Eddicks M. Überprüfung der Verträglichkeit des Salmonella Typhimurium – Lebendimpfstoffes Salmoporc® bei oraler Anwendung für drei Tage alte Saugferkel unter Berücksichtigung der Ausscheidung, Persistenz und Immunogenität des Impfstamms. München: Diss. LMU; 2006.
26. Brown WR, Kloppel TM. The liver and IgA: immunological, cell biological and clinical implications. Hepatology. 1989;5:763–84.
27. Martinoli C, Chiavelli A, Rescigno M. Entry route of Salmonella Typhimurium directs the type of induced immune response. Immunity. 2007; doi:10.1016/j.immuni.2007.10.011.
28. Wijburg OL, Uren TK, Simpfendorfer K, Johansen F, Brandtzaeg P, Strugnell RA. Innate secretory antibodies protect against natural Salmonella Typhimurium infection. J Exp Med. 2006; doi:10.1084/jem.20052093.
29. Bemark M, Hazanov H, Strömberg A, Komban R, Holmqvist J, Köster S, Mattsson J, Sikora P, Mehr R, Lycke NY. Limited clonal relatedness between gut IgA plasma cells and memory B cells after oral immunization. Nat Comms. 2016; doi:10.1038/ncomms12698.
30. Vaerman J, Langendries A, Pabst R, Rothkötter H. Contribution of serum IgA to intestinal lymph IgA, and vice versa, in minipigs. Vet Immunol Immunopathol. 1997; doi:10.1016/S0165-2427(97)00041-X.
31. Snoeck V, Peters IR, Cox E. The IgA system: a comparison of structure and function in different species. Vet Res. 2006; doi:10.1051/vetres:2006010.
32. Roesler U, Heller P, Waldmann K, Truyen U, Hensel A. Immunization of sows in an integrated pig-breeding herd using a homologous inactivated Salmonella vaccine decreases the prevalence of Salmonella Typhimurium infection in the offspring. J Vet Med Series B. 2006; doi:10.1111/j.1439-0450.2006.00951.x.

8

Immunogenicity and protective efficacy of a *Salmonella* Enteritidis *sptP* mutant as a live attenuated vaccine candidate

Zhijie Lin[1†], Peipei Tang[1†], Yang Jiao[1], Xilong Kang[1], Qiuchun Li[1], Xiulong Xu[1,3,4], Jun Sun[1,2], Zhiming Pan[1*] and Xinan Jiao[1*]

Abstract

Background: *Salmonella enterica* serovar Enteritidis (*S.* Enteritidis) is a highly adaptive pathogen in both humans and animals. As a *Salmonella* Type III secretion system (T3SS) effector, *Salmonella* protein tyrosine phosphatase (SptP) is critical for virulence in this genus. To investigate the feasibility of using C50336Δ*sptP* as a live attenuated oral vaccine in mice, we generated the *sptP* gene deletion mutant C50336Δ*sptP* in *S.* Enteritidis strain C50336 by λ-Red mediated recombination and evaluated the protective ability of the *S.* Enteritidis *sptP* mutant strain C50336Δ*sptP* against mice salmonellosis.

Results: We found that C50336Δ*sptP* was a highly immunogenic, effective, and safe vaccine in mice. Compared to wild-type C50336, C50336Δ*sptP* showed reduced virulence as confirmed by the 50% lethal dose (LD_{50}) in orally infected mice. C50336Δ*sptP* also showed decreased bacterial colonization both in vivo and in vitro. Immunization with C50336Δ*sptP* had no significant effect on body weight and did not result in obvious clinical symptoms relative to control animals treated with phosphate-buffered saline (PBS), but induced humoral and cellular immune responses at 12 and 26 days post inoculation. Immunization with 1×10^8 colony-forming units (CFU) C50336Δ*sptP* per mouse provided 100% protection against subsequent challenge with the wild-type C50336 strain, and immunized mice showed mild and temporary clinical symptoms as compared to those of control group.

Conclusions: These results demonstrate that C50336Δ*sptP* can be a live attenuated oral vaccine for salmonellosis.

Keywords: *Salmonella* Enteritidis, SptP, Vaccine, Immunogenicity, Immune protection

Background

Salmonella spp. is a Gram-negative, facultative anaerobe and intracellular pathogen in both humans and animals. Infection by *Salmonella* is a major public health problem [1], causing an estimated 93.8 million illnesses and 155,000 deaths each year worldwide [2] and more than 1 million illnesses and 350 deaths each year in the U.S. [3]. In the past 20 years, *Salmonella enterica* serovar Enteritidis (*S.* Enteritidis) has been one of the most common serotypes in salmonellosis in humans despite the implementation of control and prevention measures [4]. Humans can be infected with *Salmonella* via consumption of contaminated pork, beef, poultry, and eggs or contact with fecal matter in places with poor sanitation. Salmonellosis in humans is characterized by abdominal pain, diarrhea, nausea, vomiting, fever, and headache [5].

Salmonellosis treatment and protection strategies include antimicrobial therapy and vaccination, but emergence of multidrug-resistant strains is becoming a serious global problem [6, 7]. Vaccines based on inactivated bacteria can potentially prevent salmonellosis [8]; however, attenuated live vaccines generated by deletion of various identified *Salmonella* virulence genes have higher immunogenicity and greater efficacy than killed bacteria [9–14].

* Correspondence: zmpan@yzu.edu.cn; jiao@yzu.edu.cn
†Equal contributors
[1]Jiangsu Key Laboratory of Zoonosis, Jiangsu Co-Innovation Center for Prevention and Control of Important Animal Infectious Diseases and Zoonosis, MOA Key Laboratory of Prevention and Control of Biological Hazard Factors (Animal Origin) for Agrifood Safety and Quality, MOE Joint International Research Laboratory of Agriculture and Agri-product Safety, Yangzhou University, Yangzhou 225001, China
Full list of author information is available at the end of the article

Salmonella protein tyrosine phosphatase (SptP) is a *Salmonella* T3SS effector protein encoded in *Salmonella* pathogenicity islands (SPI)-1. The SptP protein has an N-terminal domain that acts as a GTPase-activating protein for Cdc42 and Rac1, mediating alterations in the actin cytoskeleton of host cells [15], as well as a C-terminal domain that inhibits mitogen-activated protein kinase and extracellular signal-regulated kinase signaling [16]. SptP also suppresses interleukin-8 (IL-8) production and consequently the inflammatory response in hosts, thereby promoting *Salmonella* invasion and intracellular replication [17, 18]. In a mouse infection model, SptP suppressed the degranulation of mast cells and blocked neutrophil recruitment [19].

In this study, we generated the *sptP* gene deletion mutant C50336Δ*sptP* in *S.* Enteritidis strain C50336 by λ-Red mediated recombination [20]. The growth characteristics of C50336Δ*sptP* were similar to those of wild-type C50336. We therefore investigated the feasibility of using C50336Δ*sptP* as a live attenuated oral vaccine in mice by evaluating virulence, changes in body weight and clinical symptoms, bacterial persistence, immune responses, and protective efficacy.

Methods

Bacterial strains and cells lines

The wild-type *S.* Enteritidis strain C50336 was obtained from the National Institute for the Control of Pharmaceutical and Biological Products (Beijing, China). The *sptP* deletion mutant strain C50336Δ*sptP* was constructed by λ-Red-mediated recombination as previously described [20]. Briefly, the sequence of the chloramphenicol resistance cassette (Cm^R) was amplified from plasmid pKD3, including 39-bp homology extensions at the 5′ and 3′ ends of the *sptP* gene (primers: forward 5′-tgaatcagcaggaagtgctcaaaaacatactgcaggaatgtgtaggctg-gagctgcttc -3′; reverse 5′-cttactttcagatagttctaaaagtaagc-tatgtttttaatgggaattagccatggtcc -3′). PCR products were purified and transferred into C50336 cells containing plasmid pKD46 by electroporation. Recombinant C50336-Cm^R cells grown on Luria-Bertani (LB) agar plates were selected for both Cm^R and ampicillin resistance (Amp^R). Allelic replacement of *sptP* with the Cm cassette was verified by PCR analysis (primers: forward 5′-atccgaactactttacgc-3′; reverse 5′-tgaatggtattctactgg-3′) and DNA sequencing. The cassette was then excised by introducing the Flp recombinase-expressing vector pCP20. Biochemical tests were performed using the API 20E identification kit (BioMérieux, Lyon, France) and VITEK 2 Gram-negative bacilli test (BioMérieux) according to the manufacturer's protocol. Bacteria were cultured in LB broth followed by overnight incubation at 37 °C with shaking at 180 rpm [21]. XLT4 (Difco Laboratories, San Jose, CA, USA) and 1.5% LB agar were used for bacterial culture and counts of colony-forming units (CFU).

Human epithelial cells Caco-2 BBE and mouse macrophage RAW264.7 cells were cultured and maintained in Dulbecco's modified Eagle's medium (DMEM) containing 10% fetal bovine serum (FBS), 50 μg/ml streptomycin, and 50 U/ml penicillin.

Experimental animals

Female BALB/c mice (8 weeks old) used for vaccination experiments were obtained from the Comparative Medical Center of Yangzhou University (Yangzhou, China). The animal experiments were all approved by the Animal Care and Ethics Committee of Yangzhou University, Yangzhou, China (Approval ID: SYXK [Su] 2012–0029).

Assessment of bacterial virulence

The virulence of mutant C50336Δ*sptP* and wild-type strain C50336 was evaluated in BALB/c mice by oral inoculation of the mice with various doses of the bacterial strains. The morbidity and mortality of the mice were observed as previously described [22]. Briefly, water and food were withdrawn 4 h before oral gavage with 100 μl of 5% sodium bicarbonate to neutralize stomach acid; 1 h later, mice were administered 10-fold dilutions of C50336Δ*sptP* or C50336 [1×10^8–1×10^4 CFU in 100 μl of phosphate-buffered saline (PBS)] by oral gavage. Control mice received 100 μl of PBS via the same route. All deaths of mice were recorded over the 16-day experimental period. The LD_{50} was calculated using the Karber and Behrens method [23].

Bacterial colonization in cells

Human epithelial cells Caco-2 BBE and mouse macrophage RAW264.7 were grown in DMEM with 10% FBS. At 90–100% confluence, the monolayers were washed three times with PBS, and then the cells were colonized with an equal number of the indicated bacteria for 30 min (multiplicity of infection = 100). For bacterial adhesion, the cells were washed, and then incubated with PBS containing Triton X-100 (0.5%) at 37 °C for 10 min. For bacterial invasion, 30 min after bacterial colonization, the cells were incubated for an additional 30 min in DMEM with gentamicin (100 μg/ml), washed and incubated with PBS containing Triton X-100 (0.5%) at 37 °C for 10 min [24]. Serial 10-fold dilutions of cell lysates were plated on XLT4 agar and incubated at 37 °C for 12–16 h. The number of bacteria was counted and expressed as 10^7 CFU/ml.

Bacterial colonization and persistence in organs and tissues

Bacterial colonization and persistence in the internal organs of infected mice were evaluated. Mice were administered 1×10^8 or 1×10^7 CFU of C50336Δ*sptP* by oral gavage, and six mice per day were sacrificed at 1, 3, 5, 7, 14, 21, 28, and 44 days post-immunization (DPI). Liver, spleen, and mesenteric lymphadenitis (mLN) samples were aseptically collected, weighed, and homogenized in 1 ml of PBS; Serial 10-fold dilutions of tissue homogenates (100 μl each) were plated on XLT4 agar and incubated at 37 °C for 12–16 h. Bacteria were counted and the numbers are expressed as $\log_{10}$ CFU/g.

Changes in body weight and clinical symptoms after immunization

Mice were immunized with C50336Δ*sptP* at 1×10^8 or 1×10^7 CFU in 100 μl of PBS by oral gavage (two doses of immunization at 0 and 14 DPI). Control animals received 100 μl of PBS. Body weight was recorded at 1, 3, 5, 7, 14, 21, 28, and 44 DPI. The mice were monitored from 1 to 44 DPI for clinical symptoms, including feed intake, susceptibility, depression and diarrhea.

Serum IgG test

Specific IgG antibody and IgG subtype levels were measured by enzyme-linked immunosorbent assay (ELISA) using soluble antigens prepared from *S.* Enteritidis strain C50336 (SEAgP) as the coating antigen in 96-well plates (100 μl of SEAgP at 2 μg/ml in each well). Serum samples were collected from mice at 12 and 26 DPI and diluted 1:50 for use as the primary antibody. Horseradish peroxidase (HRP)-conjugated goat anti-mouse IgG (or anti-mouse IgG1 and IgG2a for IgG subtype detection) was used as the secondary antibody (dilution 1:10,000). HRP activity was determined using 3,3′,5,5′-tetramethylbenzidine (Sigma-Aldrich, St. Louis, MO, USA). Absorbance was read at 450 nm using an automated microplate reader (Titertek Multiskan; Flow Laboratories, Lugano, Switzerland).

Lymphocyte stimulation test

The lymphocyte proliferation assay was performed using SEAgP as a stimulator. The spleen was isolated from the mice at 12 and 26 DPI and homogenized. Splenic lymphocytes were obtained by passing the homogenate through a filter with 40-μm pores (BD Biosciences, San Jose, CA, USA). Cell viability was determined based on Trypan Blue dye exclusion. Spleen mononuclear cell suspensions (1×10^7 cells/ml) were cultured in Roswell Park Memorial Institute 1640 medium containing 10% FBS, 50 μg/ml streptomycin, and 50 U/ml penicillin in 96-well tissue culture plates with 10 μg/ml SEAgP or 10 μg/ml concanavalin A (Con A, a lymphocyte mitogen) as a positive control at 37 °C in a humidified atmosphere of 5% CO_2 for 72 h. Lymphocyte proliferation was measured with a BrdU kit (Roche, Basel, Switzerland). Blastogenic responses to SEAgP are expressed as a mean stimulation index (SI) calculated based on the optical density of stimulated cultures at 450 nm, as previously described [25, 26].

Immune protection assessment of C50336Δ*sptP*

The protective efficacy of the mutant C50336Δ*sptP* was evaluated in mice immunized orally with 1×10^8 CFU (group A) in 100 μl of PBS (two doses of immunization at 0 and 14 DPI). Control mice (groups B and C, respectively) received 100 μl of PBS. At 28 DPI, group A was challenged orally with 1×10^8 CFU of wild-type strain C50336 in 100 μl of PBS, whereas group B was challenged with 5×10^5 CFU of wild-type strain C50336 in the same way. Group C received 100 μl of PBS as a blank control. The number of surviving mice and extent of bacterial colonization in internal organs were determined at 16 days post challenge. The number of CFUs recovered from tissues was replica-verified by PCR analysis (Primers: Forward 5′-atccgaactactttacgc-3′; Reverse 5′-tgaatggtattctactgg-3′). Clinical symptoms, including anorexia, diarrhea, depression, and mortality, were recorded daily.

Statistical analysis

Data are expressed as the mean ± SEM. All statistical tests were two-sided. $P < 0.05$ was considered to be statistically significant. Differences between two samples were evaluated using Student's t test. Statistical analyses were performed using SAS v.9.4 software (SAS Institute, Cary, NC, USA).

Results

Construction of a *sptP* deletion mutant C50336Δ*sptP* in *S.* Enteritidis

The *sptP* gene deletion mutant was established in *S.* Enteritidis strain C50336 by λ-Red-mediated recombination. Our PCR data showed that the *sptP* gene was deleted in the C50336Δ*sptP* mutant (Fig. 1a). The growth characteristics of the C50336Δ*sptP* mutant and wild-type C50336 cells were determined in LB liquid medium, with no significant difference observed between the mutant and wild type (Fig. 1b). Biochemical tests were performed using the API 20E identification kit (BioMérieux, Lyon, France) and VITEK 2 Gram-negative bacilli test (BioMérieux) according to the manufacturer's protocol, also showed no difference between these strains (data not shown).

C50336Δ*sptP* exhibits reduced virulence in a murine model

The virulence of *S.* Enteritidis wild-type C50336 and C50336Δ*sptP* was evaluated in BALB/c mice with oral gavage. As shown in Table 1, the LD_{50} of C50336 was

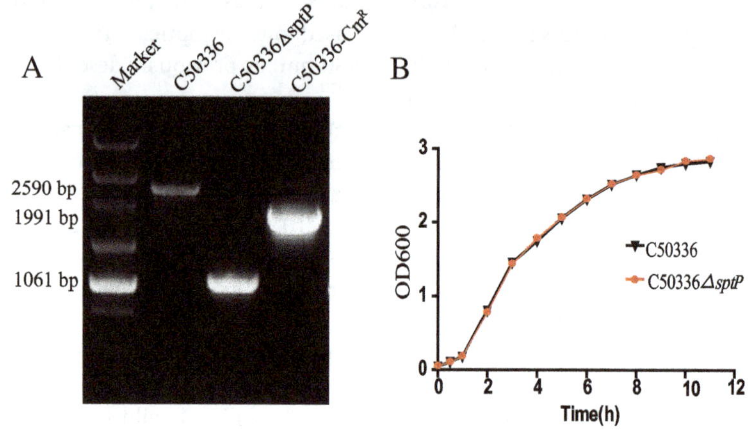

Fig. 1 Construction of *sptP* deletion mutant in *S.* Enteritidis strain C50336. **a** PCR verification of C50336Δ*sptP* and C50336-Cm^R. The wild type strain harbors the complete *sptP* gene, with a PCR product length of 2509 bp, whereas the PCR product from C50336Δ*sptP* has a length of 1061 bp, and the product from the C50336-Cm^R has a length of 1991 bp (*right*). **b** Growth curves of wild-type *S.* Enteritidis C50336 and C50336Δ*sptP*. Bacteria were grown in liquid LB medium at 37 °C for 12 h with agitation, and the OD_{600} values of triplicate cultures in LB medium were determined in 1-h intervals

3.16×10^5 CFU, but no mice died in the group challenged by C50336Δ*sptP*, indicating that the virulence of the *S.* Enteritidis mutant C50336Δ*sptP* was attenuated.

sptP deletion leads to reduced bacterial colonization in cells

The bacterial colonization in cells was determined in human epithelial Caco-2 BBE and mouse macrophage RAW264.7 cells. As shown in Fig. 2, the total number of associated bacteria was not different between C50336Δ*sptP* and C50336 in Caco-2 BBE and RAW264.7 cells. However, cells colonized with C50336Δ*sptP* showed a decreased intracellular bacterial load compared to cells colonized with C50336 (Fig. 2a & b). These results indicate that *S.* Enteritidis with *sptP* deletion has reduced bacterial colonization in vitro.

Table 1 LD_{50} of C50336Δ*sptP* in BALB/c mice

Strain	Inoculation dose (CFU)	Number of dead mice/total number of mice	LD_{50}
C50336	1.0×10^7	5/5	3.16×10^5
	1.0×10^6	4/5	
	1.0×10^5	1/5	
	1.0×10^4	0/5	
C50336Δ*sptP*	1.0×10^8	0/5	—
	1.0×10^7	0/5	
	1.0×10^6	0/5	
	1.0×10^5	0/5	
	1.0×10^4	0/5	

Colonization and persistence of *Salmonella* C50336Δ*sptP* in internal organs and tissues

The bacterial number was calculated in the liver, spleen and mLN of BALB/c mice following oral immunization with 1×10^8 CFU or 1×10^7 CFU C50336Δ*sptP*. As shown in Fig. 3, *Salmonella* colonization reached the highest level at 3 DPI (first immunization) in the liver, spleen, and mLN (Fig. 3b–d), and at 28 DPI (14 days post second immunization), two and one of the six mice were positive for *Salmonella* in the liver and spleen, respectively, in both the 1×10^8 and 1×10^7 CFU- immunized groups. In the 1×10^7 CFU immunized group, *Salmonella* was detected in the mLN of one mouse. At 44 DPI, we did not detect *Salmonella* in any tissues from immunized mice. All samples from the negative control group (PBS group) were negative for *Salmonella*.

Immunogenicity of C50336Δ*sptP*

The changes in body weight and clinical symptoms were monitored in mice following immunization with C50336Δ*sptP*. The body weights of the mice were shown in Fig. 3a. A decrease in body weight loss was noticed in the initial days of post immunization, but no statistically significant differences were observed among the three groups (immunized with 1×10^8 CFU C50336Δ*sptP*, immunized with 1×10^7 CFU C50336Δ*sptP*, and treated with PBS as a control). No significant differences were found in clinical symptoms among the three groups, although slight and temporary anorexia was observed in vaccinated mice. Clinical signs of disease such as lethargy and diarrhea were absent in all immunized mice and control mice. The procedures for immunization are shown in Fig. 4a.

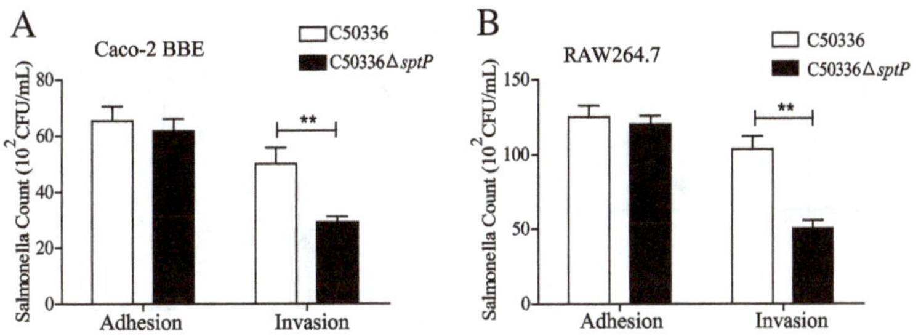

Fig. 2 Bacterial colonization in cells. *Salmonella* adhesion and invasion in the Human epithelial Caco-2 BBE cells (**a**), and mouse macrophage RAW264.7 cells (**b**). The number of *Salmonella* was determined and presented as 10^2 CFU/mL. Data are expressed as the mean ± SEM. $^{**}P \leq 0.01$

The humoral immune responses were evaluated in mice following oral immunization with C50336Δ*sptP*. Serum IgG levels were determined by indirect ELISA. As shown in Fig. 4b, mice immunized with 1 × 10^8 CFU and 1 × 10^7 CFU of C50336Δ*sptP* showed significantly higher levels of serum IgG at 12 and 26 DPI than the control group. Furthermore, the titers of the IgG1 subtype were significantly higher than those of IgG2a, demonstrating that *S.* Entertidis C50336Δ*sptP* tends to induce a Th2 immune response in mice (Fig. 4c).

The cellular immune responses in mice following oral immunization with C50336Δ*sptP* were evaluated by splenic lymphocyte proliferation assay. As shown in Fig. 4d, the SI values of immunized mice were significantly higher than control mice after stimulation with SEAgP or lymphocyte mitogen ConA at 12 and 26 DPI. This finding indicates that C50336Δ*sptP* also induces cellular immune responses in mice.

C50336Δ*sptP* protects mice against oral challenge with wild-type *S.* Enteritidis

Mice were orally vaccinated with 2 doses of 1 × 10^8 CFU of C50336Δ*sptP*, and then at 28 DPI, they were challenged with wild-type C50336. The percentage of surviving mice at 16 days post challenge is shown in Table 2. None of the immunized mice died in group A and group C, whereas ten of fifteen mice died in control group B. Slight and temporary anorexia as well as depression were observed following challenge in the immunized mice (group A) when compared the blank control group C. Severe clinical symptoms and mortality

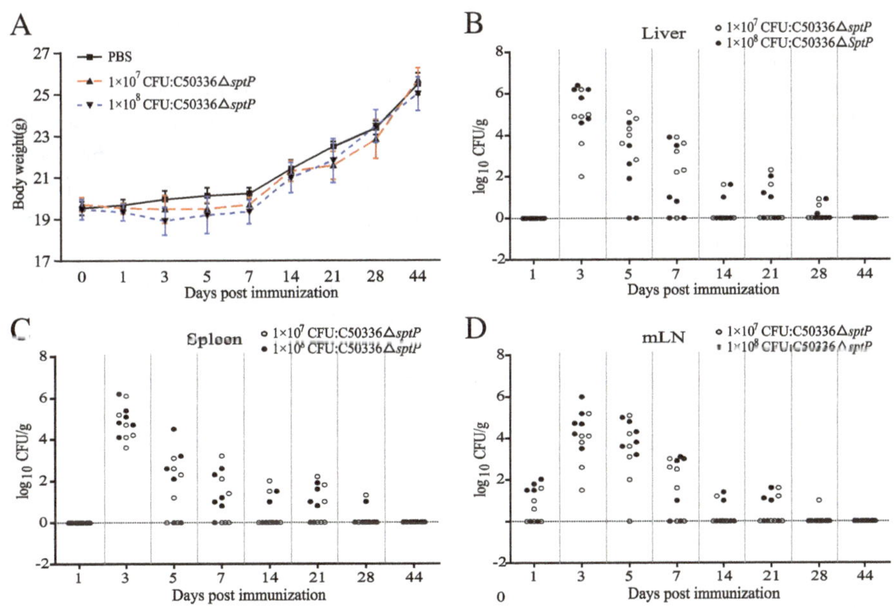

Fig. 3 Body weight (**a**) and bacterial colonization in mouse organs post immunization. *Salmonella* colonization and persistence in the liver (**b**), spleen (**c**), and mLN (**d**) of mice following oral immunization with 1 × 10^7 CFU or 1 × 10^8 CFU of C50336Δ*sptP*. Control mice received 100 μl of PBS and were negative for *Salmonella* in the liver, spleen, and mLN. The number of *Salmonella* was determined and represented as Log_{10} CFU/g

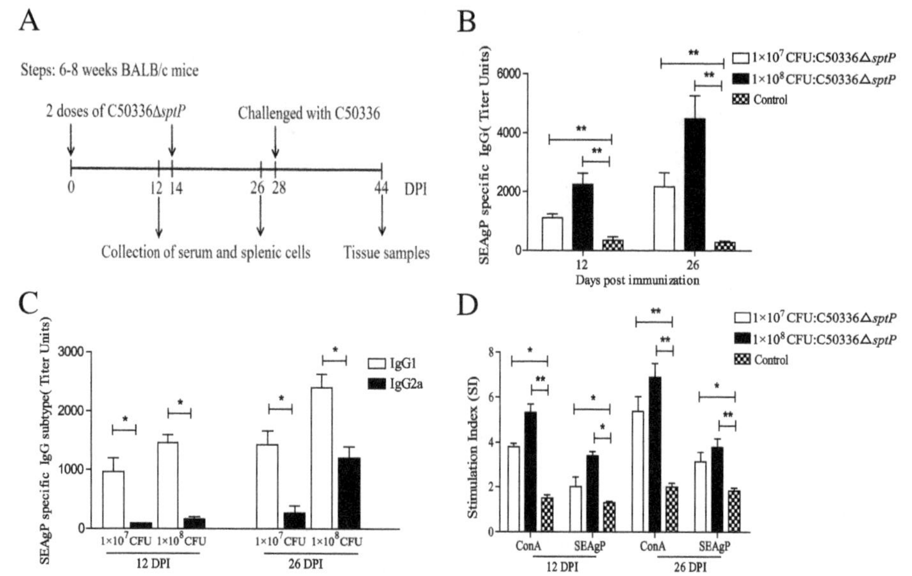

Fig. 4 Immunogenicity of C50336Δ*sptP*. Procedure for immunization (**a**). Determination of serum IgG levels (**b**) and IgG subtype levels (**c**) at 12 and 26 days post immunization. Stimulation index (SI) of mice lymphocytes determined by splenic lymphocyte proliferation assay using soluble antigen SEAgP (**d**) or lymphocyte mitogen ConA as a positive control. The vaccinated group received 1×10^7 CFU or 1×10^8 CFU of C50336Δ*sptP* orally, and the control group received 100 μl of PBS. Data are expressed as the mean ± SEM. *$P \leq 0.05$, **$P \leq 0.01$

were observed following challenge in the non-immunized mice. The survival curve is shown in Fig. 5a.

All surviving mice were sacrificed at 16 days post challenge, and tissues including the liver, spleen and cecum were sampled. As shown in Fig. 5, for the group vaccinated with 1×10^8 CFU of C50336Δ*sptP*, four of ten immunized mice carried a low level of *Salmonella* in the liver and spleen (Fig. 5b & c), and two of ten mice were positive for *Salmonella* in the cecum (Fig. 5d). The mice in group B carried a higher level of *Salmonella* in the liver, spleen, and cecum than the immunized mice from group A. All samples from the blank control group (group C) were negative for *Salmonella*.

Discussion

In current study, we constructed an *sptP* mutant in *S.* Enteritidis C50336, and evaluated the efficacy of C50336Δ*sptP* as a candidate live attenuated vaccine for *Salmonella* infection based on virulence, changes in body weight and clinical symptoms, bacterial colonization, serum IgG level, splenic lymphocyte proliferation and protective efficiency in mice. Our results showed that the body weight change of mice orally vaccinated with C50336Δ*sptP* (1×10^7 CFU or1 $\times 10^8$ CFU) was similar to that of the PBS control. After immunization with C50336Δ*sptP*, only small amounts of *Salmonella* colonized and persisted in the liver and spleen of the mice at 28 days, but strong humoral and cellular immune responses were induced to protect the mice against secondary *S.* Enteritidis challenge.

Salmonella enterica subsp. enterica includes several important serovars including Typhimurium, Enteritidis Typhi, and Paratyphi, which are the leading sources of human salmonellosis. Vaccines have been developed for one of these serovars and will prevent disease caused by *S.* Typhimurium or *S.* Enteritidis [27]. Symptoms of human Salmonellosis include abdominal pain, diarrhea, nausea, vomiting, fever, and headache [5]. *S.* Enteritidis is also increasingly reported in cases of invasive and extra-intestinal infections, such as arthritis, septicemia, meningitis, endocarditis, and urinary tract infections [28–34]. Infection with *Salmonella* is usually caused by consumption of contaminated pork and beef, poultry and eggs. It is necessary to take effective measures to

Table 2 Protective effects of C50336Δ*sptP* in mice

Group	Vaccination		Number	Challenge			Survivors/total	Survival rate (%)
	Strain	Dose (CFU)		Strain	Route	Dose (CFU)		
A	C50336Δ*sptP*	1×10^8	10	C50336	oral	1×10^8	10/10	100
B	PBS	—	10	C50336	oral	5×10^5	5/15	33
C	PBS	—	10	PBS	oral	—	5/5	100

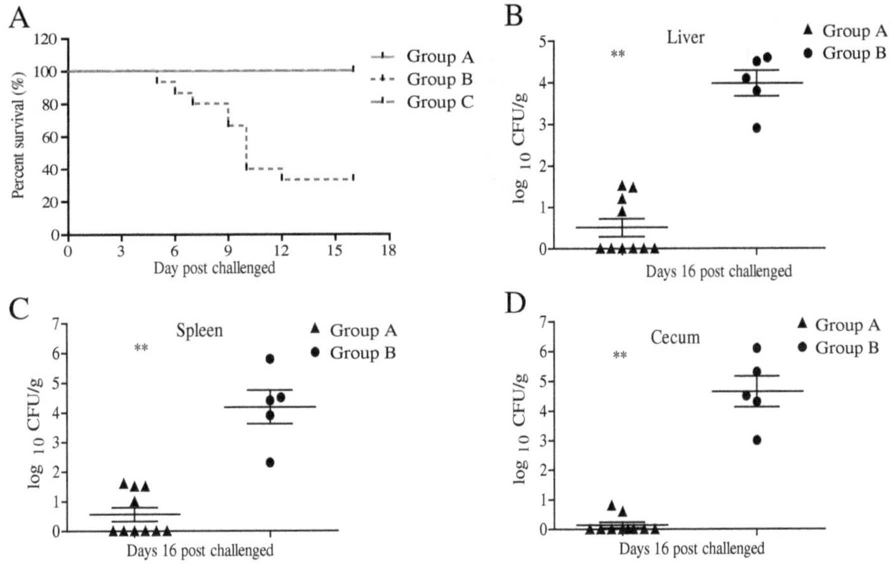

Fig. 5 Survival curve (**a**) and bacterial colonization in challenged mice. Bacterial colonization in the liver (**b**), spleen (**c**) and cecum (**d**) of challenged mice (Table 2, group A, immunized with C50336Δ*sptP* and then challenged with 1 × 10^8 CFU of C50336; group B, immunized with PBS and then challenged with 5 × 10^5 CFU of C50336). All samples from the blank control group were negative for *Salmonella* (Table 2, group C). The number of bacteria was determined and expressed as $\log_{10}$ CFU/g. Data are expressed as the mean ± SEM, $^{**}P \leq 0.01$

control and prevent *Salmonella* infection. Vaccination with live attenuated *Salmonella* may be a viable choice. Many live attenuated vaccines have been developed against *Salmonella* and have been confirmed to be generally more effective than vaccines prepared with dead bacteria [9–14].

The ideal vaccine should be avirulent, especially for live attenuated vaccines. Some *S.* Typhimurium and *S.* Enteritidis mutants with deletion of T3SS effector encoding genes or SPI-1 or SPI-2 display decreased virulence in mice, poultry, pigs, and humans [35–40]. In the current study, the LD_{50} of C50336Δ*sptP* in mice inoculated by the oral route demonstrated that the virulence of the mutant C50336Δ*sptP* was significantly decreased in comparison with that of the wild-type strain. The body weight of mice immunized with C50336Δ*sptP* was not significantly different from that of control mice and no or less clinical symptoms were observed following immunization. All of these findings show that C50336Δ*sptP* has almost no side effects in terms of growth performance in mice.

For live attenuated *Salmonella* vaccines, it is critical to stimulate the humoral and cellular immune responses in the immunized host [8, 41]. Systemic dissemination of *Salmonella* can lead to antigen presentation, resulting in high induction of specific humoral and cellular immune responses, and efficient protection against secondary infection [12, 42]. In this study, the *Salmonella*-specific serum IgG level in mice immunized with C50336Δ*sptP* at 12 and 26 DPI was significantly higher than the antibody level detected in the control group. In addition, the SI values of splenic lymphocyte proliferation in immunized mice were significantly higher than that in control mice. All of these findings indicate that strong humoral and cellular immune responses can be stimulated by C50336Δ*sptP*. In addition, the mice vaccinated with 1 × 10^8 CFU C50336Δ*sptP* showed higher levels of serum IgG and splenic lymphocyte proliferation capability than mice vaccinated with 1 × 10^7 CFU C50336Δ*sptP*.

S. Enteritidis deleted with one or several effector encoding genes provided efficacious protection against secondary *S.* Enteritidis challenge in mice [12, 13]. In our study, to evaluate the protective efficacy of C50336Δ*sptP*, we orally immunized mice with 1 × 10^8 CFU of C50336Δ*sptP*, and determined protection rates following oral challenge with 1 × 10^8 CFU of wild-type C50336. Our results show that mice immunized with 1 × 10^8 CFU of C50336Δ*sptP* developed extensive humoral and cellular immune responses and experienced 100% protection against subsequent *S.* Enteritidis challenge.

Pathogenesis of *Salmonella* is associated with a specialized ability to invade and persist within intestinal epithelial cells, where it can replicate and evade the host immune system [43]. T3SS-1 and T3SS-2 are encoded by SPI-1 and SPI-2 respectively, secreting various effector proteins that are essential for *Salmonella* colonization and intracellular persistence in the host [11, 35, 44]. SptP is a T3SS-1 effector protein that mediates the reversion of pathogen-induced changes in the actin cytoskeleton after *Salmonella* invasion

[15]. In our study, *S.* Enteritidis C50336 with deletion of *sptP* led to decreased invasion in Caco-2 BBE and RAW264.7 cells. SptP also inhibits the MAPK pathway, suppresses IL-8 production, and reduces the inflammatory response in host cells, thereby enhancing intracellular *Salmonella* replication [16–18]. In current study, deletion of *sptP* resulted in induction of strong humoral and cellular immune responses against subsequent *Salmonella* challenge.

Conclusion

Our present work demonstrates that vaccination of mice with the candidate vaccine C50336Δ*sptP* conferred development of acquired immunity and efficacious protection against experimental systemic infection. Thus, the *sptP* mutant strain of *S.* Enteritidis C50336 has the potential of being a safe, immunogenic vaccine against *Salmonella* infection.

Abbreviations

CFU: Colony-forming units; DPI: Days post-immunization; ELISA: Enzyme-linked immunosorbent assay; IL-8: Interleukin-8; LD_{50}: 50% lethal dose; mLN: mesenteric lymphadenitis; PBS: phosphate-buffered saline; *S.* Enteritidis: *Salmonella enterica* serovar Enteritidis; SI: Stimulation index; SPI-1: *Salmonella* pathogenicity islands 1; SptP: *Salmonella* protein tyrosine phosphatase; T3SS: *Salmonella* Type III secretion system

Acknowledgments

Not applicable.

Funding

This work was supported by the Projects of International Cooperation and Exchanges NSFC (31320103907); The Special Fund for Agro-Scientific Research in the Public Interest (201403054); The National Key Research and Development Program Special Project (2016YFD0501607); The Program for High-end talents of Yangzhou University; The Graduate Student Research and Innovation Project of Jiangsu Province (KYZZ_0368); The "Six Talent Peaks Program" of Jiangsu Province (NY-028); The Yangzhou University Science and Technology Innovation Team; Priority Academic Development Program of Jiangsu Higher Education Institutions.

Authors' contributions

ZP and XJ: the conception and design of the study. ZL, PT, YJ, XK, QL and XX: acquisition of data, analysis and interpretation of data. ZL, PT and JS: wrote the main manuscript text, prepared figures, statistical analysis and revised the manuscript. QL, XX and JS: technical, material support. XJ: final approval of the version to be submitted. All authors read and approved the final manuscript.

Competing interests

The authors declare that they have no competing interests.

Consent for publication

Not applicable.

Author details

[1]Jiangsu Key Laboratory of Zoonosis, Jiangsu Co-Innovation Center for Prevention and Control of Important Animal Infectious Diseases and Zoonosis, MOA Key Laboratory of Prevention and Control of Biological Hazard Factors (Animal Origin) for Agrifood Safety and Quality, MOE Joint International Research Laboratory of Agriculture and Agri-product Safety, Yangzhou University, Yangzhou 225001, China. [2]Division of Gastroenterology and Hepatology, College of Medicine, University of Illinois at Chicago, Chicago 60612, USA. [3]Center for Comparative Medicine, Animal Infectious Disease Laboratory, College of Veterinary Medicine, Yangzhou University, Yangzhou 225001, China. [4]Department of Anatomy and Cell Biology, Rush University Medical Center, Chicago 60612, USA.

References

1. Chai SJ, White PL, Lathrop SL, Solghan SM, Medus C, McGlinchey BM, et al. *Salmonella* enterica serotype Enteritidis: increasing incidence of domestically acquired infections. Clinical infectious diseases: an official publication of the Infectious Diseases Society of America. 2012;54(Suppl 5):S488–97.
2. Majowicz SE, Musto J, Scallan E, Angulo FJ, Kirk M, O'Brien SJ, et al. International collaboration on enteric disease 'Burden of illness S: the global burden of nontyphoidal Salmonella gastroenteritis. Clinical infectious diseases: an official publication of the Infectious Diseases Society of America. 2010;50(6):882–9.
3. Scallan E, Hoekstra RM, Angulo FJ, Tauxe RV, Widdowson M-A, Roy SL, et al. Foodborne illness acquired in the United States—major pathogens. Emerg Infect Dis. 2011;17(1):7–15.
4. Braden CR. *Salmonella* enterica serotype Enteritidis and eggs: a national epidemic in the United States. Clinical infectious diseases: an official publication of the Infectious Diseases Society of America. 2006;43(4):512–7.
5. CDC. *Salmonella* serotype enteritidis infections among workers producing poultry vaccine–Maine. MMWR Morb Mortal Wkly Rep 2007 Aug 31. November-December 2006;56(34):877–9.
6. Tollefson LM. Margaret Ann: antibiotic use in food animals: controlling the human health impact. J AOAC Int. 2000;83(2):245–54.
7. Whichard JM, Gay K, Stevenson JE, Joyce KJ, Cooper KL, Omondi M, et al. Human *Salmonella* and concurrent decreased susceptibility to quinolones and extended-spectrum cephalosporins. Emerg Infect Dis. 2007;13(11):1681–8.
8. Mastroeni P, Chabalgoity JA, Dunstan SJ, Maskell DJ, Dougan G. *Salmonella*: immune responses and vaccines. Vet J. 2001;161(2):132–64.
9. Geng S, Jiao X, Barrow P, Pan Z, Chen X. Virulence determinants of *Salmonella* Gallinarum biovar Pullorum identified by PCR signature-tagged mutagenesis and the spiC mutant as a candidate live attenuated vaccine. Vet Microbiol. 2014;168(2–4):388–94.
10. Haneda T, Okada N, Kikuchi Y, Takagi M, Kurotaki T, Miki T, et al. Evaluation of *Salmonella* enterica serovar Typhimurium and Choleraesuis slyA mutant strains for use in live attenuated oral vaccines. Comp Immunol Microbiol Infect Dis. 2011;34(5):399–409.
11. Bohez L, Ducatelle R, Pasmans F, Haesebrouck F, Van Immerseel F. Long-term colonisation-inhibition studies to protect broilers against colonisation with *Salmonella* Enteritidis, using *Salmonella* Pathogenicity Island 1 and 2 mutants. Vaccine. 2007;25(21):4235–43.
12. Karasova D, Sebkova A, Vrbas V, Havlickova H, Sisak F, Rychlik I. Comparative analysis of *Salmonella* enterica serovar Enteritidis mutants with a vaccine potential. Vaccine. 2009;27(38):5265–70.
13. Si W, Wang X, Liu H, Yu S, Li Z, Chen L, et al. Physiology, pathogenicity and immunogenicity of live, attenuated *Salmonella* enterica serovar Enteritidis mutants in chicks. Microb Pathog. 2015;83-84:6–11.
14. Araya DV, Quiroz TS, Tobar HE, Lizana RJ, Quezada CP, Santiviago CA, et al. Deletion of a prophage-like element causes attenuation of *Salmonella* enterica serovar Enteritidis and promotes protective immunity. Vaccine. 2010;28(33):5458–66.
15. Fu Y, Galan JE. A *Salmonella* protein antagonizes Rac-1 and Cdc42 to mediate host-cell recovery after bacterial invasion. Nature 1999;401(6750):293–7.
16. Murli S, Watson RO, Galan JE. Role of tyrosine kinases and the tyrosine phosphatase SptP in the interaction of *Salmonella* with host cells. Cell Microbiol. 2001;3(12):795–810.
17. Haraga A, Miller SI. A *Salmonella* enterica Serovar Typhimurium translocated leucine-rich repeat effector protein inhibits NF- B-dependent Gene expression. Infect Immun. 2003;71(7):4052–8.

18. Lin SL, Le TX, Cowen DS. SptP, a *Salmonella* Typhimurium type III-secreted protein, inhibits the mitogen-activated protein kinase pathway by inhibiting Raf activation. Cell Microbiol. 2003;5(4):267–75.
19. Choi HW, Brooking-Dixon R, Neupane S, Lee CJ, Miao EA, Staats HF, et al. *Salmonella* Typhimurium impedes innate immunity with a mast-cell-suppressing protein tyrosine phosphatase. SptP Immunity. 2013;39(6):1108–20.
20. Datsenko KA, Wanner BL. One-step inactivation of chromosomal genes in *Escherichia coli* K-12 using PCR products. Proc Natl Acad Sci U S A. 2000;97(12):6640–5.
21. McCormick BA. *Salmonella* Typhimurium attachment to human intestinal epithelial monolayers: transcellular signalling to subepithelial neutrophils. J Cell Biol. 1993;123(4):895–907.
22. Zhang X, Kelly SM, Bollen WS, Curtiss R 3rd. Characterization and immunogenicity of *Salmonella* Typhimurium SL1344 and UK-1 delta crp and delta cdt deletion mutants. Infect Immun. 1997;65(12):5381–7.
23. Gilles HJ. Calculation of the index of acute toxicity by the method of linear regression. Comparison with the method of "Karber and Behrens". European journal of toxicology and environmental hygiene Journal europeen de toxicologie. 1974;7(2):77–84.
24. Meng X, Meng X, Zhu C, Wang H, Wang J, Nie J, et al. The RNA chaperone Hfq regulates expression of fimbrial-related genes and virulence of *Salmonella* enterica serovar Enteritidis. FEMS Microbiol Lett. 2013;346(2):90–6.
25. Rana N, Kulshreshtha RC. Cell-mediated and humoral immune responses to a virulent plasmid-cured mutant strain of *Salmonella* enterica serotype gallinarum in broiler chickens. Vet Microbiol. 2006;115(1–3):156–62.
26. Brito JR, Hinton M, Stokes CR, Pearson GR. The humoral and cell mediated immune response of young chicks to *Salmonella* Typhimurium and S. Kedougou. The British veterinary journal. 1993;149(3):225–34.
27. Strugnell RA, Scott TA, Wang N, Yang CY, Peres N, Bedoui S, et al. *Salmonella* vaccines: lessons from the mouse model or bad teaching? Curr Opin Microbiol. 2014;17(17C):99–105.
28. Morpeth SC, Ramadhani HO, Crump JA. Invasive non-Typhi *Salmonella* disease in Africa. Clinical infectious diseases: an official publication of the Infectious Diseases Society of America. 2009;49(4):606–11.
29. Katsenos C, Anastasopoulos N, Patrani M, Mandragos C. *Salmonella* Enteritidis meningitis in a first time diagnosed AIDS patient: case report. Cases journal. 2008;1(1):5.
30. Gordon MA, Graham SM, Walsh AL, Wilson L, Phiri A, Molyneux E, et al. Epidemics of invasive *Salmonella* enterica serovar Enteritidis and S. Enterica Serovar Typhimurium infection associated with multidrug resistance among adults and children in Malawi. Clinical infectious diseases: an official publication of the Infectious Diseases Society of America. 2008;46(7):963–9.
31. Tena D, Gonzalez-Praetorius A, Bisquert J. Urinary tract infection due to non-typhoidal *Salmonella*: report of 19 cases. The Journal of infection. 2007;54(3):245–9.
32. Kobayashi H, Hall GS, Tuohy MJ, Knothe U, Procop GW, Bauer TW. Bilateral periprosthetic joint infection caused by *Salmonella* enterica serotype Enteritidis, and identification of *Salmonella* sp using molecular techniques. International journal of infectious diseases: IJID: official publication of the International Society for Infectious Diseases. 2009;13(6):e463–6.
33. Mutlu H, Babar J, Maggiore PR: Extensive Salmonella Enteritidis endocarditis involving mitral, tricuspid valves, aortic root and right ventricular wall. Journal of the American Society of Echocardiography: official publication of the American Society of Echocardiography 2009, 22(2):210. e1–3.
34. Ghosh TS, Vogt RL. Cluster of invasive salmonellosis cases in a federal prison in Colorado. Am J Infect Control. 2006;34(6):348–50.
35. Khan SA, Stratford R, Wu T, Mckelvie N, Bellaby T, Hindle Z, et al. *Salmonella* Typhi and S-Typhimurium derivatives harbouring deletions in aromatic biosynthesis and *Salmonella* Pathogenicity Island-2 (SPI-2) genes as vaccines and vectors. Vaccine. 2003;21(5–6):538–48.
36. Coombes BK, Coburn BA, Potter AA, Gomis S, Mirakhur K, Li Y, et al. Analysis of the contribution of *Salmonella* pathogenicity islands 1 and 2 to enteric disease progression using a novel bovine ileal loop model and a murine model of infectious enterocolitis. Infect Immun. 2005;73(11):7161–9.
37. Boyen F, Pasmans F, Van Immerseel F, Morgan E, Botteldoorn N, Heyndrickx M, et al. A limited role for SsrA/B in persistent *Salmonella* Typhimurium infections in pigs. Vet Microbiol. 2008;128(3–4):364–73.
38. Dieye Y, Ameiss K, Mellata M, Curtiss R 3rd. The *Salmonella* Pathogenicity Island (SPI) 1 contributes more than SPI2 to the colonization of the chicken by *Salmonella* enterica serovar Typhimurium. BMC Microbiol. 2009;9(1):1–14.
39. Karasova D, Sebkova A, Havlickova H, Sisak F, Volf J, Faldyna M, et al. Influence of 5 major *Salmonella* pathogenicity islands on NK cell depletion in mice infected with *Salmonella* enterica serovar Enteritidis. BMC Microbiol. 2010;10:75.
40. Matulova M, Havlickova H, Sisak F, Rychlik I. Vaccination of chickens with *Salmonella* Pathogenicity Island (SPI) 1 and SPI2 defective mutants of *Salmonella* enterica serovar Enteritidis. Vaccine. 2012;30(12):2090–7.
41. Collins FM, Scott MT. Effect of Corynebacterium Parvum treatment on the growth of *Salmonella* Enteritidis in mice. Infect Immun. 1974;9(5):863–9.
42. Berndt A, Wilhelm A, Jugert C, Pieper J, Sachse K, Methner U. Chicken cecum immune response to *Salmonella* enterica serovars of different levels of invasiveness. Infect Immun. 2007;75(12):5993–6007.
43. Haraga A, Ohlson MB, Miller SI. *Salmonellae* interplay with host cells. Nat Rev Microbiol. 2008;6(1):53–66.
44. Cirillo DM, Valdivia RH, Monack DM, Falkow S. Macrophage-dependent induction of the *Salmonella* pathogenicity island 2 type III secretion system and its role in intracellular survival. Mol Microbiol. 1998;30(1):175–88.

9

Vaccine resistant pseudorabies virus causes mink infection in China

Gui-sheng Wang[1,2], Yijun Du[3], Jia-qiang Wu[3], Fu-lin Tian[1], Xue-jie Yu[4] and Jin-bao Wang[2*]

Abstract

Background: Pseudorabies, a highly contagious infectious disease of swine is caused by pseudorabies virus (PRV). PRV can cause fatal infection in other animal species.

Results: We report a deadly outbreak of pseudorabies that killed 87.2% (3522/4028) minks in a farm in 2014 in Shandong Province, China. PRV was isolated by using Vero cell culture and detected in mink samples by PCR from minks died during the outbreak. Epidemiological analysis indicated that 5.8% of minks (33/566) were PCR positive to PRV in Shandong Province. Phylogenetic analysis indicated that the PRV strains isolated from minks in this study were in the same clade with the Chinese porcine PRV isolates, which are resistant to the PRV vaccine.

Conclusions: We demonstrated that pseudorabies virus caused an outbreak of minks in a farm in Shandong Province of China and the virus has a very high infection rate in minks in Shandong Province, which is a challenge for the fur industry in China.

Keywords: Minks, Pseudorabies, Pseudorabies virus, Herpesvirus, China

Background

Pseudorabies, also known as Aujeszky's disease, is caused by pseudorabies virus (PRV), a herpesvirus of genus *Varicellovirus* in the family *Herpesviridae.* PRV causes diseases in domesticated and wild animals, but only swine is considered as the reservoir and animal host of PRV because swine are the only animal species that can survive an acute infection and have a latent infection [1, 2]. Like other alphaherpesviruses, in its natural host swine, PRV first invade epithelial cells of the mucosal surfaces, then the termini of nerve fibers, and finally the peripheral ganglia and the central nervous system to establish latent infection. In piglets or immunocompromised pigs, the nonspecific immune response is delayed or ineffective and the virus spreads through the central nervous system to cause abortion in pregnant swine and high mortality rates in piglets [2–4].

Due to its serious impact on the pig industry, some countries have tried to eradicate pseudorabies in commercial swine population based on the DIVA (differentiating infected from vaccinated individuals) vaccination program [5]. Pseudorabies has been eradicated in a few developed countries including the United States, several European countries and New Zealand [6–9]. Although the DIVA vaccination programs have been used in China, pseudorabies has reemerged since 2011 in China with increased infection frequency and severity in swine and other animals [10]. In recent years, a highly virulent PRV strain appeared in China that caused high mortality rates in grown pigs [4, 9]. The new PRV variant is resistant to vaccine immunization in vaccinated swine herds in many regions of China [10].

PRV can infect a broad range of domestic and wild animals with the exception of higher-order primates [11]. The hallmark of the PRV infection in non-porcine animal species is pruritus in the infected area and it is usually fatal PRV-infected mink exhibit neurological signs and die within a few days without pruritus [12].

PRV genome is a linear double-stranded DNA, approximately 150Kb with capacity to encode approximately 70 proteins [13]. PRV genome consists of a unique long region (UL) and a unique short region (US). The US region is bracketed by inverted repeat sequences, resulting in the formation of two possible PRV genome isomers with oppositely oriented US regions [13]. PRV major protective antigens including gB, gC,

* Correspondence: 578005428@qq.com
[2]School of Life Sciences, Shandong University, 27 Shanda Road South, Jinan 250100, China
Full list of author information is available at the end of the article

gD, and gH can stimulate animals to produce viral neutralization antibody and cellular immunity against the virus [14]. gE and TK genes are major PRV virulence genes. gE mediates cell fusion, virus diffusion between cells, and virion releasing and neurotropic tropism. It is also a marker gene to distinguish natural infection from vaccination since the vaccine lacks the gE gene. TK plays important roles in viral infections in the body and viral proliferation in nervous tissue. Although PRV infects several animal species, reported natural PRV infection of minks are rare [15, 16]. In September of 2014,3522 of 4028 minks died in 1 week in a farm in Shandong Province, China with 100% (3522/3522) case fatality and 87.2% (3522/4028) mortality. The clinical symptoms of the minks were sudden onset of pneumonia like syndroms, diarrhea and lethargy. Minks started to die 2 days after onset of illness and all of the dead minks died within a week. In this study, we studied the pathogen that caused the outbreak in minks in China.

Methods

Mink samples

We randomely seleted 10 dead minks during the outbreak from the farm to determine the causative agent. After the outbreak of mink infections on the intial farm, we obtained samples of 566 dead minks in 14 farms from 14 cities in Shandong Province to determine the ditribution and infection rate of the causative agent in minks in Shandong Province (Fig. 1). Sample size was determined according to a 95% confidence level and 10% PRV infection rate. The organs of the dead minks including heart, liver, spleen, lung, kidney, brain and intestine were collected from dead minks aseptically and were homogenized using metal beads (Tissue Lyser; Qiagen) in the RLT buffer (Qiagen).

DNA and RNA extraction

Two hundred microliters of homogenized mink tissue supernatant from each organ was used for total nucleotide extraction with the MiniBEST Viral RNA/DNA Extraction Kit (Takara, Dalian, China) in accordance with the manufacturer's protocol. The nucleic acid templates were stored at −80 °C until use.

PCR and RT-PCR amplification and DNA sequencing

All the mink organs obtained above were tested for pseudorabies virus, influenza virus, parvovirus, rotavirus and porcine circovirus with PCR or RT-PCR. Porcine circovirus was amplified as previously described [17]. Pseudorabies virus, influenza virus, parvovirus, and rotavirus virus were amplified by using kit for each virus from Beijing Anheal Laboratories Co (Beijing, China) following the protocols of the manufacture.

For isolated strains of PRV, 6 genes including gB, gC, gD, gE, gH and TK were amplified by PCR (Table 1). High fidelity Taq enzyme AccuTaq™ LA DNA Polymerase (Sigma-Aldrich, Shanghai, China) was used for PCR in this study. For each reaction 1 μl of extracted DNA/RNA sample was used as template. The primers were designed in this study and the PCR cycles were the same for all primer pairs, which included a cycle of 95 °C for 3 min, 15 cycles of 95 °C for 30s, 65 °C for 30s (decreasing 1 °C each cycle) and 72 °C for 2 min, 15 cycles of 95 °C for 30s, 51 °C for 30s, and 72 °C for 2 min, and a final cycle of 72 °C for 10 min. The PCR products were electrophoresed on agarose gels and DNA bands with expected sizes were excised from the gels. The DNA purified from the gels was cloned into plasmid vector pMD18-T (Takara, Dalian, China). Three clones of each recombinant plasmid were sequenced on both stands by

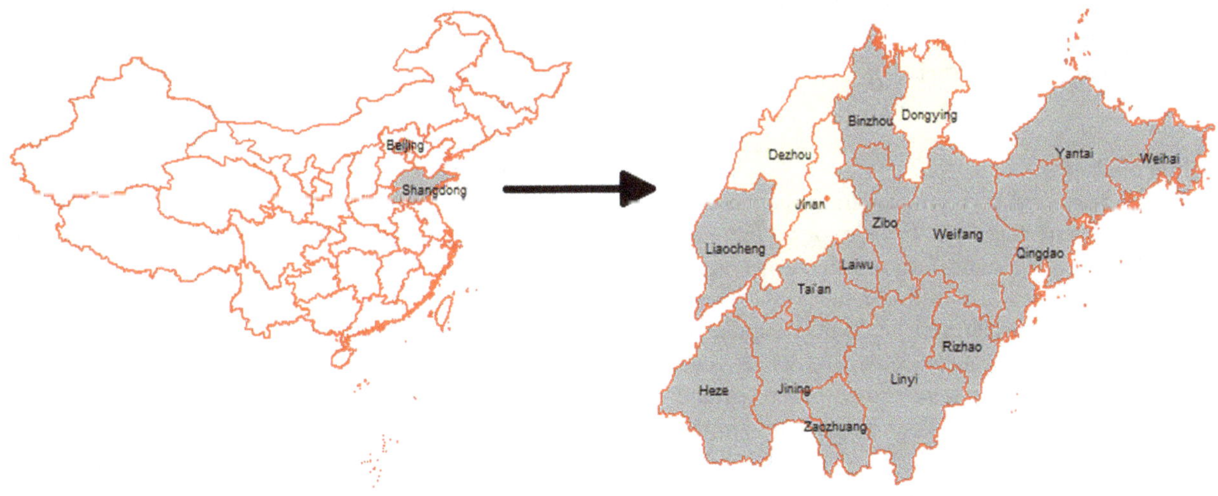

Fig. 1 Geographic location of Shandong Province of China (left) and the mink sample collection sites (right). Mink samples were collected from 14 (grey areas) of 17 cities in Shandong Province. The maps were drawn using the R Project for Statistical Computing (https://www.r-project.org/)

Table 1 Primers amplification of the entire CDS of gC, gD, gH, gE, and TK genes of PRV

Primers	Sequence	Position (bp)	Length (bp)	Annealing temperature	GenBank accession
gB-F	CTGGTGGCGGTCTTAGGCG	8–27	2738	60	KJ526439
gB-R	CTACAGGGCGTCGGGGTCC	2726–2744			
gC-F	GCTCGTGCAGGCGTACGT	53,326–53,343	1625	55	AF158090
gC-R	GCGGTCGTTTATTGATTCGG	54,950–54,931			
gD-F	CCCAGGTTCCCATACACTCAC	121,236–121,256	1258	55	AF086702
gD-R	TACTGCGGAGGCTACGGAC	122,487–126,469			
gE-F	AGACCATGCGGCCCTTTC	122,353–122,370	2710	58	AY249861
gE-R	ACGACCACTCCGTGTCCAGC	125,090–125,071			
gH-F	GGAGATGGGGGTGTGACC	59,631–59,648	3108	53	M61196
gH-R	GCGGCAGACACTTTAACTCTTG	62,701–62,680			
TK-F	AGGCGTTCGTAGAAGCGGT	59,195–59,213	1147	56	AY217095
TK-R	GGGCACGGCAAACTTTATTG	60,340–60,321			

the Biotechnology Research Center, Shandong Academy of Agricultural Sciences (Jinan, China).

Phylogenetic analysis

In order to get comparable phylogenetic results for all genes, we only selected sequences for viruses that had complete genome sequences in GenBank to do phylogenetic analysis. The DNA sequences were aligned using the Clustal W program implemented in the MEGA7.0 software. The phylogenetic trees that reflected evolutionary distances were constructed using the Maximum-likelihood method employing a Kimura 2-parameter model for nucleotides reconstructed using the same software [18].

Bacterial culture

The tissues of the brains and livers of minks were scratched with a bacterial inoculation loop and inoculated onto trypsin soy agar plates and blood agar plates. The plates were incubated at 37 °C for 48 h under aerobic and anaerobic conditions.

Isolation of virus

The frozen brain and liver samples from the minks were homogenized, centrifuged at 7168 x g for 10 min at 4 °C, filtered through disposable filters with an average pore diameter of 0.22 μm and transferred to a Vero cell monolayer. The cells were cultured in DMEM supplemented with 2% fetal bovine serum at 37 °C and 5% CO_2 condition for 72 h. The cultures were then harvested and repeatedly frozen and thawed three times. The suspension was used for passages on Vero cells. On the third passage of the cell cultures, the supernatant was tested with PCR using the PRV gB gene primers to determine infection with PRV.

Results

Bacterial pathogen detection

To determine whether the minks died of bacterial infection, their brain and liver tissue smears were stained by Gram staining and examed by microscopy. No bacterium was observered in these tissues from the Gram stain. Additionally, brain and liver samples of each mink were cultured on tryptic soy agar plates and blood agar plates. No bacterium was obtained from brain and liver tissues, suggesting that the minks were not infected with a bacterial pathogen.

PRV as the causative agent of the mink outbreak

PCR amplification of PRV gE gene indicated that 100% (10/10) minks from the farm were positive to PRV with all organs tested incluing heart, liver, spleen, lung, kidney, brain and intestine. However, none of the organs was positive to other viruses including influenza virus, Parvovirus, rotavirus and porcine circovirus by PCR or RT-PCR amplification.

Prevalence of minks to PRV

After demonstrating that the dead minks from the farm were infected with PRV, we further collected samples of 566 dead minks in 14 mink farms according to the 95% confidence level and 10% PRV infection rate. PCR amplification of gE gene showed that 5.8% (33/566) of minks were positive to PRV.

Isolation of PRV from minks

To further determine the characteristics of PRV in the minks, we isolated PRV from mink tissues. On the third passage of the mink sample innoculated cell cultures, the supernatant of the culture was amplifed with PCR by using the gB gene primers. PCR amplification indicted that cells derived from two mink samples were positive. The viruses were named W-MPRV1 and W-MPRV2, respectively. Strain W-MPRV1 was isolated from the sample of a dead mink from the farm with outbreak of pseudorabies and W-MPRV2 was isolated from a dead mink from another farm during the epidemilogic investigation.

Mink PRV sequence analysis

The entire coding region plus the 5′ and 3′ end of non-coding regions of gB (2735 bp), gC (1624 bp), gD (787 bp), gE (2724 bp), gH (3262 bp) and TK (1157 bp) of the PRV strains W-MPRV1 and W-MPRV2 were sequenced based on the PCR products of each gene. The DNA sequences of two genes (gB and TK) were 100% identical between the two mink PRV strains. The DNA sequence homology of three genes between the two mink PRV strains (gC, gE, and gH) were 99.8% to 99.9%. BLAST analysis indicated that homology of the strains W-MPRV1, W-MPRV2 and Chinese PRV isolates DL14/08(GenBank accession: KU360259), HNX (KM189912), HNB(KM189914), HN1201 (KP722022), HeN1(KP098534), TJ (KJ789182) were 99.9% to 100% for the 6 genes. The gD gene of strain W-MPRV1 was identical to strain W-MPRV2 and the Chinese PRV isolates on the 5′ end, but missed a 281 bp near the 3′ end of the gene compared to strain W-MPRV2 and the Chinese PRV isolates in GenBank (Fig. 2). The deletion

```
W-MPRV1   ACCGGGAGGTGGTGAACTACTGGTACCGCAAGAACGGCCGGACGCTCCCGCGGGCCTACG  780
          ||||||||||||||||||||||||||||||||||||||||||||||||||||||||||||
W-MPRV2   ACCGGGAGGTGGTGAACTACTGGTACCGCAAGAACGGCCGGACGCTCCCGCGGGCCTACG  780

W-MPRV1   CCGCCGC-----------------------------------------------------  787
          |||||||
W-MPRV2   CCGCCGCCACGCCGTACGCCATCGACCCCGCGCGGCCCTCGGCGGGCTCGCCGAGGCCCA  840

W-MPRV1   ------------------------------------------------------------

W-MPRV2   GGCCCCGGCCCCGGCCCAGGCCCCGGCCGAAGCCCGAGCCCGCCCCGGCGACGCCCGCGC  900

W-MPRV1   ------------------------------------------------------------

W-MPRV2   CCCCCGGCCGCCTGCCCGAGCCGGCGACGCGGGACCACGCCGCCGGGGGGCGCCCCACGC  960

W-MPRV1   ------------------------------------------------------------

W-MPRV2   CGCGACCCCCGAGGCCCGAGACGCCGCACCGCCCCTTCGCCCCGCCGGCCGTCGTGCCCA  1020

W-MPRV1   --------------------------------------------------GCCGGGCGTCT  798
                                                            |||||||||||
W-MPRV2   GCGGGTGGCCGCAGCCCGCGGAGCCGTTCCCGCCCCGGACCACCGCCGCGCCGGGCGTCT  1080

W-MPRV1   CGCGCCACCGCTCGGTGATCGTCGGCACGGGCACCGCGATGGGCGCGCTCCTGGTGGGCG  858
          ||||||||||||||||||||||||||||||||||||||||||||||||||||||||||||
W-MPRV2   CGCGCCACCGCTCGGTGATCGTCGGCACGGGCACCGCGATGGGCGCGCTCCTGGTGGGCG  1140

W-MPRV1   TGTGCGTCTACATCTTCTTCCGCCTGAGGGGGGCGAAGGGGTATCGCCTCCTGGGCGGTC  918
          ||||||||||||||||||||||||||||||||||||||||||||||||||||||||||||
W-MPRV2   TGTGCGTCTACATCTTCTTCCGCCTGAGGGGGGCGAAGGGGTATCGCCTCCTGGGCGGTC  1200

W-MPRV1   CCGCGGACGCCGACGAGCTAAAAGCGCAGCCCGGTCCGTAGCCTCCGCAGTA  978
          ||||||||||||||||||||||||||||||||||||||||||||||||||||
W-MPRV2   CCGCGGACGCCGACGAGCTAAAAGCGCAGCCCGGTCCGTAGCCTCCGCAGTA  1252
```

Fig. 2 DNA sequence alignment of gD gene of mink isolates of PRV W-MPRV1 and W-MPRV2. W-MPRV1 had a deletion of 281 nucleotides from 787 nucleotide to 1069 nucleotide of 281 nucleotides in the gD gene of W-MPRV1 caused a frameshift mutation and generated a protein with a deletion of 93 amino acids near the C-terminal (Fig. 3). The sequences generated in this study were deposited in GenBank (Accession numbers: MF940933 – MF940944).

Phylogenetic analysis

Phylogenetic analysis with each individual gene and the concatenated sequence of gB, gC, gD, gE and TK genes showed similar results and only the phylogenetic trees of gB gene and the concatenated sequence were shown in Fig. 4. The PRV strains were classified into two branches with all 6 genes or the concatenated sequences with the Chinese isolates in one branch represented by strains W-MPRV1 and W-MPRV2 and the American and European isolates in another branch represented by Becker strain (Fig. 4).

Discussion

In this study we investigated the causative agent of an outbreak of a fatal acute infectious disease in minks in a farm in Shandong Province of China, which caused a large scale of mink death with 100% cases fatality (3522 /3250) and 87.2% (3522/4028) mortality. We first screened the minks by PCR for pseudorabies virus, influenza virus, Parvovirus, rotavirus and porcine circovirus. Except for pseudorabies virus, all other viruses were negative in the mink samples. Our results indicated that PRV caused the outbreak of minks in the farm. To investigate whether PRV infection is widely distributed in Shandong Province, we subsequently collected samples of 566 minks from 14 farms in 14 cities of Shandong Province and amplified the gE gene with PCR. We found that 5.8% of 566 dead minks from all over Shandong Province were PCR positive to PRV. Our results further suggest that PRV infection of minks is widely spread in mink populations in Shandong Province.

We isolated two strains of pseudorabies virus from two dead minks from the farms. W-MPRV1 strain was isolated from a mink from the farm with pseudorabies outbreak and W-MPRV2 strain was isolated from a mink obtained in the subsequent epidemiologic investigation from another farm. Strains W-MPRV1 and W-MPRV2 were highly homologous, but not identical based on DNA sequences. They have identical sequences on gB and TK genes and 99.8% to 99.9% homology on gC, gE, and gH gene. The major difference between these two strains is that W-MPRV1 has a 281 bp deletion near the 3 end of the gD gene that generates a frameshift in gD gene resulting in a protein missing 93 amino acid near the C-terminal. Apparently the mutation in gD did not affect the virulence of W-MPRV1 to

```
                   170       180       190       200       210       220
           ---------+---------+---------+---------+---------+---------+

PRV1.pro   EGQYRRLVSVDGVNILTDFMVALPEGQECPFARVDQHRTYKFGACWSDDSFKRGVDVMRF

PRV2.pro   EGQYRRLVSVDGVNILTDFMVALPEGQECPFARVDQHRTYKFGACWSDDSFKRGVDVMRF

                   230       240       250       260       270       280
           ---------+---------+---------+---------+---------+---------+

PRV1.pro   LTPFYQQPPHREVVNYWYRKNGRTLPRAYAAA----------------------------

PRV2.pro   LTPFYQQPPHREVVNYWYRKNGRTLPRAYAAATPYAIDPARPSAGSPRPRPRPRPRPRPK

                   290       300       310       320       330       340
           ---------+---------+---------+---------+---------+---------+

PRV1.pro   ------------------------------------------------------------

PRV2.pro   PEPAPATPAPPGRLPEPATRDHAAGGRPTPRPPRPETPHRPFAPPAVVPSGWPQPAEPFP

                   350       360       370       380       390       400
           ---------+---------+---------+---------+---------+---------+

PRV1.pro   ------PGVSRHRSVIVGTGTAMGALLVGVCVYIFFRLRGAKGYRLLGGPADADELKAQP

PRV2.pro   PRTTAAPGVSRHRSVIVGTGTAMGALLVGVCVYIFFRLRGAKGYRLLGGPADADELKAQP
```

Fig. 3 Amino acid sequence alignment of gD of mink isolates of PRV W-MPRV1 and W-MPRV2. W-MPRV1 had a deletion of 93 amino acids near the C-terminal

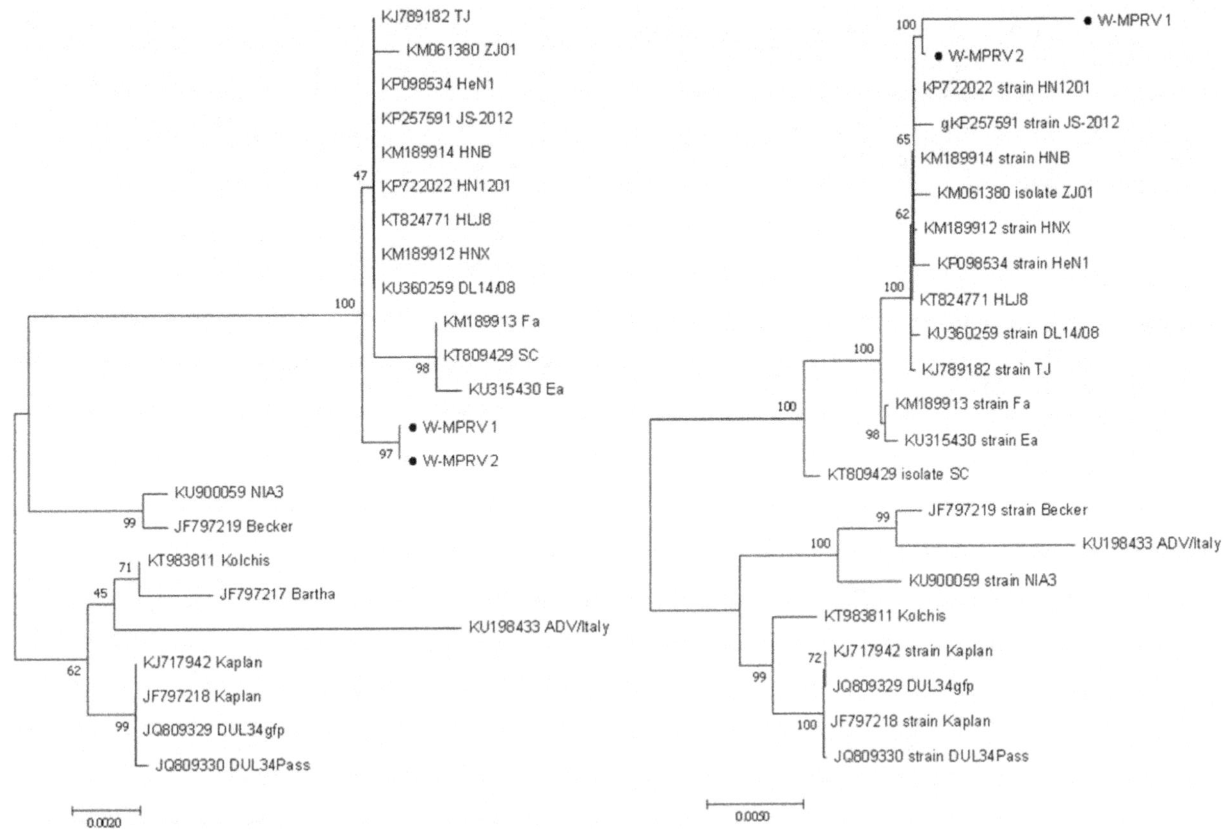

Fig. 4 Phylogenetic tree of Pseudorabies virus. The phylogenetic tree was constructed with gB gene sequence (left) and the concatenated sequence of gB, gC, gD, gE, gH and TK genes (right) using MEGA5 software with 1000 replicates for bootstrap testing. Numbers (> 50) above or below branches are posterior node probabilities. The GenBank number was labeled on each line. Dots indicated sequences obtained in this study. Scale bar indicates nucleotide substitutions per site

minks because it was isolated from a mink died in the outbreak. The gD of PRV is the viral ligand required for entry of extracellular particles [19, 20]. We do not know if the mutation generated a functional protein or not.

PRV strains from minks in this study are in the same phylogenetic clade with porcine PRV strains from China. This indicated that the mink PRV is a strain of porcine PRV. Among pigs, PRV is transmitted by contaminated secretions, excretions, aerosols, and venereal route [21]. No pig was present in the mink farm where PRV was isolated in this study and the farm was not near any pig farms. It is most likely the minks acquired PRV from meat products. A recent report indicated that farm raised foxes and domesticated dogs were infected with PRV transmitted by pork offal in China [22, 23]. A less likely possibility is that minks acquired PRV through long distance transmissions from aerosols because PRV can be transmit via the air [24]. In recent years porcine PRV infection has been a problem for pig farms in China. Bartha-K61 vaccine has been used worldwide to eradicate PRV [25]. Bartha-K61 vaccination provided complete protection against infection by the classic PRV SC strain. However, since late 2011 several highly virulent PRV strains including strains HeN1, JS-2012, and TJ have been isolated in various parts of China and the disease caused by these PRV strains is characterized by neurologic symptoms and a high mortality rate in pigs [25–27]. In protection assays, Bartha-K61 vaccine provided only partial protection against infection by strains HeN1, JS-2012, and TJ, suggesting that Bartha-K61 vaccine does not provide effective protection against new PRV strain infections in China [25–27]. The PRV strain isolate from minks in this study is phylogenetically closely related to the Bartha-K61 vaccine-resistant PRV strains, suggesting that vaccine-resistant PRV has spread widely throughout China and can cause a variety of animal infections. Eradicating pseudorabies in China under these circumstances proves challenging.

Shandong Province has the largest fur industry in China, which annually produces more than 50% of fur animals in China. In 2011, more than 30 million minks were raised in Shandong Province, with an annual increase of 20–40% [28]. This study indicated that PRV is widely distributed and can cause deadly outbreaks in minks in Shandong Province. Therefore, PRV infection of minks should be monitored and controlled in Shandong Province. Minks are primary fed fish and chicken products in Shandong Province. The source of PRV infected minks in Shandong Province is not clear. We also do not know whether PRV can establish persistent or prolonged infection in minks.

Conclusions

We suggested that pseudorabies virus could cause an outbreak of minks in a farm in Shandong Province of China and the virus has a very high infection rate in minks in Shandong Province, which is a challenge for the fur industry in China.

Abbreviation

PRV: Pseudorabies virus

Acknowledgements

We are grateful to Hao Yu (Fudan University School of Medicine) for reading the manuscript, to Xiang-rong Qin and Jian-Wei Liu (Wuhan University School of Health Sciences) for phylogenetic analysis.

Funding

This work was supported in part by a grant from the Shandong Provincial Modern Agricultural Industry Technology System (#SDAIT-21-05), a grant from Shandong Province Science and Technology Development Program (2014GSF121004), a grant from Shandong Agricultural Science and Technology Innovation Project (CXGC2016B14), and a grant from the National Nature Science Foundation of China (31570167). The funding bodies have no role in the design or conclusion of the study.

Authors' contributions

GSW, FLT, and JBW participated in the design of the study. GSW, YJD, JQW planned and performed the experiments. GSW and XJY analyzed the data and contributed to write the manuscript. All authors read and approved the final manuscript.

Consent for publication

Not applicable.

Competing interests

The authors declare that they have no competing interests.

Author details

[1]Shandong Provincial Center for Animal Disease Control and Prevention, Jinan, China. [2]School of Life Sciences, Shandong University, 27 Shanda Road South, Jinan 250100, China. [3]Shandong Key Laboratory of Animal Disease Control and Breeding, Institute of Animal Science and Veterinary Medicine, Shandong Academy of Agricultural Sciences, Jinan, China. [4]School of Health Science, Wuhan University, Wuhan, China.

References

1. Marcaccini A, López Peña M, Quiroga MI, Bermúdez R, Nieto JM, Alemañ N. Pseudorabies virus infection in mink: a host-specific pathogenesis. Vet Immunol Immunopathol 2008;124(3–4):264-73. https://doi.org/10.1016/j.vetimm.2008.03.013. Epub 2008 Apr 8. PubMed PMID: 18490062.
2. Pensaert M, Kluge JP. Pseudorabies virus (Aujeszky's disease). In: Pensaert MB, editor. Virus infections of Porcines. Amsterdam: Elsevier; 1989. p. 39–65.
3. Wohlgemuth K, Leslie PF, Reed DE, Smidt DK. Pseudorabies virus associated with abortion in swine. J Am Vet Med Assoc 1978;172(4):478-479. PubMed PMID:203566.
4. Wu R, Bai C, Sun J, Chang S, Zhang X. Emergence of virulent pseudorabies virus infection in northern China. J Vet Sci. 2013;14(3):363-365. PubMed PMID: 23820207; PubMed Central PMCID: PMC3788163.
5. van Oirschot JT. Diva vaccines that reduce virus transmission. J Biotechnol 1999; 73(2–3):195-205. Review. PubMed PMID: 10486928.
6. Davidson RM. Control and eradication of animal diseases in New Zealand. N Z Vet J 2002;50(3 Suppl):6-12. PubMed PMID: 16032229.
7. Moynagh J. Aujeszky's disease and the European Community. Vet Microbiol 1997;55(1–4):159-66. PubMed PMID: 9220609.
8. Müller T, Bätza HJ, Schlüter H, Conraths FJ, Mettenleiter TC. Eradication of Aujeszky's disease in Germany. J Vet Med B Infect Dis Vet Public Health 2003;50(5):207-13. PubMed PMID: 12864894.
9. Anderson LA. Pseudorabies (Aujeszky's disease) and its eradication: a review of the US experience 2008. United States Department of Agriculture, animal and plant health inspection service., 2008.
10. Sun Y, Luo Y, Wang CH, Yuan J, Li N, Song K, Qiu HJ. Control of swine pseudorabies in China: opportunities and limitations. Vet Microbiol 2016; 183:119-24. https://doi.org/10.1016/j.vetmic.2015.12.008. PubMed PMID: 26790944.
11. Marcaccini A, López Peña M, Quiroga MI, Bermúdez R, Nieto JM, Alemañ N. Pseudorabies virus infection in mink: a host-specific pathogenesis. Vet Immunol Immunopathol 2008;124(3–4):264-73. https://doi.org/10.1016/j.vetimm.2008.03.013. PubMed PMID: 18490062.
12. Pensaert M, Kluge JP. Pseudorabies virus (Aujeszky's disease). In: Pensaert MB. (Ed.) (1989) Virus infections of Porcines.Elsevier, Amsterdam: 39-65.
13. Klupp BG, Hengartner CJ, Mettenleiter TC, Enquist LW. Complete, annotated sequence of the Pseudorabies virus genome. J Virol. 2004;78:424–40.
14. Yin Z. In: Liu JH, editor. Animal Virology. Beijing: Science Press; 1997. p. 1000–1.
15. Liu H, Li XT, Hu B, Deng XY, Zhang L, Lian SZ, Zhang HL, Lv S, Xue XH, Lu RG, Shi N, Yan MH, Xiao PP, Yan XJ. Outbreak of severe pseudorabies virus infection in pig-offal-fed farmed mink in Liaoning Province, China. Arch Virol 2017;162(3):863-866. https://doi.org/10.1007/s00705-016-3170-7. PubMed PMID: 27885561.
16. Christodoulou T, Tsiroyiannis E, Papadopoulos O, Tsangaris T. An outbreak of Aujeszky's disease in minks. Cornell Vet 1970;60(1):65-73. PubMed PMID: 5434273.
17. Wang GS, Sun N, Tian FL, Wen YJ, Xu C, Li J, Chen Q, Wang JB. Genetic analysis of porcine circovirus type 2 from dead minks. J Gen Virol 2016;97(9): 2316-22. https://doi.org/10.1099/jgv.0.000529. PubMed PMID: 27324162.
18. Kumar S, Stecher G, Tamura K. MEGA7: molecular evolutionary genetics analysis version 7.0 for bigger datasets. Mol Biol Evol 2016 Jul;33(7):1870-4. https://doi.org/10.1093/molbev/msw054. Epub 2016 Mar 22. PubMed PMID: 27004904.
19. Ch'ng TH, Spear PG, Struyf F, Enquist LW. Glycoprotein D-independent spread of pseudorabies virus infection in cultured peripheral nervous system neurons in acompartmented system. J Virol 2007;81(19):10742-57. PubMed PMID: 17652377; PubMed Central PMCID: PMC2045490.
20. Farnsworth A, Goldsmith K, Johnson DC. Herpes simplex virus glycoproteins gD and gE/gI serve essential but redundant functions during acquisition of the virion envelope in the cytoplasm. J Virol 2003;77(15):8481-94. PubMed PMID:12857917; PubMed Central PMCID: PMC165244.
21. Romero CH, Meade PN, Shultz JE, Chung HY, Gibbs EP, Hahn EC, Lollis G. Venereal transmission of pseudorabies viruses indigenous to feral swine. J Wildl Dis 200137(2):289-96. PubMed PMID: 11310879.
22. Jin HL, Gao SM, Liu Y, Zhang SF, Hu RL. Pseudorabies in farmed foxes fed pig offal in Shandong province, China. Arch Virol 2016161(2):445-8. https://doi.org/10.1007/s00705-015-2659-9. Epub 2015 Nov 13. PubMed PMID: 26563317.
23. Zhang L, Zhong C, Wang J, Lu Z, Liu L, Yang W, Lyu Y. Pathogenesis of

natural and experimental Pseudorabies virus infections in dogs. Virol J 2015; 12:44. https://doi.org/10.1186/s12985-015-0274-8. PubMed PMID: 25889104; PubMed Central PMCID: PMC4374540.

24. Christensen LS, Mousing J, Mortensen S, Soerensen KJ, Strandbygaard SB, Henriksen CA, Andersen JB. Evidence of long distance airborne transmission of Aujeszky's disease (pseudorabies) virus. Vet Rec 1990;127(19):471-4. PubMed PMID: 1980166.
25. An TQ, Peng JM, Tian ZJ, Zhao HY, Li N, Liu YM, Chen JZ, Leng CL, Sun Y, Chang D, Tong GZ. Pseudorabies virus variant in Bartha-K61-vaccinated pigs, China, 2012. Emerg Infect Dis 2013;19(11):1749-55. https://doi.org/10.3201/eid1911.130177. PubMed PMID: 24188614; PubMed Central PMCID: PMC3837674.
26. Tong W, Liu F, Zheng H, Liang C, Zhou YJ, Jiang YF, Shan TL, Gao F, Li GX, Tong GZ. Emergence of a Pseudorabies virus variant with increased virulence to piglets. Vet Microbiol 2015;181(3–4):236-40. https://doi.org/10.1016/j.vetmic.2015.09.021. Epub 2015 Sep 30. PubMed PMID: 26507829.
27. Luo Y, Li N, Cong X, Wang CH, Du M, Li L, Zhao B, Yuan J, Liu DD, Li S, Li Y, Sun Y, Qiu HJ. Pathogenicity and genomic characterization of a pseudorabies virus variant isolated from Bartha-K61-vaccinated swine population in China. Vet Microbiol 2014;174(1–2):107-15. https://doi.org/10.1016/j.vetmic.2014.09.003. PubMed PMID: 25293398.
28. Wang GZ, Qing MJ, Zhang W. Shandong Province fur animal breeding industry problems and countermeasure strategy. Shangdong J Anim Sci Vet Med. 2014;35(8):21–2.

Efficacy of a polyvalent mastitis vaccine against *Staphylococcus aureus* on a dairy Mediterranean buffalo farm: results of two clinical field trials

Jacopo Guccione[1], Antonella Pesce[2], Massimo Pascale[3], Caterina Salzano[2], Gianni Tedeschi[4], Luigi D'Andrea[1], Angela De Rosa[1] and Paolo Ciaramella[1*]

Abstract

Background: In the last years the knowledges on Mediterranean Buffalo (MB) mastitis is remarkably improving, nevertheless the attention has been never focused on vaccination as preventive strategy for the control of mastitis in these ruminates. The aim of the current study was to assess clinical efficacy over time of two different preventive vaccination protocols against *S. aureus* mastitis, in primiparous MB.Vaccinated (VG) and not-vaccinated (N-VG) groups, of 30 MB each one, were selected from two different herds (herd A: VG1 and N-VG1; herd B: VG2 and N-VG2) of the same farm. Herd A received a double vaccination (Startvac®, 45 and 10 days before calving, protocol A), while in herd B an additional administration was performed (52 days after calving, protocol B). Bacteriological milk culture and assessment of somatic cell count (SCC) were performed at 10, 30, 60 and 90 days in milk (DIM) from composite milk samples. After 90 DIM, daily milk yields and SCC values were monthly detected until dry-off.

Results: The overall incidence of positive MB for *S. aureus* was 40.8% (49/120) in VG1 and 43.3% (52/120) in N-VG1 (Protocol A), while 45.8% (55/120) and 50.8% (61/120) in VG2 and N-VG2 (Protocol B). The latter was associated with a significant decreased in prevalence (at 90 DIM) and incidence of mastitis (animals positive for *S. aureus*, SCC > 200^10^3, with or without clinical signs) in the vaccinated MB, while no difference occurred in protocol A. Moreover, herd B showed a significant reduction in prevalence of intramammary infection (animals positive for *S. aureus*, SCC < 200^10^3, no clinical signs) in the vaccinated MB at 60 DIM while no differences were detected in herd A, at any sampling time; N-VG2 had significantly higher overall SCC values than VG2 (4.97 ± 4.75 and 4.84 ± 4.60 Log10 cells/mL ± standard deviation, respectively), while no differences were recorded in herd A.

Conclusions: The current investigation explores for the first time the clinical efficacy of vaccinations against *S. aureus* infections in MB, showing encouraging results regarding reduction in mastitis and somatic cell count; the polyvalent mastitis vaccine may be considered an additional tool for in-herd *S aureus* infection and should be associated to other control procedures to maximize its properties.

Keywords: *Staphylococcus aureus*, Vaccination, Prophylaxis, *Bubalus bubalis*, Udder health

* Correspondence: paociara@unina.it
[1]Department of Veterinary Medicine and Animal Productions, University of Napoli "Federico II", Via Delpino 1, 80137 Naples, Italy
Full list of author information is available at the end of the article

Background

Mastitis represents one of the major causes of economic loss in dairy Mediterranean buffaloes (MB) because negatively influencing milk quality and yields of the animals affected [1, 2]. In MB mastitis is mainly caused by several contagious (e.g. *Staphylococcus aureus*, *Streptococcus agalactiae*), environmental (e.g. *Streptococcus uberis* and *Streptococcus dysgalactiae*, *Escherichia coli*, *Enterobacteriaceae*, and yeasts), and opportunistic (e.g. coagulase-negative staphylococci) bacteria [3–5].

S. aureus is one of the most important pathogens, causing clinical and subclinical mastitis in dairy MB and cows all over the world [2, 6, 7]; Clinical outcomes and high within-herd prevalence were recently described in MB confirming its relevance as contagious microorganism [2]. This bacteria typically colonizes the injured skin; damage of the teat end and faulty milking encourages migration of bacteria into the udder causing intramammary infections (IMI) and sometimes persisting for extended periods [4, 8, 9]. Some strains are particularly resistant to antibiotics [4] and moderate results were reported in an our previous study exploring the effects of an antibiotic selective treatment [1]. As a consequence, similarly to dairy cows additional strategies of herd health management including treatment or culling of affected animals, implementation of biosecurity measures and hygienic milking practices, have been recommended to prevent and control udder health problems related to *S. aureus* in MB farms [2].

Although with different outcomes, great scientific attention was recently given to mastitis control by means of preventive vaccination protocols in cows [10–16]. A commercial multivalent vaccine containing inactivated *S. aureus* and *E. coli* has been available in European Union for the last years and several investigations regarding its usefulness were recently performed in cows with different results [13, 14, 17]. In MB, the awareness for mastitis are remarkably improving, although the attention has been never focused before on vaccination as preventive strategy for mastitis.

Considering the premises, the aims of the present study was to evaluate the clinical efficacy of a polyvalent commercial vaccine administered in dairy primiparous MB evaluating as outcomes (1) the prevalence and incidence of IMI and mastitis, (2) the effects on somatic cell count and (3) milk yield.

Methods

Animals and Farm Management

All the animals chosen in the present study were reared in the same breeding farm of approximately 700 dairy buffaloes, free from mandatory reportable diseases and located in Caserta area (Southern Italy). The eligible criteria for the farm were represented by 3, monthly and consecutive samplings of bulk tank milk positive for *S. aureus* before the beginning of the study, analyzed by means of PCR-based assay as described by Syring et al. [18]. No strict criteria were instead applied for bulk milk somatic cell count (SCC) or mastitis incidence. Differences observed about herd management practices were recorded during the period of the investigation (two consecutive years) to exclude possible influences on vaccination efficacy.

Farm was characterized by herringbone parlor and animals were milked twice a day. A mean of 247 ± 23-day milk yield per head of 2200 kg while mean bulk tank SCC values of $172 \times 10^3 \pm 49 \times 10^3$ and $179 \times 10^3 \pm 32 \times 10^3$ cell/mL were recorded for the whole herd during the first and the second year of investigation, respectively. All MB selected were kept in a roofed common paddock of ~ 1200 m^2 (~30 m × 40 m) As often observed in MB's farms, before parturition and until 40–50 DIM, all the *primiparous* MB were housed separated from the *pluriparous*. Milking was performed in the same milking parlor, although the *primiparous* animals were milked first. After 50 DIM, *primiparous* were mixed with the *pluriparous* animals, including milking time. The barn was characterized by a common bedded area (with dried manure solids), a loafing area and a feeding alley with solid non-grooved concrete floor (cleaned twice a day). The entire herd was fed a total mixed ratio including hay, silage and a multi-vitamin integrator three times a day; free access to the protected water trough was always guaranteed.

Study design

Two herds (A and B) were enrolled in the current study. Sixty *primiparous* for each herd were subdivided into two groups of 30 MB: vaccinated and not-vaccinated (herd A: VG1 and N-VG1; herd B: VG2 and N-VG2). Animals were chosen from the same farm in two consecutive lactations (herd A: I year, December 2012 to November 2013 - herd B: II year, December 2013 to November 2014). Every year the animals were chosen by means convenience sampling from 80 *primiparous* in good health having 4 functional quarters, teats free of significant lesions, and with an estimated calving date to allow vaccination at predicted times before calving. Samples size was calculated by using the formula proposed by Thrusfield [19] considering the following values: study population (pregnant primiparous MB in farm, ~14% of entire herd – approximately stable parameter in both years considered), expected prevalence of positive primiparous MB for *S. aureus* (55%) [1], confidence interval 95% and desired absolute precision (5%).

All the animals were individually submitted to a complete clinical examination with particular focus on the udder health status following the clinical procedure described by Ciaramella [20].

For each herd the progressive vaccination was performed on 50 MB were chosen by means of simple randomization; out of the latter, the first 30 animals reaching the entire vaccination protocol were enrolled as VG. The other 30 not vaccinated subjects were selected as N-VG.

On sampling day, local and systemic signs and changes in milk appearance, such us overall appearance of depression, udder swelling and pain, off-color and watery appearance of milk, and presence of flakes, clots or pus, were recorded. California Mastitis Test (CMT) was routinely performed from each composite milk sample, with values ≥1 interpreted as positive [2] (data not shown).

Vaccine

Commercial polyvalent mastitis vaccine (*STARTVAC*®, HIPRA Spain Co. Ltd, Girona) containing inactivated *E. coli* J5 and inactivated *S. aureus* (CP8) strains SP 140, expressing slime-associated antigenic complex (SAAC) was used [21].

The farmer was previously informed about the purposes and methods of the two clinical field-trials and the study received the approval by the Ethical Animal Care and Use Committee of University of Studies of Naples "Federico II". During the present investigation each herd was submitted to a different vaccination protocol: the first (protocol A - herd A) was based on two intramuscular vaccine injections located at the medium third of the neck (2 mL each one) and performed at 45 and 10 days before the estimated date of calving on VG1; the second one (protocol B - herd B), instead included an additional administration on VG2 at 52 days in milk (DIM).

Milk Samples

All milk samples were aseptically collected in sterile test tubes immediately before regular evening milking, as described by National Mastitis Council [22] for dairy cows. At 10, 30, 60 and 90 DIM, a sample from each quarter was collected; a composite milk sample was created by mixing equal amounts of milk (50 mL) from all 4 quarters into a sterile test tube (BD Vacutainer, Oxford, UK) and used to perform bacteriological milk culture (BMC) and determine the SCC; finally, milk yields were also recorded during the same samplings time using automatic dedicated software (Afifarm, Afimilk, Kibbutz Afikim, Israel). After 90 DIM, milk yield and SCC values were evaluated at 150 and 240 DIM (close to dry off). As described by a previous study [1], a great variability to achieve the supposed drying-off time (daily milk yield < 0.5 L/day) was detected in the enrolled animals (from 240 to 260 DIM), as consequence, the last sample considered useful for the statistical and economic analysis was collected at 240 DIM.

Definition of Udder Health Status

Following the classification reported in previous studies [1, 23], the animals enrolled were defined as negative for *S. aureus*, affected by IMI or mastitis considering: presence/absence of clinical signs, SCC values, and microbiological status; briefly, MB producing milk with SCC below the threshold of 200×10^3 cells/mL and associated with BMC negative to *S. aureus* were considered and hereafter referred to as "healthy udder"; animals with analogous SCC values and positive BMC caused by *S. aureus* have been instead considered affected by IMI; moreover, buffaloes producing milk with SCC upon the threshold of 200×10^3 and positive BMC for *S. aureus* have been defined as affected by mastitis, with (clinical mastitis - CM) or without clinical signs (subclinical mastitis - SCM) [1, 23]. All the MB affected by mastitis (CM and/or SCM) due to *S. aureus* were considered in end-point phase and excluded from the study.

Cytological and bacteriological investigations

Composite milk samples were placed in a cool box (4 °C) and brought to the reference laboratory within 1 h (h) of collection, where they were submitted to SCC analysis and BMC within 2 h of collection. SCC was determined using an automatic analyzer, approved for buffalo milk (Fossomatic 5000, Foss Electric, Hillerod, Denmark) [24]. The BMC and bacteriological identification were performed according to guidelines of the National Mastitis Council [25]. Briefly, 10 μL of each milk sample was streaked on one quarter of a blood-agar plate (Merck KGaA, Darmstadt, Germany), incubated at 37 °C for up to 48 h and examined two time (at 24 and 48 h of incubation). Bacterial colonies were tentatively identified on gross morphology; number and types of colonies were also recorded. As described in previous studies [2], when 3 or more dissimilar colony types were isolated on the plate, the sample was considered contaminated. Gram staining and catalase testing were performed to differentiate between streptococci and staphylococci, and tube coagulase testing using rabbit plasma to differentiate between coagulase-positive and coagulase-negative staphylococci. A final identification of microorganisms was performed using the colorimetric automated identification system (Vitek 2 XL 120; bioMerieux Inc., Hazelwood, MO), according to the manufacturer's instructions. Enterobacteriaceae were grown on MacConkey agar (Oxoid, Basingstoke, UK) and identified using the same automated system. Isolates identified with confidence levels greater than 0.90 were considered identified mastitis pathogens at species level; otherwise, they were identified at genus level.). All the laboratory procedures were performed without previous informations about the results of the clinical examination of the udder (physical and CMT).

Statistical analysis

Different animal health status, SCC, and milk yields were analyzed by standard descriptive statistics and normality was assessed using histograms, normal probability plots and Shapiro Wilk tests. Data were expressed as absolute numbers, percentage, or mean ± SD. Log- transformation was applied to variable not normally distributed. Untransformed and log-transformed continuous variables (SCC and milk yields) were compared using Student's *t*-test. Significant differences between expected and observed frequencies of categorical data (i.e. vaccine efficacy: VG1 vs. N-VG1 and VG2 vs. N-VG2) were assessed by means of contingency tables, using χ^2-test. Fisher's exact test was performed in case of low expected frequencies (<5). *P*robabilities <0.05 were considered significant. Moreover, a mixed models were also used to investigate the direct effects of the vaccination intra- and inter-protocols. The final model included fixed time effect, fixed group effect, fixed interaction time*group and buffalo as random effect. For statistical analysis of the outcomes a mixed linear models was used for continuous data (SCC and milk yield); Bonferroni correction was used to set *P*-value for multiple statistical test; the threshold for statistical significance in our analysis was $P = 0.0052$, the null hypothesis was rejected for $P < 0.01$.

For categorical data (presence/absence of mastitis) a mixed logistic models based only on fixed group effects and buffalo-specific random effect was performed because otherwise the function to be maximized was not concave due to the small amount of observations. Data inter-protocols (absolute values) were combined in the model including time and group as fixed effects. *P*robabilities <0.05 were considered significant. All the statistical data were analyzed using dedicated software (STATA 12.0, StataCorp LP, Collage Station, Texas, USA).

Results

Course of the study and prevalence of udder pathogens

No general or local adverse reactions to the use of the vaccine was observed in all the buffaloes of both the protocols after the administrations. The request number of vaccinated animals was reached in 1.5 months in herd A and in 2 months in herd B. Vaccinations were performed 45.8 ± 4.1 and 11.1 ± 2.4 days pre-calving in VG1, while 46.2 ± 4.6 and 10.3 ± 2.2 days-pre calving in VG2; the additional vaccination expected for protocol B was instead administered 52.2 ± 1.1 days post-calving. During the two years of study, no differences about all the aspects of herd management practices (e.g. feeding and housing system, milking routine, dairy workers, therapeutic protocols for mastitis, etc.) were detected.

Throughout the study, 480 composite milk samples were collected and submitted to BMC. All udder pathogens isolated during the first 90 DIM in vaccinated and not-vaccinated groups of the two herds and their relative incidence are reported in Table 1. Briefly, the most commonly isolated pathogens in both the groups of the two herds, were *S. aureus* followed by coagulase-negative staphylococci. Positive-culture status for *S. aureus* was detected in 30.2% (49/162) and 32.5% (52/160) of the overall bacteriological results in VG1 and N-VG1, respectively; it was instead recorded in 41.9% (55/131) and 50.4% (61/121) of the samples in VG2 and N-VG2, respectively. *E. coli* was only detected in both groups of herd B (VG2: 1 time, 0.8% and N-VG2: 2 times, 1.7%, Table 1) and associated with not severe CM (mild milk change, CMT ≥2).

The overall percentage of positive samples for other udder pathogens, except for *S. aureus* and *E. coli,* was 29.6% (48/162) in VG1 and 30.6% (49/160) in N-VG1, while it was 35.9% (47/131) and 23.9% (29/121) in VG2 and N-VG2, respectively.

Negative-culture status was observed in 40.1% (65/162) and 36.9% (59/160) of the all bacteriological results observed in VG1 and N-VG1, respectively; 21.4% (28/131) and 24.0% (29/121) were instead recorded in VG2 and N-VG2, respectively.

Vaccine effects

Protocol A

The 40.8% (49/120) and 43.3% (52/120) of the samples collected were positive for *S. aureus* in VG1 and N-VG1. No bacteria were detected at 10 DIM (0/30) in VG1, while their presence increased up to 16.7% (5/30), 60.0% (18/30) and 89.2% (25/28) at 30, 60 and 90 DIM, respectively; in N-VG1 the prevalence of positive-cultures for *S. aureus* was instead of 3.3% (1/30), 33.3% (10/30), 53.6% (15/28) and 92.8% (26/28) at 10, 30, 60 and 90 DIM, respectively; no statistically significant difference was found regarding this variable between VG1 and N-VG1 at any sampling time.

Details regarding of the effects of *S. aureus* on udder health are reported in Table 2. Briefly, two CM due to *S. aureus* were recorded both in VG1 (6.6%, 2/30) and N-VG1 (6.6%, 2/30), at 60 and 30 DIM, respectively. During the investigation, no SCM due to *S. aureus* were detected between 10 and 60 DIM in both groups, while they were observed both in VG1 (14.3%, 4/28) and N-VG1(10.7%,3/28) at 90 DIM. No statistically significant difference between prevalence of mastitis in VG1 and N-VG1 was observed. During the first 90 DIM, no statistically significant difference was recorded between the incidence of mastitic animals in VG1 (20.0%, 6/30) and

Table 1 Bacteriological results of all samples collected in both the herds of *primiparous* Mediterranean buffalo during the first 90 days in milk of investigation. Percentages represent the proportion calculate on the total number bacteriological results

	Herd A				Herd B			
	VG1		N-VG1		VG2		N-VG2	
Pathogens	No.	Percent	No.	Percent	No.	Percent	No.	Percent
Staphylococcus aureus	49	30.2	52	32.5	55	41.9	61	50.4
Coagulase-negative staphylococci	32	19.9	32	19.3	41	31.3	16	13.1
Enterococcus faecalis	2	1.2	2	1.3	1	0.8	1	0.8
Aerococcus viridans	4	2.5	4	2.5	2	1.5	4	3.3
Streptococcus dysgalactiae	2	1.2	1	0.6	0	0	2	1.7
Streptococcus thoraltensis	2	1.2	2	1.3	0	0	1	0.8
Other gram-positive pathogens (not *S. aureus*)	2	1.2	5	3.1	3	2.3	2	1.7
Escherichia coli	0	0	0	0	1	0.8	2	1.7
Acinetobacter lwoffii	4	2.5	3	1.9	0	0	2	1.7
Bacillus spp.	0	0	0	0	0	0	1	0.8
Culture negative	65	40.1	59	36.9	28	21.4	29	24.0
Total	162	100	160	100	131	100	121	100

No = number; VG1 and N-VG1 = Vaccinate Group1 and Not-Vaccinated Group1, respectively; VG2 and N-VG2 = Vaccinate Group1 and Not-Vaccinated Group2, respectively. Herd A: received two doses of vaccine pre-calving; Herd B: received two doses of vaccine pre-calving and one post-calving

Table 2 Udder health status in primiparous Mediterranean buffalos within the two study herds (A and B) in association with *Staphylococcus aureus* detection in composite milk samples

Herd A									
		10 DIM		30 DIM		60 DIM		90 DIM	
Udder health status	Groups	No.	Percent	No.	Percent	No.	Percent	No.	Percent
CM	VG1	0/30	0	0/30	0	2/30	6.6	0/28	0
	N-VG1	0/30	0	2/30	6.6	0/28	0	0/28	0
SCM	VG1	0/30	0	0/30	0	0/30	0	4/28	14.3
	N-VG1	0/30	0	0/30	0	0/28	0	3/28	10.7
IMI	VG1	0/30	0	5/30	16.7	16/30	53.3	22/28	78.6
	N-VG1	1/30	3.3	8/30	26.6	15/28	53.6	23/28	82.1
Healthy	VG1	30/30	100	25/30	83.3	12/30	40.0	2/28	7.1
	N-VG1	29/30	96.7	20/30	66.7	13/28	46.4	2/28	7.1
Herd B									
CM	VG2	0/30	0	0/30	0	0/28	0	0/27	0
	N-VG2	0/30	0	0/27	0	0/23	0	0/20	0
SCM	VG2	0/30	0	2/30	6.6	1/28	3.6	3/27^{a}	11.1
	N-VG2	3/30	10.0	4/27	14.8	3/23	13.0	5/20^{b}	25.0
IMI	VG2	2/30	6.6	12/30	40.0	14/28^{a}	50.0	21/27	77.8
	N-VG2	1/30	3.3	15/27	55.5	20/23^{b}	86.9	13/20	65.0
Healthy	VG2	28/30	93.3	16/30	53.3	13/28^{c}	19.1	3/27	11.1
	N-VG2	26/30	86.7	8/27	29.3	0/23^{d}	0	2/20	10.0

VG1 and N-VG1 = Vaccinate Group1 and Not-Vaccinated Group1, respectively; VG2 and N-VG2 = Vaccinate Group1 and Not-Vaccinated Group2, respectively. CM = Clinical Mastitis; SCM = Subclinical Mastitis; IMI = Intramammary infection; DIM = Days in Milk. Herd A: received two doses of vaccine pre-calving; Herd B: received two doses of vaccine pre-calving and one post-calving. Animals affected by mastitis (SCM or CM) were considered in end- point. $^{a,b}P$ <0.01, $^{c,d}P$ <0.001

N-VG2 (16.7%, 5/30). Regarding the prevalence of MB affected by IMI or with healthy udder, data are reported in detail in Table 2; no statistically significant difference between prevalence of IMI or healthy udder was found in VG1 and N-VG1 at any sampling time.

Details regarding of the effects on SCC and milk yield are reported in Table 3. Briefly, during the protocol A, the overall averages of Log_{10} SSC values observed during the whole lactation were 4.93 ± 4.71 Log_{10} cells/mL in VG1 and 4.95 ± 4.78 Log_{10} cells/mL in N-VG1 (IMI + healthy udder MB); no statistically significant difference was found between the two values as well as between the daily mean values of SCC recorded at all sampling times in VG1 and N-VG1. Regarding the milk yields, the overall mean values observed in the same animals (IMI + healthy udder MB) during the entire investigation were 9.70 ± 2.07 L/day in VG1 and 9.35 ± 1.57 L/day in N-VG1; no statistically significant difference was recorded for this parameter at any sampling time.

Protocol B

The 45.8% (55/120) and 50.8% (61/120) of the samples cultured were positive for *S. aureus* in VG2 and N-VG2, respectively. The prevalence of positive-cultures for *S. aureus* in VG2 was 6.6% (2/30) at 10 DIM and increased up to 46.7% (14/30), 53.6% (15/28) and 88.9% (24/27) at 30, 60 and 90 DIM, respectively; in N-VG2 it was instead of 13.3% (4/30), 70.4% (19/27), 100% (23/23) and 90.0% (18/20) at 10, 30, 60 and 90 DIM, respectively; a statistically significant difference was found between VG2 and N-VG2 at 60 DIM ($P < 0.001$).

Details regarding of the effects of *S. aureus* on udder health are reported in detail in Table 2. No CM due to *S. aureus* were recorded during the entire protocol in both groups (VG2 and N-VG2). SCM were detected at 30, (6.6%, 2/30), 60 (3.6%,1/28) and 90 DIM (11.1%,3/27) in VG2, while in N-VG2, they were detected at each sampling time with a prevalence ranged between 10% and 25%. A statistically significant difference was found at 90 DIM (P <0.01). During the first 90 DIM, a statistically significant difference between the incidence of animals affected by mastitis in was also recorded (VG2: 20.0% - 6/30 and N-VG2: 50.0% - 15/30, P <0.05). According to the mixed logistic model the VG2 animals had less 23% of probability to develop mastitis compared to N-VG2 (P <0.001). Regarding the prevalence of MB affected by IMI and with healthy udder a statistically significant difference between prevalence of MB affected by IMI in VG2 and N-VG2 was found at 60 DIM (P <0.01), while between healthy udder at 60 DIM (P <0.001).

Details regarding of the effects on SCC and milk yield are reported in Table 3. Briefly, during the protocol B, the overall average of Log_{10} SSC values observed during the whole lactation were 4.84 ± 4.60 Log_{10} cells/mL in VG2 and 4.97 ± 4.75 Log_{10} cells/mL in N-VG2 (IMI + healthy udder MB); a statistically significant difference was found between the two values (P <0.05). A statistically significant difference was also recorded between daily mean values of SCC in VG2 and N-VG2 at 10 (P <0.05), 30 (P <0.05), 150 (P <0.05) and 240 DIM (P <0.01). Regarding the milk yields, the overall mean values observed in the same animals during the entire investigation were 10.37 ± 2.18 L/d in VG2 and 10.03 ± 2.28 L/d in N-VG2; no statistically significant difference was recorded at any sampling time between the two groups. The mixed linear model confirmed a significant

Table 3 Daily means somatic cell count values (Log_{10} cells/mL ± SD) and milk yields (Litres ± SD) detected in VGs and N-VGs in both the herds of *primiparous* Mediterranean buffalo during 240 days in milk of study

	DIM					
Item	10	30	60	90	150	240
Herd A -Log_{10} SCC						
VG1	4.84 (±4.51)	4.73 (±4.62)	4.82 (±4.54)	5.10 (±4.75)	5.02 (±4.90)	5.08 (±4.95)
N-VG1	4.88 (±4.65)	4.80 (±4.68)	4.87 (±4.77)	5.05 (±4.92)	4.98 (±4.89)	5.09 (±4.78)
Herd B -Log_{10} SCC						
VG2	4.86 (±4.60)^{a}	4.67 (±4.45)^{a}	4.86 (±4.71)	4.97 (±4.66)	4.84 (±4.51)^{a}	4.85 (±4.67)^{c}
N-VG2	4.99 (±4.74)^{b}	4.94 (±5.01)^{b}	4.87 (±4.69)	4.87 (±4.73)	4.98 (±4.67)^{b}	5.15 (±4.64)^{d}
Herd A –Milk Yields						
VG1	7.85 (±0.85)	13.10 (±2.56)	13.04 (±2.77)	12.19 (±2.59)	8.63 (±2.13)	3.37 (±1.51)
N-VG1	7.31 (±2.36)	12.89 (±2.20)	13.20 (±2.21)	11.63 (±1.48)	8.01 (±0.56)	3.05 (±0.59)
Herd B –Milk Yields						
VG2	8.50 (±2.04)	13.39 (±2.27)	13.66 (±2.15)	13.87 (±2.89)	8.84 (±1.94)	3.98 (±1.77)
N-VG2	7.7 (±2.12)	13.08 (±2.53)	13.10 (±2.83)	12.41 (±2.34)	9.57 (±4.89)	4.34 (±1.57)

VG1 and N-VG1 = Vaccinate Group1 and Not-Vaccinated Group1, respectively; VG2 and N-VG2 = Vaccinate Group1 and Not-Vaccinated Group2, respectively; DIM = days in milk; $^{a,b}P$ <0.05,$^{c,d}P$ <0.01. Herd A: received two doses of vaccine pre-calving; Herd B: received two doses of vaccine pre-calving and one post-calving difference between mean SCC of VG2 and N-VG2 at 150 (−66611.1, $P<0.001$) and 240 (−76444.4, $P<0.01$) DIM. No difference where instead detected regarding milk yields.

Finally, combining the two field trial, the mean difference of SCC between VG2 and N-VG2 was significantly higher than the analogous difference between VG1 and N-VG1 (−19778.06, $P<0.05$). No significant differences were instead observed regarding the milk yields.

Discussion

For the purposes of the analysis outlined in this paper, the efficacy of two different regimens of vaccination, based on the use of a multivalent commercial inactivated bovine vaccine against *S. aureus* mastitis, was compared for the first time in MB during the lactation. Estimation of vaccine effects against contagious infections and mastitis under field conditions is an interesting challenge in species like MB where the knowledges regarding the preventions of mastitis are truly rare.

The high prevalence of mastitis due to *S. aureus* mono-infection reported in these ruminants [1], has been confirmed also in the present investigation. In this context, the influence of the dilution effects of *S. aureus* due to composite milk samples use has been not considered substantial, as described for cows [26]. Instead, the lack of quarter milk samples could represent a restriction of the present study because of lower sensibility of IMI detection and loss of useful information on quarter level (e.g. new infection rate, bacteriological cure rate, duration of the infections).

During the survey, only *primiparous* MB were enrolled because our previous studies showed a high-frequency isolation of *S. aureus* in first lactating animals between 30 and 90 DIM [1, 2, 5] and also to exclude the potential negative influence of a poor management of dry period. The complete lack of previous knowledge concerning preventive vaccination against mastitis in MB, lead the authors in a careful and methodical approach for the evaluation of the outcomes of a vaccine produced in origin for dairy cows; for this reason, two different regimens were carried out according to the manufacturer's instructions verifying the tolerance of the animals to the product, the effects on udder health, the milk quality and yields.

As described by Schukken et al. [13] for cows, also for MB the analysis of the data regarding the efficacy estimates was focused on the animals that received the full vaccination protocols; despite the ambition to vaccinate the animals according to the vaccination schemes planned, some difficulties were detected to achieve the necessary number of vaccine doses planned because of a continuous and precise scheduling required, inaccurate estimation of duration of pregnancy, early loss of pregnancy, abortions or MB calving pretermly. Given that incomplete vaccination due to the reasons described could be a common finding also in many MB herds, it is possible that our estimates of vaccine efficacy could be overestimated compared with the efficacy observed under true field conditions.

The importance of *S. aureus* as a contagious pathogen has been widely recognized both in dairy buffaloes and cows because cause of mastitis and relevant economic losses due to its negative influence on milk quality and yields [2, 6]. A previous study investigating clinical relevance and genotype of *S. aureus* in MB, elucidated that (1) genotype B was the only one detected, (2) it was associated to high within-herd prevalence (up to 55%) and incidence (up to 20.4%, during the whole lactation period), (3) it was responsible of contagious mastitis [2]. As well established also for cows, some strains of *S. aureus* (e.g. genotype B) are related to high contagiousness, causing herd problems with a within-herd prevalence of up to 87% [27]. A high prevalence and incidence of positive MB for *S. aureus* was also detected in both protocols and groups of the current investigation confirming the high-frequency isolation of this pathogen. Moreover, considering the overall cultured milk samples, *S. aureus* was also the most frequently isolated bacterium in both the herds and groups followed by coagulase-negative staphylococci. The result confirms a similar findings recently observed both in MB [2] and cows herds [28] where the percentage of isolation of coagulase-negative staphylococci and *Streptococci* were indeed considerably lower in herds positive for *S. aureus* showing high contagiousness and pathogenicity.

A significant difference in the overall rate of mastitis, comparing unvaccinated and vaccinated MB, was observed only in herd B. The administrations of 3 doses of vaccine, may significantly reduce the incidence of mastitis within the herd; the difference seems to be related to the lower prevalence of SCM detected at any sampling time in the VG2 than N-VG2 and achieving a significant peak at 90 DIM. Therefore, the novel contribution of the current study has been to show encouraging results regarding the efficacy of the inactivate vaccine on MB, in contrast with some previous similar studies on staphylococcal vaccination in dairy cows described relatively low vaccine efficacy or no vaccine efficacy at all [15, 17]. However, it is necessary to underline that another of the restrictions of the present investigation may be represented by the chosen study design: indeed only the direct vaccine effects, without attempt to estimate the overall population estimates, were described; as a consequence, it possible that our outcomes may be overestimated if compared with the truly observed vaccine efficacy under overall population conditions. Furthermore, the presence of CM in herd A (VG and CG) suggests that the protocol based on 2 vaccine administrations had not effect to prevent the appearance of clinical signs; on the contrary, in herd B, no difference has been found in both the groups considered overtime and therefore it has been not possible to evaluate this effect. The finding merits further scientific attention, because of the small number of animals enrolled and the lack of previous studies performed on MB useful to compare the results observed.

Regarding IMI due to *S. aureus,* a high prevalence of MB infected was recorded in both the protocols although lower rate of infection was observed in VGs than N-VGs in almost all the samplings. During the investigation a higher prevalence of infections was always observed between 60 and 90 DIM in both the protocols and groups; these effects may have been caused by mixing *primiparous* with *pluriparous* animals in the herds, as initiated by the farmer between 40 and 50 DIM. It is interesting to highlight how the administration of the third dose seems to decrease significantly the prevalence of IMI between VG2 and N-VG2 at 60 DIM, conversely to the use of two doses. Moreover, the moderate reduction of IMI observed in this sampling time, may have consequently reduced the mastitis prevalence observed in the successive control time; the finding described may be also supported by the significant higher percentages of healthy udder MB recorded in VG2 than N-VG2 at 60 DIM. The results observed seem less encouraging than those recently described for cows where vaccination resulted in moderate reduction in incidence of new infections and more pronounced reduction in duration although in presence of an efficacy for transmission still relatively low [13]. As reported by several studies in cows [27–29], also in our investigation the vaccine effects on IMI may be influenced by farm-specific characteristics, such as strain types and farm management practices, and not be only ascribed to the vaccine's properties. Excellent preventive herd management strategies may contribute to significantly reduce the overall herd exposure to *S. aureus* both in MB and cows [2, 13, 30], resulting in an important contribution to indirect vaccine efficacy.

Regarding the effects of vaccination on milk yield and quality, no significant differences were observed between the overall mean milk yields and daily mean production between the two groups of both protocols, while a significant difference between the two regimens was observed regarding SCC. As reported in Table 3, the protocol A was not able to positively influence SCC values in VG1 compared with N-VG1, differently from the protocol B, in which the additional vaccine's dose may have produced an additional immunization of VG able to reduce *S. aureus* multiplication in the mammary gland as reported also for cows [15]; therefore, the additional administration seems to significantly decrease SCC values in the successive days in milk and take part in the significant difference observed on overall SCC mean values. Moreover, the decrease of *S. aureus*' negative effects seems to be also confirmed by the lower prevalence of mastitis recorded from 30 to 90 DIM in VG2 than N-VG2.

Conclusions

The current study represents the first investigation evaluating direct effects of vaccination against *S. aureus* in dairy Mediterranean Buffalo. Even though this study included only a small number of animals, the use of inactivated vaccine by means of the protocol B (based on label use) shows encouraging results because associated with significant lower prevalence and incidence of mastitis as well as lower SCC values, than the protocol A (based on two doses). Nevertheless, the lack of large-scale effects against IMI highlights that vaccination in MB, as in cow, may be considered only an additional tool in the control of *S. aureus* infections on farms and that its use should be always associated with excellent farm management practices to successfully improve the infections control within the herd. The assessment of its effects on the entire dairy MB herd under field conditions, as well as the in-depth analysis of the infectious dynamics, warrant further scientific attention with the goal to fully understand the potentialities of this inactivated vaccine in dairy buffalo management.

Abbreviations

BMC: Bacteriological milk culture; Cell: Cellules; CM: Clinical mastitis; CMT: California mastitis test; DIM: Days in milk; *E. coli*: *Escherichia coli*; h: Hour; IMI: Intramammary infection; MB: Mediterranean buffaloes; mL: Milliliter; N-VG: Not-vaccinated group; SAAC: Slime-associated antigenic complex; SCC: Somatic cell count; SCM: Subclinical mastitis; *S. aureus*: *Staphylococcus aureus*; VG: Vaccinated group

Acknowledgements

The Authors acknowledge the precious collaboration of farmer during both the clinical trials.

Funding

The study was financially supported by Hipra (Rovato, Italy). The funding company participated in the conceptual aspect and design of the study and reviewing of the final version of the manuscript.

Authors' contributions

JG, AP, MP, GT & PC participated in the conceptual aspect and design of the study. JG, MP, LDA, ADR & PC involved in samples and data collection. JG, AP & CS performed the samples analysis. JG, AP & PC statistical evaluation and data interpretation. All authors provided consultation and coordination. JG, AP & PC wrote the first draft of the manuscript, with all authors involved in reviewing. All authors read and approved the final version of the manuscript.

Competing interests

The authors declare that they have no competing interests. The author affiliated with the private company did not influence in anyway the outcomes of the study. He was only involved in conceptual aspect and design of the study and reviewing of the final version of the manuscript. The company that he represents adheres to the Good Publication Practice guidelines for pharmaceutical companies (GPP3) ensuring that the publication is produced in a responsible and ethical manner.

Consent for publication

Not applicable.

Author details

[1]Department of Veterinary Medicine and Animal Productions, University of Napoli "Federico II", Via Delpino 1, 80137 Naples, Italy. [2]Istituto Zooprofilattico del Mezzogiorno, Via A. Jervolino 19, 81100, Tuoro, Caserta District, Italy. [3]Veterinary practitioner, Caserta District 81100, Italy. [4]Hipra Italia s.r.l., Via Franciacorta 74, 25038 Rovato, Italy.

References

1. Guccione J, Cosandey A, Pesce A, Di Loria A, Pascale M, Piantedosi D, et al. Clinical outcomes and molecular genotyping of *Staphylococcus aureus* isolated from milk samples of dairy primiparous Mediterranean buffaloes (Bubalus bubalis). J Dairy Sci. 2014;97:7606–13.
2. Guccione J, Pesce A, Pascale M, Tommasini N, Garofalo F, Di Loria A, et al. Short communication: Effects of systemic treatment with *penethamate hydriodide* on udder health and milk yields in dry primiparous Mediterranean buffaloes (Bubalus bubalis). J Dairy Sci. 2014;97:2219–25.
3. Moroni P, Rossi CS, Pisoni G, Bronzo V, Castiglioni B, Boettcher PJ. Relationships between Somatic Cell Count and Intramammary Infection in Buffaloes. J Dairy Sci. 2006;89:998–1003.
4. Fagiolo A, Lai O. Mastitis in buffalo. Ital J Anim Sci. 2007;6:200–6.
5. Guccione J, Perreten V, Steiner A, Thomann A, Pesce A, Ciaramella P, et al. Short communication: Role of *Streptococcus pluranimalium* in Mediterranean buffaloes (Bubalus bubalis) with different udder health statuses. J Dairy Sci. 2016;99:2945–9.
6. Sears PM, McCarthy KK. Management and treatment of staphylococcal mastitis. Vet Clin North Am Food Anim Pract. 2003;19:171–85.
7. Barkema HW, Schukken YH, Zadoks RH. Invited review: The role of cow, pathogen, and treatment regimen in the therapeutic success of bovine *Staphylococcus aureus* mastitis. J Dairy Sci. 2006;89:1877–95.
8. Barkema HW, Green MJ, Bradley AJ, Zadoks RN. Invited review: The role of contagious disease in udder health. J Dairy Sci. 2009;92:4717–29.
9. Keefe G. Update on control of *Staphylococcus aureus* and *Streptococcus agalactiae* for management of mastitis. Vet Clin North Am Food Anim Pract. 2012;28:203–16.
10. Pérez MM, Prenafeta A, Valle J, Penadés J, Rota C, Solano C, et al. Protection from Staphylococcus aureus mastitis associated with poly-N-acetyl beta-1,6 glucosamine specific antibody production using biofilm-embedded bacteria. Vaccine. 2009;27:2379–86.
11. Pereira UP, Oliveira DG, Mesquita LR, Costa GM, Pereira LJ. Efficacy of Staphylococcus aureus vaccines for bovine mastitis: A systematic review. Vet Microbiol. 2011;148:117–24.
12. Daum RS, Spellberg B. Progress toward a Staphylococcus aureus vaccine. Clin Infect Dis. 2012;54:560–7.
13. Schukken YH, Bronzo V, Locatelli C, Pollera C, Rota N, Casula A, et al. 2014. Efficacy of vaccination on Staphylococcus aureus and coagulase-negative staphylococci intramammary infection dynamics in 2 dairy herds. J Dairy Sci. 2014;97:5250–64.
14. Bradley AJ, Breen JE, Payne B, White V, Green MJ. An investigation of the efficacy of a polyvalent mastitis vaccine using different vaccination regimens under field conditions in the United Kingdom. J Dairy Sci. 2015;98: 1706–20.
15. Middleton JR, Luby CD, Adams DS. Efficacy of vaccination against staphylococcal mastitis: A review and new data. Vet Microbiol. 2009;134:192–8.
16. Freick M, Frank Y, Steinert K, Hamedy A, Passarge O, Sobiraj A. Mastitis vaccination using a commercial polyvalent vaccine or a herd-specific *Staphylococcus aureus* vaccine. Results of a controlled field trial on a dairy farm. Tierarztl Prax Ausg G Grosstiere Nutztiere. 2016;44:219–29.
17. Landin H, Mörk MJ, Larsson M, Waller KP. Vaccination against *Staphylococcus aureus* mastitis in two Swedish dairy herds. Acta Vet Scand. 2015;57:81.
18. Syring C, Boss R, Reist M, Bodmer M, Hummerjohann J, Gehrig P, et al. Bovine mastitis: The diagnostic properties of a PCR-based assay to monitor the *Staphylococcus aureus* genotype B status of a herd, using bulk tank milk. J Dairy Sci. 2012;95:3674–82.
19. Thrusfield M. Surveys. In: Thrusfield M, editor. Veterinary epidemiology. London: UK: Blackwell science Ltd; 2007. p. 228–42.
20. Ciaramella P, Guccione J. Esame del buffalo di razza mediterranea italiana. In: Ciaramella P, editor. Semeiologia Clinica Veterinaria. Milano, Italy.: Poletto Editore srl; 2014. p. 524–32.
21. European Medicine Agency®, Science medicine health. London 2012. http://www.ema.europa.eu/ema/index.jsp?curl=pages/medicines/veterinary/medicines/000130/vet_med_000187.jsp&mid=WC0b01ac058008d7a8. Accessed 25 Sept 2016.
22. National Mastitis Council. Procedures for Collecting Milk Samples in Microbiological Procedures for the Diagnosis of Bovine Udder Infection and Determination of Milk Quality. Madison, WI: National Mastitis Council Inc; 2004.
23. Tripaldi C, Paolacci G, Mairelli M, Catta M, Orlandini S, Amatiste S, et al. Effects of mastitis on buffalo milk quality. Asian-australas J Anim Sci. 2010; 23:1319–24.
24. Fossomatic™ FC. Somatic cell count. Hilleroed Denmark 2012 http://www.foss.dk/industry-solution/central-milk-testing/brochures-and-data-sheets. Accessed 01 October 2012.
25. National Mastitis Council. Laboratory Handbook on Bovine Mastitis. Rev. ed. National Mastitis Council Inc., Madison, WI. 1999.
26. Lam TJ, Van Vliet JH, Schukken YH, Grommers FJ, Van Velden-Russcher A, Barkema HW, et al. The effect of discontinuation of postmilking teat disinfection in low somatic cell count herds. II. Dynamics of intramammary infections. Vet Q. 1997;19:47–53.
27. Michel A, Syring C, Steiner A, Graber HU. Intramammary infections with the contagious *Staphylococcus aureus* genotype B in Swiss dairy cows are associated with low prevalence of coagulase-negative staphylococci and *Streptococcus* spp. Vet J. 2011;188:313–7.
28. Lam TJGM, van Wuijckhuise LA, Franken P, Morselt ML, Hartman EG, Schukken YH. Use of composite milk samples for diagnosis of Staphylococcus aureus mastitis in dairy cattle. J Am Vet Med Assoc. 1996; 208:1705–8.
29. Barlow JW, Zadoks RN, Schukken YH. Effect of lactation therapy on Staphylococcus aureus transmission dynamics in two commercial dairy herds. BMC Vet Res. 2013;9:28–40.
30. Guccione J, Carcasole C, Alsaaod M, D'Andrea L, Di Loria A, De Rosa A, Ciaramella P, Steiner A. Assessment of foot health and animal welfare: clinical findings in 229 dairy Mediterranean Buffaloes (Bubalus bubalis) affected by foot disorders. BMC Vet Res. 2016;12:(1).

Serological response and protection level evaluation in chickens exposed to grains coated with I2 Newcastle disease virus for effective oral vaccination of village chickens

Reta D. Abdi[1,2*†], Kasahun Amsalu[3†], Olana Merera[4], Yilkal Asfaw[1], Eseyas Gelaye[5], Marta Yami[5] and Teshale Sori[1]

Abstract

Background: Conventional Newcastle disease (ND) vaccination strategies in village chicken production settings is impractical due to shortage of cold-chain, unsuitability of vaccine administration routes and demanding trained personnel and hence affected its adoption. Results from earlier works elsewhere showed that the heat stable vaccines such as NDI_2 are thought to be promising for village chickens. This study investigated the suitability and efficacy of Ethiopian cereal grains as carriers for the orally administrated NDI_2 vaccine in chickens.

Results: Of the 15 treatment groups, drinking water, cracked maize and parboiled barley induced significantly higher HI antibody titer than the other carrier grains and naive control. The higher mean HI titer of chickens in drinking-water, cracked maize and parboiled barley group resulted in 100 % survival rate. In general, there was an inverse relationship between chicken mortality (%) and mean HI titer. Chickens with higher HI antibody titers had better survival rate to the challenge experiment. Booster vaccination at age of day 35 and 105 induced progressively higher HI antibodies titers in all treatment groups.

Conclusions: Vaccine coated parboiled grains could be a good carrier followed by cracked grains while untreated vaccine carrier grains had lower serological responses and protection levels. The current finding gives insights on suitable vaccine delivery system in villages with weak health and transportation infrastructure, unreliable electricity, and minimally trained health workers without catching chickens individually.

Keyword: Cereal grains, Chicken, Vaccination, Newcastle disease, Ethiopia

Background

Ethiopia has several diverse indigenous chicken ecotypes. Their diversity is revealed in genetic diversity [1], morphology [2] and production performance [3]. Ethiopia has greater than 42.9 million chickens, with the majority (95 %) kept in village scavenging systems [4]. Chickens in scavenging production systems in rural settings exist with little human input and are constrained by feed, management and disease problems [3]. Newcastle disease (ND) is a devastating disease of both commercial farms and village chickens [5].

In village chickens, different ND virus strains and velogenic pathotypes have been identified in clinically affected and apparently healthy chickens [6]. Therefore, village chickens may serve as a reservoir to disseminate ND virus to the nearby commercial poultry farms [7]. The control of ND in village chickens, therefore, not only reduces the impact of the disease within the village but may also prevent spread to nearby poultry commercial farms. Historically, annual

* Correspondence: retaduguma@gmail.com; rabdi@utk.edu
†Equal contributors
[1]Clinical Studies Department, College of Veterinary Medicine and Agriculture, Addis Ababa University, P.O. Box 34, Bishoftu, Ethiopia
[2]Department of Animal Science, University of Tennessee, 2506 River Drive, Knoxville, USA
Full list of author information is available at the end of the article

ND outbreaks with high mortality are thought to have deterred the potential of owners to rear village chicken [8]. Effective ND control could, therefore, improve rural farmers' confidence in the profitability of village chickens production, and in turn play a role in the rural poverty reduction strategy [5]. Vaccination is an effective control strategy against ND [9].

However, the adoption of conventional vaccine strategies in a village production setting faces many challenges. Such challenges include the dependency on cold-chain, large dose preparation per vial and vaccine administration methods (i.e. eye drop and aerosol) developed for a commercial setting [10]. For village chickens, heat stable, non-pathogenic ND strains (I2 and V4) have been identified as an innovate alternatives to traditional vaccines [11]. Heat stable vaccines, such as NDI_2, are cheaper to produce, do not rely on a cold-chain and can be easily administered with feed grain or water without catching individual bird, and are thought to be suitable and fit for village chickens [12]. The reports from other countries indicated that NDI_2 vaccine retains potency in the absence of a cold chain, for eight weeks when stored in a cool, dark condition, or at 28 °C in a freeze-dried form [13]. A standard dose of $10^6 EID_{50}$/bird can protect birds of all age categories when administered via eye-drop, drinking water, certain feeds or injection [13]. Water-based oral delivery system of NDI_2 vaccine appeared to be constrained by variability in water mineral composition (hard water + high chlorine) at different locations. Hence, carrier grains are preferred to water. Carrier grains adsorb the virus from an aqueous suspension and release it in a viable form in the digestive tract of chickens [13]. Further treatment of grains particularly parboiling could probably remove some deleterious substances from the grain that hampers viability of the I2 virus, thus preserves NDI_2 [10, 13]. Oral administration of the vaccine, using a common chicken feed as a carrier, is well suited to village chicken production systems.

Feed cultivated in different regions within the same country or different countries have unique characteristic and differ in the capacity to be utilized as vaccine carriers [14]. Therefore, vaccine carriers need to be validated for each local environment. Preliminary work has been undertaken to explore the most suitable carrier grain for the NDI_2 vaccine in Ethiopia. Although this study led to promising protection [15], only two carrier grains (parboiled barley and sorghum) were investigated despite the large variety of cereal and pulse crops in Ethiopia. Therefore, the current experimental study aimed to determine the suitability and efficacy of five different Ethiopian grains as a carrier for the heat stable NDI_2 vaccine for oral immunization of rural chickens.

Methods

Experimental site

The study was conducted in the College of Veterinary Medicine and Agriculture, Addis Ababa University, Bishoftu, Oromia Regional State, Ethiopia. The College is located 45 km southeast of Addis Ababa at an altitude of 1900 m above sea level. The average annual rainfall is 851 mm and the minimum and maximum temperature is 8.9 °C and 26.2 °C, respectively. The average humidity level is 58.6 %.

Preparation of experimental house

An experimental house with an area of 16 m × 5 m was constructed. The ceiling, walls and floor of the house were disinfected using 1 % formalin. Clean, disinfected *teff* straw was spread over the floor for bedding. Equipment including drinker, feeder and buckets were cleaned, disinfected and introduced to the houses. The house was kept close for 40 days before the chickens were introduced.

Experimental management

A total of 400 fertilized Bovans brown chicken eggs were obtained from Genesis Farms PLC and hatched at National Veterinary Institute mini-hatchery room. Eggs were cleaned, fumigated and incubated. Finally, 300 chicks were hatched and collected at the 21st and 22nd day of incubation. Of these, the experimental study utilized 225 chicks.

The 225 experimental chicks were brooded together until 14 days in a pen with infrared bulbs for heating and *teff* straw for bedding. On the 14th day the chicks were randomly split into the 15 treatment groups as described under study design below (Fig. 1). The chickens were fed on purchased starter commercial ration for 2 months, grower ration the next 3–5 months, and layer ration from 5 months onwards. Water was given *ad libitum*. Antibiotic (oxytetracycline), minerals and vitamins mix in a sachet (i.e. Vytlet) was purchased and supplied for 3 days after each bleeding (Fig. 1). Chickens showing signs of disease (suspected infectious coryza and coccidiosis) were given 20 % oxytetracycline and amprolium. Mortality was recorded daily.

Experimental design and sample size

Chicken care and experimental procedures were performed under approval from the Animal Ethical Committee (AEC permit No. 6–2010) of the College of Veterinary Medicine and Agriculture of the Addis Ababa University.

A complete randomised design (CRD) was employed. Each chick was identified using wing tag and randomly assigned to one of the 15 pens. Accordingly, a total of 225 chickens were randomly assigned to 15 pens with 15

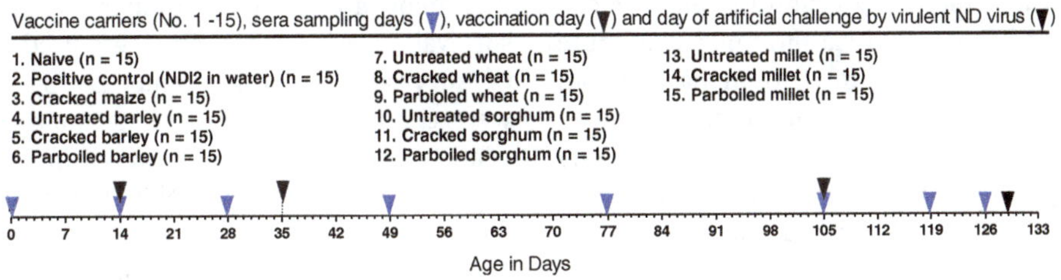

Fig. 1 Study design of the experimental NDI2 vaccine trial in Bovans brown chickens. Vaccine carrier groups (experimental units) were listed from No. 1 -15 in this figure. Sera collection was performed across age in days (indicator, blue color) to get 1ml sera per chick at each sampling day from wing vein until day 119. However, for chickens of barely and cracked maize group the last sampling was made on day 126, not on day 119. Vaccination was given at a rate of 107 EID50 NDV I 2 per dose per chick three times (indicator, black color). The value of vaccination by each grain carrier was measured by monitoring antibody production post vaccination in the regularly collected sera and by survival rate of the chickens post artificial inoculation of a virulent local Alemaya strain ND virus at a rate of 0.5 × 106.5 EID50 per chick of all experimental units intramuscularly at breast muscle at day129 (indicator, red color)

chicks per pen. The study involved 15 different treatment groups: mock vaccinated (naïve), NDI_2 vaccine administered in drinking water (conventional delivery as positive control) and NDI_2 vaccine administered with each of the 13 different carrier grains. The 15 different treatment groups were randomly assigned to the 15 pens as shown on Fig. 1. The sample size per group ($n = 15$ chickens) was calculated by setting type I error at 5 % and type II error at 20 % (80 % power); assumed survival for vaccinated (80 %) and for non-vaccinated chickens (20 %) as described by Chan [16].

Preparation of carrier grains

All carrier grains were purchased, washed, sun dried and stored at room temperature until use. About 2Kg of each grain was cracked to small size to improve the swallowing by the chicks. About 2 kg of each grain was parboiled grains according to Cumming [17]. The grains were added to boiling water at ratio of 1 kg per 3 l and boiled for two minutes, rinsed with cool distilled water, drained and sun dried.

Vaccine and coating of grains with the vaccine

Vials of freeze dried NDI_2 vaccine (300 doses per vial) were purchased from National Veterinary Institute (NVI) located in Bishoftu. Vials were reconstituted in 150 ml of clean, sterile, non-chlorinated distilled water (manufacturer's instruction). About 48.5 ml of clean, non-chlorinated water was added to the grain first to wet it. Subsequently, for each treatment group ($n = 15$ chickens) 7.5 ml of vaccine suspension (0.5 ml per chick) was mixed with 150 g of carrier grain (10 g per chick) to deliver one dose (10^7 EID_{50}) as described by Wambura et al. [18]. The final suspension of vaccine was stored at room temperature for 6 h. Prior to vaccination, feed was withheld for 7 h, after which the chickens were given the grains coated with the vaccine. Commercial feed was not provided until the chickens consumed the coated grains completely.

NDI_2 vaccination interval and sera collection

Vaccination of the chickens was administered on day 14, 35, and 105 as shown on Fig. 1. Sera were collected for haemagglutination inhibition (HI) assay. At every bleeding, sera were collected on day 0, 14, 28, 49, 77, 105 and on day 119 or 126 from the 225 chicken's wing vein aseptically. Bleeding of maize and barley treatment group transferred to day 126 from 119 due to shortage of syringes and Eppendorf tube for sera storage.

Haemagglutination inhibition (HI) assay

HI assay was conducted within serology laboratory of NVI. Serum prepared from sequential blood collections (Fig. 1) was heat inactivated at 56 °C for 30 min and stored at −20 °C. The level of ND virus antibodies in serum samples were determined using the HI test as described by OIE [5]. The HI test has 98 % specificity and 69–98 % sensitivity [19]. HI titration was made to determine the right HI concentration via 2-fold serial dilution of 25 μl sera in 25 μl PBS followed by 25 μl loading of viral antigen per well. Then, after 30 min 25 μl of 1 % RBC per well was loaded and kept for 45 min to determine the end point of haemagglutination. The antibody level for each serum sample was expressed as a log to the base two and recorded. For convenience, the titer was recorded as just the log index. For example, the titer of $\log_2^2$ was recorded as two. The geometric mean titers (GM) were calculated. In this study we used the published cut off value for the protective HI antibody titer (HI titer $\geq \log_2^3$ i.e. GM ≥ 3) for ND vaccination in chickens [5, 13, 20].

Experimental challenge by virulent ND virus

All the vaccinated and non-vaccinated chickens were challenged by lethal dose ($0.5 \times 10^{6.5}$ ELD_{50} based on viral titration). Local virulent ND Alamya strain was obtained from NVI and inoculated via intramuscular route into the breast muscle. The Alamya strain has a mean embryonic death time of 51.1 h, an intracerebral pathogenicity index of 1.84 and an intravenous pathogenicity index of 2.51 [15]. The challenge time was at the age of 129 which was 3 weeks after the 3rd vaccination.

Post challenge, the chickens were examined daily for 4 weeks until the age of 160 day for clinical signs and death due to ND.

Statistical analysis

The mean value and standard deviation (SD) of HI antibody titers were determined and classified according to treatment groups. The post vaccination mean HI antibody titers were compared by General Linear model of SPSS version 15. Where the HI results were significant, least square difference (LSD) was used to compare antibody response via pair-wise treatment comparisons. Proportion of chickens with HI antibody titer $\geq \log_2^3$ between treatment groups was used as a cut-off value to compare and decide the protective level [5, 13, 20]. Serology (HI) was to predict level of protection. However, real level of protection was evaluated using challenge experiment. Subsequently, the time to death among treatment groups was compared using Kaplan-Meier survival curve with log rank test used to assess equality of survival distribution among the groups. Chickens were censored in Kaplan-Meier survival analysis whose death was not related to events of interest (i.e. death due to any other causes than ND challenge). Significant differences set at 5 % alpha and at 95 % confidence interval. The relationship between chicken mortality (%) and % of chicken with HI titer above cut-off value were compared to the mean HI titer and statistically tested by Pearson correlation.

Results

Serological analysis

The base line antibody titer

The eggs were collected from the same ND vaccinated parents of Bovans brown. The mean maternal antibody (geometric mean ± SD) titer of the 225 study chickens at day old age was 3.3 ± 0.5 and reduced over time during 14 days to 1.5 ± 0.6 at time of vaccination (Fig. 2).

Serological response to vaccination

There was a significant variation in the HI response between the different treatment groups (Table 1, Table 2 and Fig. 2). Drinking water, cracked maize and parboiled

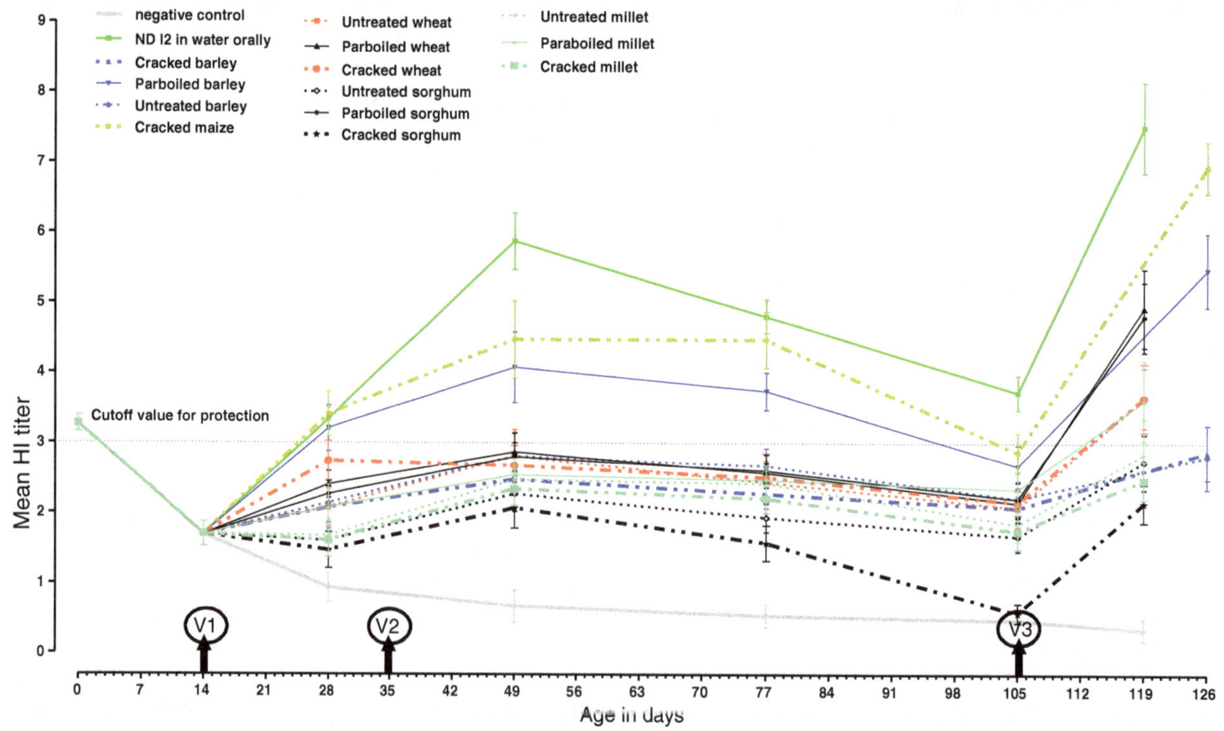

Fig. 2 Geometric mean $(\log 2^2)$ ± SE of HI antibody titer of chicken vaccinated by coating on 13 different types of grains in comparison to vaccination via water (positive control) and negative control. Red arrows labeled with V1, V2 and V3 on top indicated the day of vaccination. Maternal antibody at day old was high but reduced at day 14. One time vaccination using different carrier grains induced HI titer differently. Second and third round vaccination (booster) upgraded the induction of HI titer significantly ($p < 0.05$) but at varying level depending on the types of grain used as vaccine carrier

Table 1 Post vaccination geometric mean (mean ± SD) antibody titers of chickens increased over time by booster vaccination with disparity in titer between vaccine carrier types used

Vaccine carrier type	Post vaccination GM ± SD HI antibody titer (log2) chickens vaccinated by different methods at different ages in days (*N* = 15)					
	Day 28	Day 49	Day 77	Day 105	Day 119	Day 126
Naive	<1^{f}	<1^{ab}	<1^{g}	<1^{d}	<1^{c}	no
NDI2 in water	3.2 ± 0.6 (15)^{a}	5.7 ± 1.6 (15)c	4.7 ± 0.9 (15)^{ac}	3.6 ± 0.9 (14)^{ab}	7.1 ± 2.4 (14)a	no
Untreated Wheat	1.6 ± 1.0 (15)^{b}	2.4 ± 1.5 (15)^{d}	1.8 ± 1.3 (15)^{bd}	1.7 ± 0.9 (14)^{e}	3.3 ± 1.2 (14)^{f}	no
Parboiled Wheat	2.3 ± 0.7 (15)^{b}	2.6 ± 1.1 (15)^{d}	2.1 ± 0.8 (15)^{bd}	1.9 ± 0.8 (14)^{e}	4.5 ± 2.1 (14)^{f}	no
Cracked Wheat	2.3 ± 1.0 (15)b	2.4 ± 1.1 (15)^{d}	2.1 ± 1.4 (15)^{bd}	2.0 ± 0.7 (14)^{e}	3.3 ± 1.8 (14)^{f}	no
Untreated Sorghum	1.4 ± 0.6 (15)^{f}	2.2 ± 0.8 (15)^{d}	1.8 ± 0.8 (15)^{bd}	1.4 ± 0.8 (15)^{e}	2.4 ± 1.5 (15)^{ed}	no
Parboiled Sorghum	2.1 ± 0.7 (15)^{b}	2.7 ± 0.8 (15)^{d}	2.4 ± 0.9 (15)^{bd}	1.5 ± 0.9 (15)^{e}	4.4 ± 1.9 (15)^{f}	no
Cracked Sorghum	1.2 ± 1.0 (15)^{f}	1.6 ± 1.1 (14)^{d}	1.1 ± 0.9 (14)^{bd}	0.4 ± 0.5 (14)^{gb}	1.9 + 1.0 (14)^{ed}	no
Untreated Millet	1.3 ± 0.8 (15)^{b}	2.4 ± 0.5 (13)^{d}	2.3 ± 0.7 (13)^{bd}	1.7 ± 0.8 (12)^{e}	2.4 ± 1.8 (12)^{ed}	no
Parboiled Millet	1.4 ± 1.3 (15)^{b}	2.4 ± 0.9 (15)^{d}	2.3 ± 0.8 (15)^{bd}	2.1 ± 0.9 (15)^{e}	3.2 ± 2.0 (15)^{f}	no
Cracked millet	1.3 ± 0.5 (15)^{f}	1.5 ± 0.6 (15)^{d}	1.3 ± 1.0 (15)^{bd}	2.1 ± 0.9 (15)^{e}	2.5 ± 0.8 (14)^{ed}	no
Cracked Barely	1.6 ± 1.2 (15)b	2.4 ± 0.6 (15)^{d}	1.7 ± 0.9 (15)^{bd}	1.5 ± 0.9 (15)^{e}	no	2.5 ± 1.4 (15)^{ed}
Parboiled barely	3.0 ± 1.3 (15)^{a}	3.7 ± 1.9 (15)^{ab}	3.6 ± 1.0 (15)^{e}	2.4 ± 1.2 (15)^{fc}	no	5.1 ± 2.0 (15)g
Untreated Barely	1.7 ± 1.0 (15)b	2.5 ± 1.3 (15)^{d}	2.4 ± 1.0 (15)^{bd}	2.0 ± 1.0 (15)^{d}	no	2.8 ± 1.8 (15)^{ed}
Cracked Maize	3.2 ± 1.2 (15)^{a}	4.2. ± 2.1 (15)^{ab}	3.9 ± 1.6 (15)^{ac}	2.7 ± 1.1 (15)^{fc}	no	6.8 ± 1.4 (15)g

Means with the same letters in the same column are not significantly different at 0.05 confidence level, "no" = sera not collected

barley coated with NDI_2 vaccine induced significantly ($p < 0.05$) higher antibody titers than the other treatment groups. Parboiled sorghum, parboiled wheat, parboiled millet, untreated wheat and cracked wheat coated with the same vaccine induced moderate antibody titers.

After one booster vaccination (i.e. day 14 and 35), the chickens in most of the treatment groups had a mean HI titer between ($\log_2^2$) and ($\log_2^3$) until day 105. The administration of the 2nd booster at day 105, further increased HI titer significantly. Therefore, not only the 1st

Table 2 GLM least square difference for pair-wise comparison of HI titers among 15 different vaccine carrier grain types at day 28 (below diagonal), day 126 for barely and maize and day 119 for the rest grains (above diagonal) for significance test at 95 % CI

Grain	1	2	3	4	5	6	7	8	9	10	11	12	13	14	15
1	-	0.000	0.000	0.000	0.000	0.000	0.000	0.000	0.000	0.000	0.000	0.000	0.000	0.000	0.000
2	0.000	-	0.000	0.000	0.000	0.000	0.000	0.000	0.000	0.000	0.000	0.000	0.358	0.001	0.000
3	0.003	0.000	-	0.04	1	0.14	0.06	0.017	0.215	0.945	0.056	0.208	0.000	0.003	0.172
4	0.000	0.012	0.247	-	0.04	0.000	0.835	0.000	0.001	0.031	0.000	0.001	0.001	0.383	0.001
5	0.000	0.082	0.054	0.44	-	0.14	0.06	0.017	0.215	0.945	0.056	0.208	0.000	0.003	0.172
6	0.062	0.000	0.271	0.023	0.002	-	0.001	0.338	0.876	0.152	0.66	0.826	0.000	0.000	0.912
7	0.000	0.003	0.463	0.656	0.218	0.062	-	0.000	0.002	0.048	0.000	0.001	0.000	0.271	0.001
8	0.119	0.000	0.177	0.012	0.001	0.783	0.035	-	0.29	0.018	0.599	0.24	0.000	0.000	0.286
9	0.031	0.000	0.516	0.078	0.012	0.692	0.173	0.516	-	0.233	0.568	0.959	0.000	0.000	0.959
10	0.002	0.000	0.855	0.32	0.075	0.192	0.576	0.119	0.404	-	0.061	0.226	0.000	0.002	0.187
11	0.062	0.000	0.271	0.023	0.002	1	0.062	0.783	0.692	0.192	-	0.509	0.000	0.000	0.582
12	0.002	0.000	0.855	0.32	0.075	0.192	0.576	0.119	0.404	1	0.192	-	0.000	0.000	0.912
13	0.000	0.906	0.000	0.008	0.059	0.000	0.002	0.000	0.000	0.000	0.000	0.000	-	0.015	0.000
14	0.000	0.666	0.001	0.034	0.182	0.000	0.009	0.000	0.000	0.002	0.000	0.002	0.576	-	0.000
15	0.001	0.001	0.714	0.417	0.11	0.136	0.709	0.082	0.312	0.852	0.136	0.852	0.000	0.003	-

Keys: 1 = Naïve; 2 = ND I2 in water; 3 = Untreated wheat; 4 = Parboiled wheat; 5 = Cracked wheat; 6 = untreated sorghum; 7 = Parboiled sorghum; 8 = Cracked sorghum; 9 = Untreated millet; 10 = Parboiled millet; 11 = Cracked millet; 12 = Cracked barley; 13 = Cracked maize; 14 = Parboiled barley; 15 = Untreated barley
The pair-wise GLM least square difference significant level was conducted but not included for day 49, 77 and 105 of the HI assay in this document

booster (day 35) but also the 2nd booster (day 105) vaccination increased the induction of HI antibody progressively as shown in Table 1 and Fig. 2.

Three of the 15 treatment groups had the HI titer above $\log_2^3$ throughout the study until day 105. The assay on day 119 indicated that eight of the treatment groups had HI titer above $\log_2^3$. This implies that the 2nd booster vaccination (day 105) induced higher HI antibody in chickens of five more treatment groups (HI > $\log_2^3$). NDI_2 in water, cracked maize and parboiled barley had significantly ($p < 0.05$) higher HI titer than the others groups but no significant difference was observed among three of them ($p > 0.05$). ND I2 vaccine coated parboiled wheat and parboiled sorghum had comparable antibody titer of $\log_2^{4.5}$ and $\log_2^{4.1}$, respectively. Throughout the study period ND I2 coated cracked sorghum induced lower HI antibody response (Table 1, Table 2 and Fig. 2).

Percentage of chickens with HI titer above $\log_2^3$ (cut-off value for protection)

The percentage of chickens with a protective level (HI titers ≥ $\log_2^3$) of antibodies varied with the type of vaccine carrier grain used and frequency of vaccinations (Table 3).

Following the 1st vaccination, HI titer of ≥ $\log_2^3$ was detected in 80 % of chickens vaccinated via conventional (water) and cracked maize. It was 66.7 % in the parboiled barley treatment group and 50 % in the parboiled wheat, cracked wheat, untreated wheat and parboiled millet treatment groups. The percentage of chickens' with HI titer ≥ $\log_2^3$ was less in the cracked sorghum and untreated sorghum coated treatment groups (Table 3). After the first booster vaccination, there was an increase in the proportion of chickens with HI titer above (> $\log_2^3$) in comparison to the first vaccination. The highest percentage was observed in chicken vaccinated via conventional method (100 %), followed by cracked maize (86.7 %), parboiled barley (75 %) and parboiled wheat (73 %) in that order, as shown in Table 3. The cracked sorghum and untreated sorghum coated with vaccine had lowest titer but they scored better than their titer induced during the first vaccination. After the 2nd booster vaccination, all (100 %) of the vaccinated chickens via conventional (water) and cracked maize had HI titer ≥ $\log_2^3$. In the naive control chicken, none (0 %) of the chickens had HI titer ≥ $\log_2^3$ throughout the study period as shown in Table 3.

Monitoring the survival rate of chickens following artificial challenge

The mean HI titer and mortality (%) were inversely correlated as shown on Fig. 3 ($r = -0.938$, $p < 0.000$). The mean HI titer above $\log_2^5$ corresponds to a 100 % survival rate as shown in chickens vaccinated by conventional (water), cracked maize and parboiled wheat coated vaccine. The HI titer between $\log_2^{(3-5)}$ corresponded to survival rates between 70–80 %. The HI titer between $\log_2^2 - \log_2^3$ corresponded to survival rates of 35–60 % as shown in chickens vaccinated by cracked sorghum, untreated millet, untreated sorghum, cracked millet and cracked barley coated vaccine (Table 4, Fig. 3, left y-axis).

Table 3 The percentage of chickens with HI titers above the protective titer (≥ $\log_2 2^3$) related to the types of vaccine carrier used

	Number of chickens (%) with HI log2) ≥ 3.0 of all chicks ($N = 15$)					
Vaccine carrier type	Day 28	Day 49	Day 77[¥]	Day 105	Day 119	Day 126
Naive	0(0.0)	0(0.0)	0(0.0)	0(0.0)	0(0.0)	no
NDI2 in water	12(80)	15(100)	15(100)	10(66.7)	15(100)	no
Untreated Wheat	7(46.7)	8(53.3)	6 (40)	5(33.3)	10 (71.4)	no
Parboiled Wheat	8(53.3)	11(73)	7(46.7)	5(35.5)	11(78.5)	no
Cracked Wheat	7(46.7)	9(60)	5(33.3)	4(28.5)	9 (60)	no
Untreated Sorghum	1(6.6)	6(40)	4(26.7)	2(13.3)	7(46.7)	no
Parboiled Sorghum	6(40)	8(53.3)	6(40)	5(33.5)	9(60)	no
Cracked Sorghum	2(13.3)	5(33.3)	2(13.3)	0(0.0)	3(20)	no
Untreated Millet	4(26.7)	6(50)	5(41.7)	3(25)	7(58.3)	no
Parboiled Millet	8(53.3)	10(66.7)	7(46.7)	5(30)	11(73.3)	no
Cracked millet	4(26.7)	7(46.7)	5(33.3)	3(30)	8(53.3)	no
Cracked Barely	7(46.7)	9(60)	6(40)	4(26.7)	no[a]	0(53.3)
Parboiled barely	10(66.7)	12 (75)	8(53.3)	9(60)	no	13(86.7)
Untreated Barely	6(40)	9(60)	5(33.3)	6 (40)	no	8 (53.3)
Cracked Maize	11(73)	13(86.7)	10(66.7)	9(60)	no	15(100)

[a]no = represented sera not collected. Figures outside the brackets indicated number of chickens in each group having HI titer above cut off value whereas figures in brackets indicated percentages

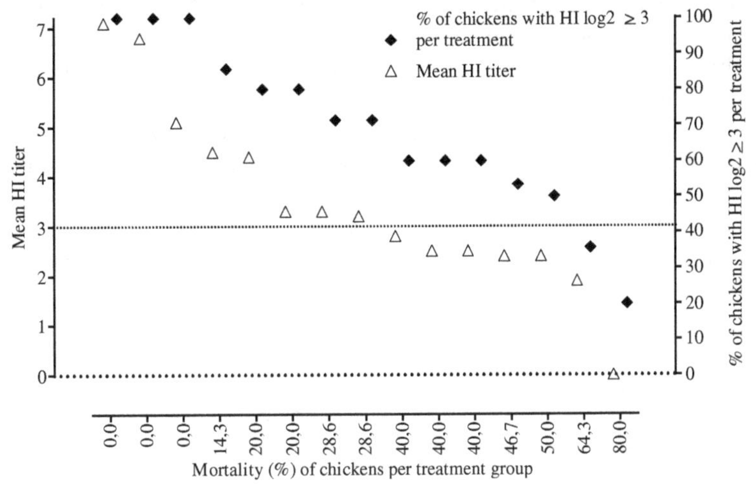

Fig. 3 The inverse relationship between chicken mortality rate (%) vs. mean HI titre (left y-axis) and % of chicken with HI titre above cut-off value (right y-axis). Each bullet points represented each treatment group of the 15 treatments. Each bullet points represents each treatment group of the 15 treatments

Figure 3 (right y-axis) indicated that when more than 80 % of the chickens in a treatment group had HI titer above cut-off value, the mortality (%) in that treatment group was nearly 0 %. In parboiled wheat, the mortality (%) was nearly 15 % while 78.5 % of the chickens in this treatment group had HI titre above cut-off value for protection. In this study, more than 50 % of the chickens in majority of the treatment groups had HI titre above cut-off value for protection that that subsequently resulted in mortality below 50 %. However, in cracked sorghum group mortality was higher (i.e. 64.3 %) as only 20 % of the chickens had HI titer above the cut-off value.

Survival analysis

The overall differences in mortality (%) were statistically significant (Log-rank = 77.35, D.F. = 14, $p < 0.0000$)

Table 4 Dependency of morbidity, mortality and survival rate of chickens on types of vaccine carrier used to resist virulent strain ND virus challenge after three times vaccination

Vaccine carrier type	Chicks N†	Mean HI titer	# morbidity (%)	# death total	#mortality[a] (%)	Lower 95 % CI	Upper 95 % CI	# Survival (%)
NDI2 in water	15	7.1	0(0.0)	0	0(0.0)	0	0	15(100)
Cracked maize	15	6.8	0 (0)	0	0(0.0)	0	0	15(100)
Parboiled barley	15	5.1	0(0.0)	0	0(0.0)	0	0	15(100)
Parboiled wheat	14	4.5	5(30.0)	2	2(14.3)	0	32.6	12(85.7)
Untreated wheat	15	3.3	6 (40.0)	3	3(20.0)	0	40.2	12(80.0)
Parboiled sorghum	15	4.4	6(26.7)	3	3(20.0)	0	40.2	12 (80.0)
Cracked wheat	14	3.3	8(53.3)	4	4(28.6)	4.9	52.2	10(71.4)
Parboiled millet	14	3.2	7(46.7)	4	4(28.6)	4.9	52.2	10(71.4)
Cracked millet	15	2.5	10(66.7)	6	6(40.0)	15.2	64.8	9(60.0)
Untreated barley	15	2.8	8(53.3)	6	6(40.0)	15.2	64.8	9(60.0)
Cracked barley	15	2.5	7(46.7)	6	6(40.0)	15.2	64.8	9(60.0)
Untreated sorghum	15	2.4	10(66.7)	7	7(46.7)	21.4	71.9	8(53.3)
Untreated millet	12	2.4	8(53.3)	6	6 (50)	21.7	78.3	6 (50.0)
Cracked sorghum	14	1.9	11(73.3)	9	9(64.3)	39.2	89.4	5(35.7)
Naïve	15	0.0	14 (93.3)	12	12(80.0)	59.8	100	3 (20.0)

N[†] represented number of chickens present in each group at age of 129 day (onset of the challenge). Figures outside the brackets indicated number of chickens in each group whereas figures in brackets indicated percentages. [a] Chickens in the treatment groups listed up to parboiled millet had significantly ($p < 0.0001$) higher survival rate compared to the naïve group. The lower and upper 95 % confidence interval (CI) of mortality of chickens per each treatment group was shown in the table among the treatment groups (Fig. 4). A small number of chickens from untreated ($n = 3$) and parboiled millet ($n = 1$), cracked sorghum ($n = 1$), parboiled ($n = 1$) and cracked wheat ($n = 1$) died due to other disease than ND at different days during the study. Infectious cryza and coccidiosis were suspected and treated long ago (about 2 months) before the inoculation of the velogenic ND viral challenge. The dead chickens were censored in Kaplan-Meier survival analysis as their death was happened before the inoculation of the virulent ND virus challenge. Post-challenge with ND virus, mortality occurred only during the first 14 days; no mortality was observed during days 15 to 30 of the follow up period (Table 4; Fig. 4). The death of chickens due to the challenge started at fourth days post challenge and persisted up to 13th days with the median survival time of 7 days among the dead chickens by the challenge.

Discussion

The control of ND in village chickens can make a vital contribution to the improvement of household food security and poverty reduction in Ethiopia. Intensive commercial poultry farmers in Ethiopia vaccinate chickens routinely, but village chicken farmers do not [3]. In the current study, five cereal grain species, in 3 different forms, were evaluated for suitability and efficacy as a carrier for the NDI_2 vaccine as a way forward for developing suitable vaccine delivery system for village chicken production system. The carrier grains have been shown to adsorb the virus from an aqueous suspension and release it in a viable form in the digestive tract of chickens [13]. However, the virus adsorption and releasing capacity of cereal grains varies among grain species and forms of preparation [13]. Grain based vaccine efficacy could be assessed via (i) monitoring sero-conversion, (ii) post vaccination challenge and (iii) survival rate as recommended by Spradbrow [13, 21, 22]. In this study, five different cereal grains were evaluated for their suitability and efficacy as vaccine carrier using the above mentioned three assessment methods.

Maternal HI antibody titer

At day old, chicks included in this study have HI antibody titer above $\log_2^3$. Such high maternal antibody titer in the baby chicks is deleterious to vaccination [5]. Thus, we waited until it declined to $\log_2^{1.5}$ titer at 14 days to overcome the risk of its interference with the vaccine. In line with this, it has been well established that chicks from immunized parents possess high level of maternal antibody which protects the chicks against virulent virus and interferes with vaccine antigens [23, 24].

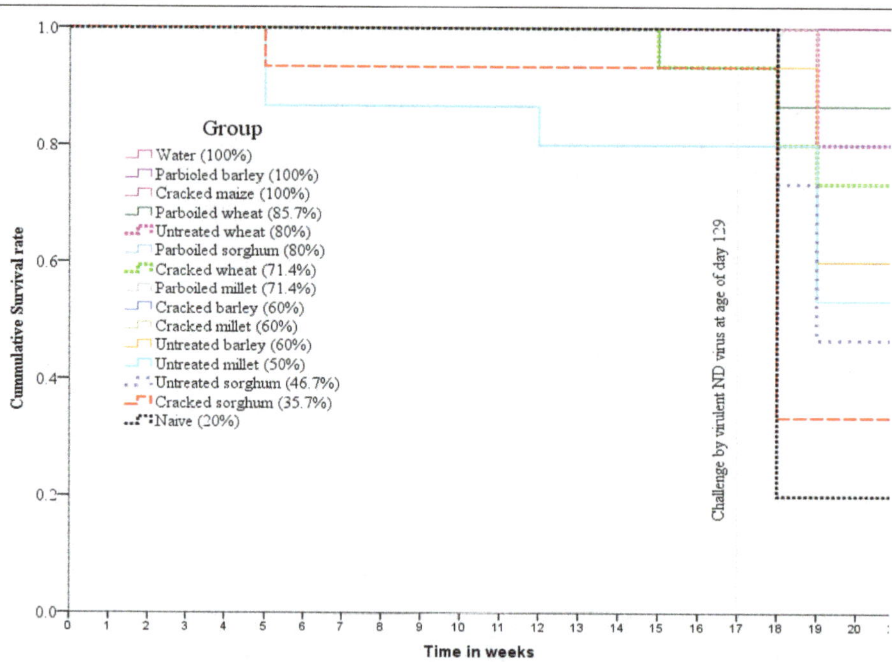

Fig. 4 Kaplan-Meier survival analysis of chickens vaccinated by NDI2 via different grain carriers as assessed before and after ND virus challenge by virulent strain at age of day 129. Morbidity was started on day 3 and severe mortality prevailed up to 14 days post challenge during 30 days of follow up. Vaccination using any type of vaccine carrier grain had an impact better than the naïve for survival rate of the chickens. However, different vaccine carrier grains had different survival rates in the range of 35.7 - 100% whilst 20% in naïve. The survival rate was significantly different among the treatment groups (Log-rank = 77.3498, D.F. = 14, $p < 0.0000$). For example, oral vaccination using water, parboiled barley and cracked maize induced 100% survival until end of the experimental period i.e. week 21

Monitoring serological response using HI antibody titer

An HI titer of $\geq \log_2^3$ following vaccination has been considered protective against virulent ND virus. HI titers lower than $\log_2^3$ have been associated with lower levels of protection [13, 20]. The results of the current study showed that administration of 2nd and 3rd booster vaccination significantly and progressively increased HI antibody titer in all treatment groups except the naïve control. Furthermore, different grains induced different level of HI antibody titer. This implies the presence of inherent variation in virus carrying capacity of different grains. This is an opportunity to screen grains of different species and varieties. Interestingly, treating grains (either cracking or parboiling) increased their efficacy as vaccine carrier, evident by induction of higher HI antibody titer than that was induced by untreated form. Similar results have been reported in Nigeria by Olabode [25] as to the efficacy of treated grain particularly maize compared to untreated grain. Grains have been known to contain tannins, anthraquinone, cardiac glycosides and alkaloids. Some of these chemicals have been shown to have antiviral properties [22, 26]. The higher HI titer induced by treated grains than untreated ones could be due to the fact that cracking grains increase the surface area of the grains to adsorb the vaccine virus [10, 13, 14, 18, 22, 25, 26]. Likewise, parboiling might destroy the antiviral factors from the seed of the grains [22, 26]. Hence, both cracking and parboiling grains would induce better HI antibody titer via adsorbing and releasing live virus in the gut. However, inconsistent results were observed for sorghum in which cracked, untreated and parboiled sorghum induced HI titer of $\geq \log_2^3$ in 20 %, 46.7 % and 60 % of chickens, respectively, after the 3rd booster vaccination.

This implies that repeated vaccination induces progressively higher HI titer that could correspond to high levels of protection. Moreover, different grain species as well as their preparations in different forms have induced different level of HI antibody titers. Treatment of grains (parboiling or cracking) renders the grains suitable for vaccine carrier for oral vaccination as evident from their corresponding improved antibody response. Higher HI antibody titer corresponded to higher protection level for most grain carriers in the order of parboiled, cracked and untreated grains. This, however, is not the case for sorghum particularly untreated form was found to be better than cracked form in HI titer and post challenge survival. Exceptionally, the parboiled and untreated sorghum induced higher HI titer than the cracked sorghum. Cracking in sorghum might have released anti-viral factors (tannins) and enzymes that probably inactivated the virus. To this end anthraquinone, alkaloids and cardiac glycosides were reported to be abundant in sorghum [26].

Despite low HI antibody titer induced by some grains (sorghum), unexpectedly higher survival % was observed following the challenge. This perhaps highlights the weak correlation between low HI titer and protection for sorghum and the difficulties of using serum antibodies to determine protection to respiratory pathogens [27, 28]. In addition to serum antibody, secretory antibody (IgA) at mucosal surfaces and cell mediated immunity are thought to play a role in resistance to challenge [29]. In general, however, this study showed a negative correlation between mean HI titer and mortality % at the group level (Fig. 3).

Other than the treatment (grain type for vaccine delivery) that of the pen effect has been handled by grouping of the chickens by randomization. However, pens are not replicated due to shortage of space in the experimental house and finance to account for the pen effect on immune response. We believe that the variance among pens is generally less than the variance of chickens within pens due to treatment effect.

Protection assessment following artificial viral challenge

In the current study, intramuscular route of the breast muscle was used to challenge the chickens. Intramuscular route was preferred as it allows birds to receive equal doses of the challenge virus. Water, cracked maize and parboiled barley were found to be carriers of NDI_2 vaccine than the others. They protected 100 % (15/15) of the chickens against virulent challenge with ND strain compared to 20 % protection in the naïve group (3/15). In agreement with this results of full protection (100 %) using the NDI_2 vaccination via drinking water and parboiled barley was previously reported in Ethiopia [15]. Another similar heat stable vaccine ($NDV_{4)}$ coated cracked maize has also been reported to induce high levels of protection in Nigeria [25] which is similar to our NDI_2 results. The 80 % protection achieved using parboiled sorghum currently is, however, in disagreement with previous results report in Ethiopia [15], Nigeria [30] and Tanzania [31].

It is widely accepted that the recommended protection level of ND vaccination is 80 % [32]. However, we have achieved 100 % protection using NDI_2 in water, cracked maize and parboiled barley at on-station condition.

The survival rate for the chickens vaccinated with untreated and cracked millet is 60 %, but 73.3 % for the parboiled millet. Our current finding is comparable to the 70 % survival rate reported elsewhere among chicken vaccinated with NDI_2 using parboiledand broken millet [33].

The chicken survival rate is 71.4 % for cracked wheat, 80 % for untreated wheat and 85.7 % for parboiled wheat group. The untreated barley as carrier for NDI_2 in the current study had 60 % survival rate. This is far lower than the previous work in Ethiopia [15] and what was reported elsewhere with 100 % protection [34]. This variation in serological response between and within grain forms could be explained by (i) differences in the contents of anti-viral factors in the grains, (ii) variability in vaccine carrying capacity among different grains, (iii) difference in agro-ecology and soil characteristics that can have different effect on physico- chemical characteristics of the grains. Oakeley [22] suggested that grains grown in different agro-ecology and on different soil characteristics tend to vary in their vaccine virus carrying capacity due to variation in the grains' physico-chemical characteristics, especially their surface properties and chlorine content [22].

In general, parboiled grains, followed by cracked ones, induced higher serological response and protection level than intact (untreated) grains. Heating, soaking, washing and cracking grains might be useful in developing a successful vaccine carrier feed. Similar findings have been reported from other countries [17, 35]. Cracked maize and parboiled barley are found to be better vaccine carriers under Ethiopian context. Our promising finding on wheat was consistent with Spradbrow [13]. Thus, cracked maize, parboiled barley or parboiled wheat should be the base for a large scale grain screening and oral based ND vaccination program. They can be used widely as carrier for oral NDI_2 vaccination. However, it should be noted that the protection level of the grain based NDI_2 vaccine varies under laboratory conditions i.e. > 90 % protection [36] and under real village conditions i.e. < 60 % [37] and with vaccine delivered by farmers [36]. This signals the necessity of pilot field trial at village level to evaluate the results of the current on-station study at real village conditions.

Durability of the virus in the grains and at room temperature

In the current study, the vaccine virus coated on grains was highly immunogenic after 6 h of exposure to room temperature; hence it could be used to vaccinate village chicken against ND. We haven't measured the upper limit of the time when it is still efficacious in order to enable central vaccine production and then distribution to rural villages. A very important condition for successful development and use of any chosen feed as vaccine carrier is the ability to allow firm binding or adherence of the coated vaccine virus without interfering with the survival of the vaccine virus. In this regard different results have been reported from different countries. According to Tu et al. [12], the NDI_2 in grains has substantial infectivity and induction of immunity in chickens under laboratory conditionsafter storage for 17 days and in village conditions after storage for 21 days. Echeonwu et al. [30] reported that the virus coated feed without additive remained stable and immunogenic for 3 weeks (millet); 3.5 weeks (sorghum) and 5 weeks for maize at room temperature. Nassir et al. [15] recovered viable vaccine virus after 14 h at room temperature on parboiled barley.

Conclusion

Chickens fed on NDI_2 vaccine coated grains induced higher HI antibody than the naïve control and in most cases protected chickens from virulent ND virus challenge. Significant variation was detected between the types and forms of grains and the use of booster vaccinations. Cracked maize, parboiled barley, untreated and parboiled wheat in addition to parboiled sorghum would be promising suitable carriers for large scale administration of NDI_2 vaccine under Ethiopian field (village) conditions. Procedures of an on-going vaccine efficacy evaluation would be needed using grain carriers under field conditions. In addition, region based large scale grain screening using cracked maize, parboiled barley and parboiled wheat as a reference for oral based ND vaccination program is suggested.

Abbreviations

EID, embryo infective dose; ELD, embro lethal dose; GM, geometric mean titers; HI, heamagglutination inhibition; LSD, least square difference; ND, newcastle disease; NVI, national veterinary institute; OIE, world organization for animal health; PBS, phosphate buffered saline; RBC, red blood cell

Acknowledgements

This study was financed by the World Bank and CIDA as channeled via Ethiopian Institute of Agricultural Research under National Agricultural Research Fund Project. Ethiopian Ministry of Science and Technology also co-funded. Addis Ababa University College of Veterinary Medicine and Agriculture hosted the implementation of the study activities within its premises. The virulent Alemaya (local) strain of ND virus for the challenge experiment was granted by National Veterinary Institute. Professor Rob Christley and Dr Stacey Lynch of Liverpool University commented this manuscript.

Authors' contributions

RD won the research grant. RD and MY conceived and designed the experiments during execution. RD, KA, YA, EG and TS performed the experiments. RD, KA, OM, MY and TS Analyzed the data. RD, YA, EG, MY and TS contributed reagents/materials/analysis tools. RD, KA, OM and MY wrote the paper. RD and OM improved and corrected the manuscript. All authors read and approved the final manuscript.

Competing interest

The authors declare that they have no competing interests.

Author details

[1]Clinical Studies Department, College of Veterinary Medicine and Agriculture, Addis Ababa University, P.O. Box 34, Bishoftu, Ethiopia. [2]Department of Animal Science, University of Tennessee, 2506 River Drive, Knoxville, USA. [3]College of Veterinary Science, Mekelle University, Mekelle, Ethiopia. [4]College of Veterinary Medicine and Agriculture, Samara University, P.O. Box 132, Samara, Ethiopia. [5]National Veterinary Institute, P.O. Box 19, Bishoftu, Ethiopia.

References

1. Goraga Z, Weigend S, Brockmann G. Genetic diversity and population structure of five Ethiopian chicken ecotypes. Anim Genet. 2011;43(4):454–7.

2. Duguma R. Phenotypic characterization of some indigenous chicken ecotypes of Ethiopia. LRRD. 2006;18(131): http://www.lrrd.org/lrrd18/9/dugu18131.htm. Accessed 2 Feb 2016.
3. Duguma R. Understanding the role of indigenous chicken during the long walk to food security in Ethiopia. LRRD. 2009;21(116): http://www.lrrd.org/lrrd21/8/dugu21116.htm. Accessed 2 Feb 2016.
4. Wilson RT. Poultry production and performance in the Federal Democratic Republic of Ethiopia. World Poultry Sci J. 2010;66:441–54.
5. OIE. Newcastle disease. In: OIE manual for diagnostic tests and vaccines for terrestrial animals. 5th ed. 2004;1: 270–283.
6. Alexander DJ. The classification, host range, and distribution of avian paramyxoviruses. In: Acute virus infections of Poultry. Edited by Mcferran, JB, McNulty MS. Martininus Nijhoff. Dordrecht, The Netherlands: Martinus Nijhoff Publishers; 1986. p. 52–66.
7. Bell JG, Mouloudi S. A reservoir of virulent Newcastle disease virus in village children flocks. Prev Vet Med. 1988;8:291–4.
8. Allan WH, Lancaster JE, Toth B. Newcastle disease vaccines–their production and use. FAO Animal Production Series Rome. 1978:10;1-163.
9. Palya V. Manual for the production of Marek's disease, Gumboro disease and inactivated Newcastle disease vaccines. Technical Centre for Agricultural and Rural Cooperation. FAO Anim Prod Health Pap. 1991;89:1–25.
10. Alders R, Spradbrow P. Controlling ND in village chickens. ACIAR Monograph. 2001;82:112.
11. Spradbrow PB, Ibrahim AC, Mustaffa-Bajee A, Kim SJ. Use of an avirulent Australia of Newcastle Disease Virus (NDV) as a vaccine. Avian Dis. 1977;22(2):329–35.
12. Tu TD, Phuc KV, Dinh NTK, Quoc DN, Spradbrow PB. Vietnamese trials with a thermostable Newcastle disease vaccine (strain I-2) in experimental and village chickens. Prev Vet Med. 1998;34:205–14.
13. Spradbrow PB. Newcastle Disease in village chickens. Poultry Science Review. 1993/4;5: 57–96.
14. Grimes ES. A basic laboratory manual for the small-scale production and testing I2 Newcastle disease vaccine. Bangkok, Thailand: FAO-APHCA; 2002. p. 103.
15. Nassir M, Lohr EJ, Mebratu YG, Zessin HK, Baumann OPM, Ademe Z. Oral Newcastle disease vaccination trials in Ethiopia. Avian Pathol. 2000;29:27–34.
16. Chan YH. Randomised controlled trials (RCTs) – sample size: The magic number? Singapore Med J. 2003;44(4):172–4.
17. Cumming RB. Newcastle disease research at the University of New England. In: Newcastle Disease in Village chickens. ACIAR Proceedings. 1992;39: 84–85.
18. Wambura PN, Meers J, Spradbrow P. Survival of avirulent thermostable Newcastle disease virus (strain I-2) in raw, baked, oiled, and cooked white rice at ambient temperatures. J Vet Sci. 2007;8:303–5.
19. de Wit JJ, van de Sande HWA, Counotte GHM, Wellenberg GJ. Analyses of the results of different test systems in the 2005 global proficiency testing schemes for infectious bursal disease virus and Newcastle disease virus antibody detection in chicken serum. Avian Pathol. 2007;36(2):177–83.
20. Alexander DJ, Bell JG, Alders RG. Technology Review: Newcastle Disease. Rome: FAO Animal Production and Health Paper; 2004. p. 1–26.
21. Oakeley RD. Emergency assistance for the control of Newcastle disease. Consultancy Report on Rural Poultry Production-Socio-Economy, FAO, Rome. 1998: 12–22.
22. Oakeley RD. The limitation of a feed/water based heat-stable vaccine delivery system for Newcastle disease control strategies for backyard poultry flocks in sub-Saharan Africa. Prev Vet Med. 2000;47:271–9.
23. Saeed Z, Ahmad S, Rizvi AR, Ajmal M. Role of maternal antibody in determination of an effective Newcastle disease vaccination programme. Pak J Vet Res. 1988;1:18–20.
24. Rahman MM, Bari ASM, Giasudin MJ, Islam RM, Sil AC. Evaluation of maternal and humoral immunity against Newcastle disease virus in chicken. Int J Poult Sci. 2002;1:161–3.
25. Olabode AO, James A, Ndako GON, Echeonwu OON, Anthony AC. Use of cracked maize as a carrier for NDV4 vaccine in experimental vaccination of chickens. Virol J. 2010;7(67):1–5.
26. Musa U, Abdu PA, Mera UM, Emmenna PE, Ahmed MS. Vaccination with Newcastle disease vaccines strain I2 and LaSota in commercial and local chickens in Plateau state Nigeria. N V J. 2010;31(1):46–55.
27. Ibrahim AL, Chulan U, Mustaffa-Babjee AM. The assessment of the Australian V4 strain of NDV as a vaccine by spray, aerosol and drinking water administration. Aust Vet J. 1981;57:277–80.
28. Holmes HC. Resistance of the respiratory tract of chickens to Newcastle disease virus infection following vaccination: the effect of passively acquired antibody on its development. J Comp Pathol. 1997;89:11–20.
29. Alexander DDJ. Newcastle and other Avian Paramixoviruses. In: Sairf YM, editor. Disease of poultry. 11th ed. Ames, Iowa: Iowa State press; 2003. p. 63–87.
30. Echeonwu BC, Ngele MB, Echeonwu GON, Joannis TM, Onovoh EM, Paul G. Response of chickens to oral vaccination with Newcastle disease virus vaccine strain I2 coated on maize offal. Afr J Biotechnol. 2008;7(10):1594–9.
31. Foster A, Chitukuro HR, Tuppa E, Mwanjala T, Kusila C. Thermostable Newcastle disease vaccines in Tanzania. Vet Microbiol. 1999;68:127–30.
32. Tizard IR. Vaccinations and vaccines. Veterinary Immunology an introduction. 6th ed. Philadelphia, Pennsylvannia: W B Saunders Company; 2000. p. 110–9.
33. Echeonwu GON, Iroegbu CU, Echeonwu BC, Ngene A, Olabode AO, Okeke OI, Ndako J, Paul G, Onovoh EM, Junaid SA, Nwankiti O. Delivery of thermostable Newcastle disease (ND) vaccine to chickens with broken millet grains as the vehicle. Afr J Biotechnol. 2007;6(23):2694–9.
34. Rushton J. Assistance to rural women in protecting their chicken flocks against Newcastel disease. Consultancy report on rural poultry production-socio-Economy, December 1995, FAO, Rome. 1995:55–56.
35. Jackson ARB. Observations on some difficulties encountered in trials with oral Newcastle disease vaccine. ACIAR Proc. Canberra, Australia. 1992;39: 15–17.
36. Aini I, Ibrahim AL, Spradbrow PB. Field trials of a food-based vaccine to protect village chickens against Newcastle disease. Res Vet Sci. 1990;49:216–9.
37. Aini I, Ibrahim AL, Spradbrow PB. Efficacy of food pellet Newcastle disease vaccine: Simulated village experiments. J Vet Med Malaysia. 1992;4:81–6.

12

"Why won't they just vaccinate?" Horse owner risk perception and uptake of the Hendra virus vaccine

J. Manyweathers[1,2*], H. Field[3], N. Longnecker[2,4], K. Agho[5], C. Smith[6] and M. Taylor[1,7*]

Abstract

Background: Hendra virus is a paramyxovirus that causes periodic serious disease and fatalities in horses and humans in Australia first identified in 1994. Pteropid bats (commonly known as flying-foxes) are the natural host of the virus, and the putative route of infection in horses is by ingestion or inhalation of material contaminated by flying-fox urine or other bodily fluids. Humans become infected after close contact with infected horses. Horse owners in Australia are encouraged to vaccinate their horses against Hendra virus to reduce the risk of Hendra virus infection, and to prevent potential transmission to humans. After the vaccine was released in 2012, uptake by horse owners was slow, with some estimated 11-17% of horses in Australia vaccinated. This study was commissioned to examine barriers to vaccine uptake and potential drivers to future adoption of vaccination by horse owners.

Methods: This study examined qualitative comments from respondents to an on-line survey, reporting reasons for not vaccinating their horses. The study also investigated scenarios in which respondents felt they might consider vaccinating their horses.

Results: Self-reported barriers to uptake of the Hendra virus vaccine by horse owners (N = 150) included concerns about vaccine safety, cost, and effectiveness. Reduction in vaccination costs and perception of immediacy of Hendra virus risk were reported as being likely to change future behaviour. However, the data also indicated that horse owners generally would not reconsider vaccinating their horses if advised by their veterinarian.

Conclusion: While changes to vaccine costs and the availability data supporting vaccine safety and efficacy may encourage more horse owners to vaccinate, this study highlights the importance of protecting the relationship between veterinarians and horse owners within the risk management strategies around Hendra virus. Interactions and trust between veterinarians and animal owners has important implications for management of and communication around Hendra virus and other zoonotic disease outbreaks.

Keywords: Risk mitigation, Biosecurity, Trust, Protection motivation theory, Hendra virus, Vaccination, zoonosis, Vaccine hesitancy

Background

During infectious disease outbreaks, risk decisions and management by all stakeholders are compelled by temporal, cultural and social factors [1]. For those involved in managing disease outbreaks, it is fundamental to have a clear understanding of all factors at play in people's adoption and adaption of officially recommended risk management strategies [2]. Research into risk has long been challenging, largely because of how risk is defined [3, 4]. Scientists, researchers and risk analysts, identified here as "salaried experts", define risk as a consideration of magnitude of the risk event and the probability of its occurrence using a mathematical approach [5, 6]. However, when considering how people respond to risk, it has been suggested that there is little benefit in discussing the risk itself [7]. Instead, the very different concept of risk perception needs to be considered. Risk perception is influenced by various social and psychological factors, including trust [8], worldview ([9]; Manyweathers, Taylor,

* Correspondence: jmanyweathers@csu.edu.au; mel.taylor@mq.edu.au
[1]Centre for Health Research, Western Sydney University, Sydney, Australia
Full list of author information is available at the end of the article

Longnecker, unpublished observations], emotion and affect [10, 11], and the effect of social and cultural processes [12]. Consequently, when examining people's decisions about health protective behaviours, an appropriate framework should include consideration of these factors.

The Cultural Theory of Risk posits that risk perceptions reflect and maintain an individual's preferred type of social organisation and cultural way of life [13]. Within the theory, risk perception is further defined by the extent to which an individual associates their identity within a particular social group and the extent to which they accept a formal hierarchical system of rules [13–15]. The Cultural Theory of Risk considers the social environment, the stakeholders and the bases on which decision are made around risk as part of one holistic process [16]. Therefore, actions taken to avoid some dangers and ignore, or not act upon, others are made within the framework of social arrangements, and these decisions and choices of how to live are taken together [16]. Because salaried experts and lay people alike lack complete knowledge and foresight, decisions required to navigate through complex risk situations are made by relying on affective and mental shortcuts, known as heuristic reasoning [17]. This reasoning is aimed at maximising desired future outcomes in risk situations. But rather than these outcomes reflecting a united goal for all stakeholders, the mental and affective shortcuts adopted by those at risk reflect an individual's worldview, their sense of who should have control and what should matter [16, 18]. Their subsequent actions are directed at protecting and maintaining this position [10]. Consequently, the spectrum of responses by stakeholders towards the risk surrounding emerging disease infections is vast and requires careful consideration.

Hendra virus (family *Paramyxoviridae*, genus *Henipavirus*) causes periodic respiratory and neurological disease and subsequent fatalities in horses and humans. Flying-foxes (family *Pteropodidae*, genus *Pteropus*) are the natural host of the virus [19, 20], with the Spectacled and Black flying-foxes evidently the most competent host species [21, 22]. The virus was first isolated and identified after the death of more than 20 horses and their trainer in 1994. Horses are thought to become infected via ingestion or inhalation of virus from pasture, water or surfaces contaminated with flying-fox excreta, with recent research suggesting that flying-fox urine is the most likely transmission medium [22]. Infection via direct contamination of mucous membranes may also occur [22–24]. Of the seven human cases of Hendra virus infection, four (57%) have been fatal [21]. All human cases arose following close and direct contact with infected horses [25].

Between 1994 and 2010, there were 14 reported Hendra virus events, including the seven human cases. In 2011, however, 18 Hendra virus events involving over 20 horses across an expanded geographic area were reported in a single three-month period [25]. This unprecedented and alarming scenario added impetus and urgency to the development of a vaccine for horses to prevent infection and transmission to humans [25]. In November 2012, a vaccine based on a viral G glycoprotein, required by the virus for binding to host cells was released. Antibodies against this protein were found to neutralise the virus and prevent disease [25]. The vaccine was initially released under a restricted permit use pending full registration with the Australian Pesticides and Veterinary Medicines Association (APVMA), the government body responsible for the registration of all agricultural and veterinary chemicals in Australia. The permit enabled the vaccine to be used under strict conditions, including administration by a trained and accredited veterinary surgeon to horses that were uniquely identified by microchip, the details of which were recorded on a national online registry. Since its release, the permit for Hendra virus vaccination has undergone several amendments and included instructions for six-monthly boosters. In August 2015, the vaccine became fully registered, with 12 monthly boosters approved in May 2016.

Despite recommendation by the main state government agencies responsible for Hendra virus policy - Queensland Department for Agriculture and Fisheries (QDAF) and New South Wales Department of Primary Industries (NSW DPI) - that vaccination is *'the single most effective way of reducing the risk of Hendra virus infection in horses'* [26], uptake of the vaccine has been slow [27]. Whilst there is no national registry of horses in Australia, and thus the total number of horses is unknown, it is estimated that the majority of horses remain unvaccinated, with vaccine rates estimated to be around 11-17% [28].

Other risk mitigation strategies aim at property management practices, reducing the possibility of contact between horses and flying-foxes. These include covering food and water sources in the paddock, removing horses from pasture when bats are most active and removing access by horses to fruiting and flowering trees [26]. However, research has highlighted the problematic nature of these approaches, with some horse owners reporting that they find the recommended strategies ineffective and impractical [29].

To implement inclusive and engaging risk management strategies, it is necessary to adopt a holistic consideration of people's perception of risk and the adoption of protective health behaviours in zoonotic disease outbreaks [30–33]. For the successful implementation of effective public health interventions, providing information about protective strategies and even the production of a vaccine, while necessary, are not enough to ensure adoption of protective behaviours [34, 35]. In fact, previous research suggests that the observed non-compliant behaviours of horse owners around Hendra virus and the vaccine release should have been anticipated [17, 30, 36] and could possibly have been avoided [37]. Research into vaccine hesitancy around human vaccines is growing [38, 39] and could provide insight into possible outcomes for vaccine roll out and uptake in animals.

In order to facilitate a deeper understanding of how horse owners perceive the risk of Hendra virus infection in horses and how this affects decisions around adoption of protective behaviours, the *Hendra Virus Infection and Transmission Dynamics – Conversation with Industry* project was launched, commissioned by the intergovernmental National Hendra Virus Taskforce [40]. Funding was provided by Australian State and Federal departments and the taskforce identified priority areas for research. The current study was tasked with three main aims:

1. To identify factors associated with the uptake of protective strategies to reduce the risk of Hendra virus infection.
2. To identify reasons for non-vaccination of horses against Hendra virus.
3. To consider how engagement with horse owners and uptake of management strategies may be improved.

In order to address the first two aims of the project and more fully understand horse owners' responses to Hendra virus and to the vaccine, a mixed method approach was adopted [41, 42]. A survey containing open ended questions provided qualitative data: self-reported reasons given by horse owners for not vaccinating their horses against Hendra virus. Quantitative data from the survey was also analysed to consider factors involved in potential uptake of risk mitigation strategies. Results from analysis of these data are reported here. Research examining how engagement with horse owners might be improved is reported elsewhere (Manyweathers, Taylor, Longnecker, unpublished observations).

Methods

An online survey was designed to explore risk mitigation practices, risk perception, and attitudes to Hendra virus risk of horse owners using both open and closed questions. The survey was directed at horse owners who had elected not to vaccinate their horses against Hendra virus and were living geographically close to the location of a previous Hendra virus case. A qualifying question was used to screen respondents in order that only those respondents that had not vaccinated all or any of their horses could proceed with the survey.

The survey comprised 38 questions with an opportunity to leave contact details for a follow up interview in the second phase of the study. Data collected from the latter are reported elsewhere (Manyweathers, Taylor, Longnecker, unpublished observations).

Respondents were asked about their reasons for not vaccinating their horse(s) and situations that might make them reconsider. Questions concerning perceived barriers to uptake of vaccination were also included, using Likert scales for responses.

The survey was developed and administered using the online hosting software SurveyMonkey™, after piloting with three horse owners and four veterinary professionals, recruited through the first author's veterinary practice. After the piloting process, demographic questions were altered slightly to ensure that all possible variations of horse ownership, management and current vaccination status were included. The survey is included as a Additional file 1. Ethics approval for the study was provided by the Human Research Ethics Committee of the University of Western Sydney (Protocol No. H10643).

The survey link was posted on the Facebook pages of 26 veterinary hospitals in areas where Hendra virus cases had previously been confirmed: far north New South Wales, South East, Central, and Far North Queensland. The survey was open for six weeks, with three postings on the Facebook page, from January 22nd until March 10th 2015. Because of the uncontrolled nature of social media posting, the location of respondents was determined using a question regarding distance to nearest Hendra virus case and confirmed using respondents' postcode.

Cross posting from veterinary hospital Facebook groups included a dressage club based in an area where a significant number of Hendra virus cases occurred and a Facebook group with an active presence in the discourse around Hendra virus vaccine.

Sample characteristics were determined by simple descriptive statistics. Descriptive analysis was also used to present data highlighting factors that might influence horse owners to reconsider vaccinating their horses against Hendra virus. Data were managed using IBM SPSS V22. Qualitative data were managed using NVivo and were coded to investigate the reasons for non-vaccination. The analysis was undertaken using the following approach modified from Braun and Clarke [41, 43]. Data familiarisation was undertaken by reading survey responses in detail. Initial codes were considered across the set of surveys until no new codes were required to represent responses, then relevant data were collated for each code. The codes were then grouped into potential themes, defined and named. Quotations from the raw data were used to narrate the themes, illustrating the unique characteristics of the respondent's perceptions. Respondents' spelling was corrected and minor grammatical adjustments made for ease of reading. Clarifications from the first author are included in bold square brackets.

Results

Sample characteristics

In total 210 respondents associated with 17 veterinary practices completed the survey and qualified for analysis by reporting having unvaccinated horses. Approximately half the sample (50%, n = 106) were aged 44 or younger. While some respondents (7%, n = 15) reported earning their main source of income from horse related business or activity, just over a quarter (23%, n = 49) earned some income from their horse involvement. A cross section of sectors of horse involvement (multiple responses allowed) were represented in the responses, with 62% (n = 131) involved in the competitive/equestrian sector, 57% (n = 120) involved in the recreational sector, and 19% involved in the working/farming/stock horse sector.

Barriers to uptake of vaccination

Just under three quarters of the sample responded to the question concerning their reason for not vaccinating, or withdrawing from the vaccination program (71%, n = 150). Each respondent gave, on average, two to three reasons for not adopting vaccination as a protective strategy. A total of 424 comments were coded to explore the reasons given for non-vaccination or not continuing with the six-monthly booster required to be compliant with the recommended vaccination protocol. Three main themes were identified from the coding structure: 'attitude towards the vaccine', 'attitude towards authorities', including veterinarians and the pharmaceutical company that produces the vaccine, and 'risk assessment'. The 'attitude towards the vaccine' theme reflected people's concerns, including the potential for side effects, the protocol at the time of data collection requiring six monthly boosters, and the cost and the perceived safety of the vaccine. The 'Risk assessment' theme included evidence of people's own risk assessment of their horses and property and the risk of vaccinating a horse that was unwell. The theme 'attitude to authorities' reflected consideration given by horse owners to the nature of the relationship between them and those in authority and the relationship between authorities. Comments consisted of a mixture of one word answers and more in-depth responses. Table 1 summarises the coding and themes.

Theme 1: Attitude to the vaccine

The majority of coded responses (310 comments) identified an aspect of the vaccine as the driver behind the decision not to vaccinate. Concern regarding side effects of the vaccine was the single most frequently given reason for non-vaccination. Some respondents reported a first-hand experience with a vaccine side effect, while others recorded anecdotal evidence.

> *I only vaccinated due to pressures from vets but am now reconsidering due to risk factors and my horse's reaction to the vaccine each time it was given.* (R23)

> *One of my horses died after receiving the vaccine which has been investigated. I've also heard far too many have bad reactions that have left them permanently damaged.* (R45)
> *There have been more cases of a reaction to the vaccine than there is of a horse contracting the virus. The reactions I've heard or read about are quite confronting and scary, which made me reconsider.* (R11)
> *Concerns from social media with side effects means that at present I have not done our miniature horse.* (R30)

The fact that the vaccine was being used under a restricted permit and was not fully registered at the time of the survey was frequently reported as proof that the vaccine was unsafe and insufficiently tested (43 comments).

> *Because the vaccine is not registered, it's unsafe and has been known to cause adverse reactions to horses and in some cases cause death. I would not give my human child a vaccine that puts them at risks like this so I won't do it to me horses!* (R75)

> *I believe that the vaccination was rushed to get out onto the market and that we do not know all of the possible side effects. I also believe that if it was safe, we'd have a similar vaccine for humans.* (R24)

The cost of the vaccine was the fourth most frequently given single response (39 comments) but is only mentioned by eight respondents as their sole reason for not vaccinating. The cost was mentioned in parallel with the protocol at the time requiring six monthly boosters and veterinary administration.

> *Also the cost to get them all done every six months by our vet.* (R47)
> *High cost of repeated treatments required. If it was a one off vaccine it would be easier to wear the once off cost of the vaccine.* (R67)

Theme 2: Risk assessment

Respondents' comments were coded for references to their consideration of the risk to them of Hendra virus infection, or Hendra virus vaccine side effects (80 comments). References to underlying horse health issues as a barrier to vaccination were included (14 comments). Biosecurity measures adopted in place of vaccination were mentioned in 10 responses.

Table 1 Reasons for non-vaccination or withdrawal from the vaccination protocol

Theme	Code	N	Description	Example Comments
Attitude towards vaccine (n = 310)	Side effects	91	Reference to side effects, whether general or specific	The amount of horses either having a reaction or death from vaccination. (R17)
	Cost	39	Reference to the cost of vaccination	The cost of the vaccine. (R7)
	Testing	40	Reference to the need for more testing of the vaccine or the lack of testing	I'm not willing to vaccinate against Hendra until more testing is done on the vaccine (R14) Not enough research and the way it was rushed to market. (R41)
	Safety	20	Reference to the safety of the vaccine	Until it has been proved for 5 years I am not convinced it is safe. (R54)
	Efficacy	13	Reference to the vaccine not working,	Current vaccination is not proved sufficiently (R13)
	Animal use	17	Reference to breeding animals and lack of safety, or issues with exporting vaccinated horses	Have not heard any proof if safe to use in breeding animals (R12)
	Hendra virus vaccine protocol	21	Reference to concern regarding the protocol, number of vaccines required, vet involvement	The number of vaccines required and the frequency of them. (R21)
	Licence	43	Reference to concern regarding the restricted licence for the vaccine	Unregistered Vaccine. (R17)
	Future intention	13	Indication that vaccination maybe reconsidered in the future	If this is sorted in the future I will consider it more readily. (R14)
	Attitude to vaccination	11	Indications of attitudes to vaccination in general or other vaccines for horses	I do however regularly vaccinate for strangles and tetanus which I see as a bigger threat having had one of my horse contract strangles even after vaccinating. (R28)
	Freedom of choice	2	Indication of desire to make own choice about whether to vaccinate	I believe in pro-choice. (R46)
Risk assessment (n = 94)	Risk assessment	70	Evidence of risk assessment, weighing up the odds, insights into where respondents feel the risk lies, includes the risk of side effects from the vaccine and the risk of Hendra virus infection	They are not in contact with other horses. (R8) The chance of reaction is higher than the chance of catching Hendra when precautions are taken. (R43)
	Biosecurity	10	Evidence of adoption or consideration of biosecurity practices	Extremely low flying fox/bat population in our area and no contact with horse from neighbouring properties. Removal of all fruiting trees and regular monitoring of blossoming/flower native trees which coincide with paddock rotations. (R34)
	Horse health	14	Reference to underlying horse health issues which precludes the vaccine being able to be used.	One is not vaccinated as she is elderly and the risk of infection and contact with people is very low. (R32)
Attitude towards authorities (n = 36)	Authorities	36	Reference to authorities, whether veterinarians or pharmaceutical companies, their behaviour, motivation	Horses have died from this vaccine and the authorities are not acknowledging this fact!! (R142)
Other (n = 1)	Other	1	Comments that do not fit in to current categories but still need to be considered.	Availability (work full time during the week and compete full time on the weekends). (R22)

The virus is a very weak one and strong hygiene practices on the home front can do a lot to mitigate any related risk. (R144)

Minute risk of a Hendra incident in my horses as assessed by myself and my vet. (R141)
I believe that the infection rate of both horses and humans to be statistically insignificant. The virus has been around for ever, why the panic now? Does someone know something I don't? Awareness and PPE covers risks. (R132)
I have two older horses and a mare I plan to breed with. Having heard of several severe reactions in vaccinated horses (particularly those with pre-existing heart and neurological conditions) I have concluded that the risk of death or serious illness from the vaccination is much higher than from Hendra in my area. Particularly, since one of my older horses has neurological and heart conditions, the risk would be too large for her. (R73)
... good biosecurity practice with ANY sick animal is a more sensible approach to take. (R96)

Some responses were indicative of where respondents perceived the risk of Hendra virus infection would most likely come from. This included infection from contact with other horses (nine comments), and unhygienic stabling conditions (two comments). Flying-foxes were mentioned in five comments.

Because the risk is very small in our area. We are not transporting our horses to events like shows only to mates' properties for mustering where the risk is also minimal. If one of our horses gets it we will put them down and aim in protecting the others in all means possible. (R25)

The risk is so low, and my experience with the conditions I witnessed at the clinic that experienced the outbreak have left me confident that my horses will not be exposed to this virus, and are not going to die. We had horses for a long time without knowing about Hendra, and nothing has changed other than in my opinion, people keeping horses in unsuitable conditions. (R04)
Low risk (no large mobs of flying foxes seen), horses do not travel or have contact with other horses. (R62)
Not necessary as in the history of this virus not one horse at any event or well cared for establishment has ever had a case that is not transmitted by poor hygiene and unsafe veterinary practices. (R134)

There was also mention of the fact that Hendra virus has been around for a while and therefore perhaps does not warrant the intense pressure of immediate and extreme action.

The virus has been around for ever and only come to light 20 years ago. (R64)

Hendra virus is hard to catch and it has been around for centuries. (R93)

Some responses indicated that horse owners are making informed choices in regard to the permit and the appropriateness of vaccination in their situation.

Not recommended for PPID [Pituitary Pars intermedia Dysfunction – Cushing's disease] cases. (R104)

One of my horses does not meet the vaccination criteria as stated on the minor use permit. (R112)

There were some comments (n = 16) that raised the issue of a Hendra virus area and vaccination not being necessary due to their geographical location relative the Hendra virus or flying-foxes.

I don't live in a Hendra area. I won't put my horses at risk of an on-trial only vac...(R28)
Willing to take the risk as not in high flying fox area. (R06)
Extremely low flying fox/bat population in our area and no contact with horses from neighbouring properties. (R34)

Theme 3: Attitude to authorities

A general sense of anger and resentment towards authorities, including veterinarians and pharmaceutical representatives, was evident in 36 comments from different individuals.

The fact people are trying to force us to vaccinate. Vets are refusing to treat horses that are unvaccinated; some grounds will not allow horses that are unvaccinated /the amount of things being swept under the rug and the lies being toted around by the Vaccination Company and vets that are reading from the same song sheet. (R17)

We have chosen not to due to the way it has been handled and the lack of truthful information. (R29)

Most of these comments indicate that horse owners connected veterinarians and the vaccine manufacturer as working together. This is evident when respondents comment on feeling forced into vaccination and bullied.

I also will not be bullied into it by the government or vets making it mandatory. (R14)

The drug company is all about money and is pushing the vets' hands so they won't come out to unvaccinated horses. (R64)

I do not support the bullying and scaremongering tactics of vets and [vaccine manufacturer] to push this vaccine! (R59)

Respondents were angered by their perception that veterinarians were using their professional power to force people to vaccinate by withholding their services if the horses were unvaccinated.

Being Forced to choose a vaccine that is Unproven to work in order to gain veterinary care. (R148)

DISGUSTED at vets refusing to attend unvaccinated horse unless to vaccinate or to put to sleep. (R115)
I think the vets have over reacted to the extreme which also makes me so angry that I would rather shoot my horse than give them money to come out and refuse treatment. (R108)

Respondents identify a lack of transparency in how their complaints and concerns were dealt with as a driver for not adopting vaccinations.

Despite the attempts to cover up the amount of horses that have died following vaccination and others that have been rendered unrideable, not to mention the adverse reactions. The truth is the truth and this vaccine in its current form is not safe for horses in its current form. Veterinarians are not reporting all reactions and are using it for a cash cow and forcing it upon people who live in low risk areas. (R81)

During the investigation into the death of my horse [vaccine manufacturer] rep attempted to intimidate me, tried to guilt trip me and lied many times which he was caught out doing. (R45)
Reactions which [vaccine manufacturer] decides if it is a reaction or not. (R136)

Overall, the comments from some horse owners when asked why they were electing not to vaccinate their horses reflect a lack of trust in the pharmaceutical company and veterinarians.

Something here is NOT right! Too many cover ups in regards to reactions & deaths from the vaccine itself. (148)
As before it has been pushed onto the market with very poor research regardless of the spin they try to put on it. Too many reactions are not acknowledged and reports just disappear. I am not anti-vaccine of any kind. But I am strongly anti Hendra vaccine. (R126)
The fact that there is SO MUCH MISINFORMATION propagated by [vaccine manufacturer] who do not report the facts on reactions (but all horse owners know them) and vets who have a vested interest in pushing the vaccine for kickbacks is disgusting. (R114)

Factors influencing the potential uptake of vaccination

Respondents were asked to consider a series of situations and indicate whether the situations would cause them to reconsider vaccinating their horses against Hendra virus. Figure 1 summarises these findings.

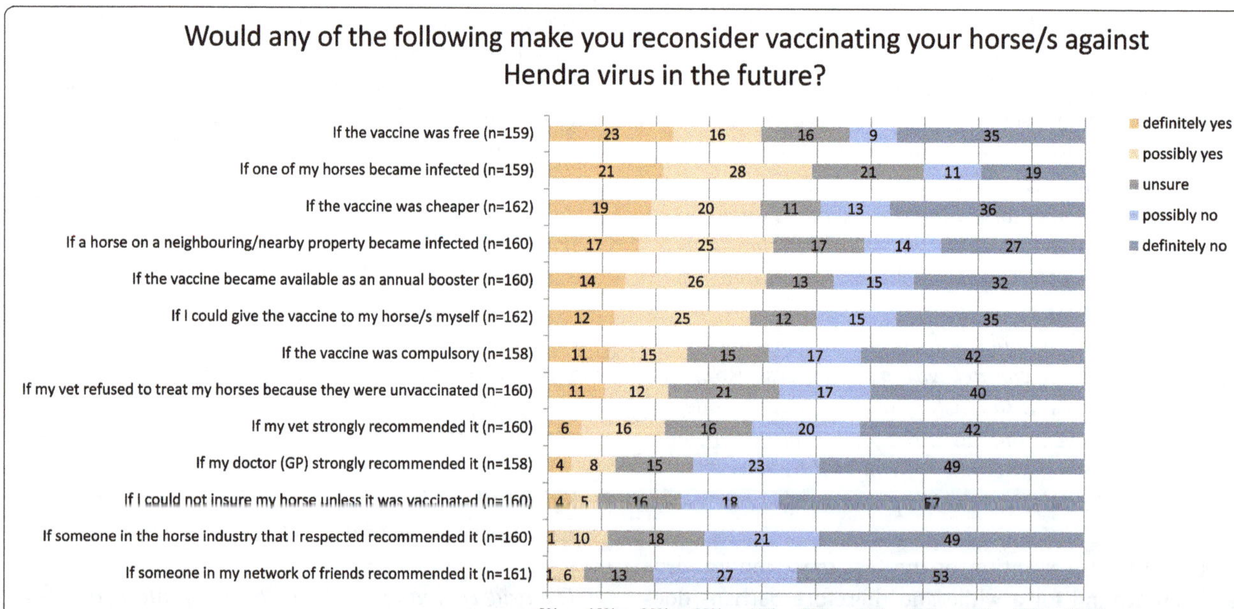

Fig. 1 Factors that would influence uptake of Hendra virus vaccination. Data has been rounded

In the top six influencing factors, 37 to 49% of respondents would reconsider vaccinating their horse(s). Issues of cost, convenience, immediacy of Hendra virus risk and personal control were features that linked more strongly to reconsideration of vaccination. Policy issues were reported to be less influential, with 23 to 26% of respondents saying they would reconsider vaccination in response to policy changes which made the vaccination compulsory, or veterinary policy changes to refuse treatment to unvaccinated horses. Recommendations from veterinarians and medical doctors were next down the list of self-reported influencers with 12- 22% saying they would reconsider vaccination following advice from them. The factors reported to be least likely to influence vaccination decisions were requirements for insurance (9%) and recommendations by others in the industry and friends (7 – 11%).

Discussion

The single most frequent reason given for non-adoption of vaccination was concern about side effects from the vaccine. Many respondents felt that the risk of side effects from the vaccine outweighed the perceived risk of Hendra virus infection. Lack of trust and confidence in veterinarians and the pharmaceutical company also featured prominently in comments as drivers for the non-adoption of the vaccine for horses. Comments suggested that the perceived lack of testing of the vaccine, and feeling that their horses were being used as 'guinea pigs' also resulted in an unwillingness to vaccinate their horses against Hendra virus. Responses regarding side effects that were thought to be inappropriately acknowledged by the pharmaceutical company also figured significantly. The results will be discussed in the context of the themes identified.

Barriers to uptake of vaccination

Theme 1: Attitude to the vaccine

Historically, attempts to claim that a technology is free from risk have sometimes resulted in a perception of increased likelihood of that risk [44, 45]. This may increase the lack of trust felt by those on the receiving end of the technology [46]. At the time of this study the discourse surrounding Hendra virus and the vaccine was further complicated because the vaccine was still being used under a restricted permit. This was perceived by some horse owners as evidence that there was something wrong with the vaccine and that adequate pre-release trials had not been carried out. Subsequent to our study data being collected, the vaccine became fully registered in August 2015 [47]. A summary of adverse experience reports by the Australian Pesticides and Veterinary Medicines Authority (APVMA), the agency responsible for assessment and registration of the vaccine, reported the adverse reaction rate at 0.001% in an estimated 100,000 horses vaccinated [48, 49] may not be sufficient to rebuild trust by horse owners that their concerns are being heard.

Some comments highlight the sense that the concerns of the horse owners are not being addressed or even acknowledged. Discounting by salaried experts of views that differ from the accepted scientific approach, or expressions of uncertainty around the risk of Hendra virus and the vaccine, may limit the opportunity for frank and open discussion. Acknowledgement of such expressions might enhance direct and transparent discourse around Hendra virus [50, 51] and continue into improved acceptance of recommended strategies. Open knowledge, or uncertainty sharing, could play a role in including horse owners as participants or stakeholders in the communication process and may help in the attenuation of risk perception surrounding Hendra virus and the vaccine, and enhance trust within stakeholder relationships [52]. Such uncertainty within scientific research is generally well considered by stakeholders and allows for resources to be invested in risk management strategies that focus on what is being done to reduce the uncertainty [53].

Theme 2: Risk assessment

Lay risk assessment is often considered to be based on ignorance or originating from faulty mental processing in regards to scientific information [10, 54]. Instead, the data collected provides evidence of careful consideration and a scientific approach to biosecurity. Some respondents cited the vaccine permit and the restrictions placed on vaccinating sick or immunocompromised horses [47] as their reason for not vaccinating. If this response is considered as noncompliant, then it does appear to make nonsense of the permit and the restrictions that are in place around the vaccine use.

Comments that indicated respondents were undertaking a personal risk assessment based on identifying areas as being more or less likely to have a Hendra virus case are of concern. Research has identified that while some areas have had more Hendra virus cases historically, given the flying-foxes' spatiotemporal distribution across Australia, it is difficult to predict where cases might occur [27]. The possibility of direct transmission from flying-fox urine to horses also suggests that even small numbers of flying-foxes may dramatically increase the risk of an infection in horses [22, 24]. Therefore, it is important to address the uncertainty surrounding Hendra virus cases and ensure that all stakeholders are fully aware of the changing nature of flying-fox distribution, and consequently risk of infection with Hendra virus, over time and space.

The comments suggesting that Hendra virus has been around for a long time are accurate [55] and should not be dismissed. However, the connection made by respondents between the historical nature of the virus and the lack of need for a vaccine would benefit from further consideration.

Theme 3: Attitude to authorities

The role of veterinarians in the provision of information and communication around animal welfare and health, and their influence on horse owner behaviour is even more crucial in the context of Hendra virus, given the potential for human infection and its high morbidity and mortality in horses and people. This reinforces the urgent need to ensure that the veterinarian-owner relationship is protected and supported in the current Hendra virus discourse. A breakdown in trust and credibility could have long-lasting and far-reaching consequences in any future emergency animal disease response [46].

There was a strong perception amongst some respondents of a conspiracy between the pharmaceutical company that manufactures the vaccine and veterinarians who must administer it and hence benefit financially. When information and recommendations are provided by sources that have commercial interests in the uptake of such information, the reliability of such material may be doubted [56]. Such complications surrounding the release of the Hendra virus vaccine communication should have been anticipated [46].

Some respondents' comments reflect an egalitarian worldview, one in which value is placed on a society free from stratification about who can offer instruction and direction [57]. This is in contrast with the traditional hierarchical worldview on which science is founded. Consideration by veterinarians of the role that worldview plays in their approach to risk, as well as in their clients' decision making may assist in creating opportunities for more open and participatory communication.

As previously discussed, the Hendra virus vaccine was initially released under a restricted permit. This meant that all Hendra virus vaccine marketing and advertising, as well as administration, could only be carried out by veterinarians, further cementing the connection between the vaccination and the profits of those administering it. Other horse vaccines in Australia can be purchased from a veterinarian by their regular clients and administered to the horse by their owner. It perhaps should have been anticipated that a dramatic change in vaccine administration would cause concern and suspicion amongst horse owners within the climate of uncertainty surrounding an emerging zoonotic virus.

Factors influencing the potential uptake of vaccination

In the final section of the study, factors that might influence horse owners to reconsider vaccinating their horses in the future were considered. A first hand or near miss experience with Hendra virus infection was most commonly reported as likely to influence potential adoption of vaccination. While this is useful and hardly surprising data, it does not inform changes in communication policy or appear to offer practical changes that can be implemented by horse owners or veterinarians, except to wait for the next infection. This phenomenon is however, supported by anecdotal reports from veterinarians in areas where there have been previous Hendra virus cases followed up a rapid increase in uptake of vaccination [58], and by peaks in laboratory submissions and visits to government Hendra virus websites following reported cases [59].

Reduction of cost was reported as a likely influencer of increased uptake, with free vaccine, cheaper vaccine, less frequent booster doses and owner-administration potentially increasing vaccine uptake. Similarly, the potential for government subsidy for the vaccine was viewed favourably. Since the vaccine's release, incentives have been used to increase uptake of vaccination. These include free second vaccine doses offered by the vaccine manufacturer, and locally arranged events with 'bulk vaccination' to reduce veterinary costs. These appear to be effective and successful approaches, although no published data are available to verify this. On the other hand, to a sizable group of respondents in this research, these offers make no difference to their stated intended uptake and, in fact, may fuel further suspicions of pressure to vaccinate for profit driven or other sinister reasons.

The influence of veterinarians, medical doctors, respected others, and friends appeared less likely than other factors examined to influence decisions regarding the uptake of vaccination and this should not be surprising. Data from the equine influenza outbreak in Australia in 2007-08 identified the importance of veterinary and other horse health professionals' infection control support in horse owner perceptions of outbreak management and effectiveness of biosecurity measures [60, 61].It is also clear that for the majority of respondents in this study, recommendations from health professionals and networks do not play a strong role in decisions around the uptake of Hendra virus vaccine. Research confirms that individuals (salaried experts and lay people alike) will align themselves with people that support their worldview while making decisions that support and maintain this identity [17]. Those who consider themselves as equally qualified with a salaried expert are less inclined to take advice from so-called "experts" [13].

This study provides an insight into the risk perception and practices of an important target audience for animal health agencies in Australia. In order to better assess its effectiveness, consideration of the limitations of the study should be undertaken. Given there is no large or reliable database of Australian horse owners from which to draw a representative sample, it is most common to adopt a self-selected approach to collect cross-sectoral industry data [29, 62]. The survey sample is also limited to those who access Facebook and either 'like' one of the participating veterinary clinic's Facebook pages or have social networks that have these links. This approach allows access to horse owners with a level of connection to a veterinary clinic in a target region. However, it does not limit the sample only to those who are registered with one of these practices. In fact, cross posting could be traced to various side groups including a dressage club.

Another pertinent issue is that given the current climate of the discourse around Hendra virus and vaccination in horses, it is possible that respondents may have held certain biases and had different motives to respond (or not) to the survey. Those who chose not to respond may have considered the survey part of a 'push' for vaccination, and those who did respond may have felt it was an opportunity to vent frustrations. Although issues of responder bias cannot be dismissed the data collected appear to be comparable to other similar studies in terms of sample demographics [29]. The deliberate selection of those who have not vaccinated would be expected to attract respondents with more negative and/or less trusting, and more questioning views of vaccination and possibly government agencies and other stakeholders. Such views are of direct relevance to the study and are therefore not viewed as a study weakness.

Conclusion

Horse owners in Australia are encouraged to vaccinate their horses against Hendra virus and to adopt a number of on-property risk mitigation practices. Both pharmaceutical and property management strategies are aimed at reducing the probability of infection from flying-foxes of horses on pasture. This research identifies self-reported reasons for the rejection of Hendra virus vaccination and seeks to identify perspectives that inform better communication and policy that may encourage or promote uptake of the vaccine.

Increased vaccination uptake could be encouraged by reducing vaccination costs and lowering concerns about the vaccine's safety and effectiveness. The latter approach is challenging; more time and data may be required to convince a sceptical or distrusting audience. The qualitative and quantitative evidence that veterinarians are not trusted within this discourse is of concern. The need to rebuild and protect good relationships between horse owners and veterinarians should be highlighted as a priority issue, as veterinarians have the most direct and frequent contact with owners, particularly during disease outbreaks. Once lost, trust in veterinarians will be hard to win back.

Tasked with improving the general understanding of horse owners' risk perception and their responses to Hendra virus risk, this research highlights the fundamental paradigm shift that is required for policy makers, veterinarians, and researchers to fully understand and participate in the Hendra virus discourse. Such a discourse requires scientific facts but also needs, perhaps more urgently, a reconsideration of how risk perception, trust and decision making are considered.

Qualitative analysis of these data illustrated the complex nature of decision making around risk and the adoption of protective behaviours. Previous research into risk perception generally and zoonotic disease management specifically has highlighted the importance of avoiding the assumption that any one research approach is unambiguous or empirically pure [18, 35]. Rather, as relationships and identities are dynamic, incomplete and always context specific, so too values, beliefs and responses can change as meaning is made [1]. Beliefs cannot be captured as discrete, measurable and static entities. Adoption of traditional quantitative research approaches alone, while able to report on the 'who is doing what', may obscure the 'how' and 'why'. Within such a discourse, the inherent assumptions on which quantitative research is based can render the more useful and significant social aspects of the risk discourse invisible. This often results in development of programs and risk management approaches that misfire, inflame the discourse and fail. Considering decisions around risk as being based solely on logic and information is misguided. Likewise, labelling noncompliant behaviour as irrational and faulty and subsequently disqualifying it from the discourse is unhelpful and counterproductive. Instead, by understanding that salaried experts and lay people alike make decisions in disease risk situations based on mental and affective shortcuts, founded on how they view the world and who should have control and make decisions could increase mutual understanding of the multitude of factors involved in these complex decisions. Promotion of transparent discussion with all stakeholders, including those actually at risk can result in a more robust and progressive dynamic discourse that is able to adapt within the changing face of an emerging infectious disease and responsive technologies that follow.

Acknowledgement

Prof Graeme Martin (University of Western Australia) has provided invaluable support to the first author during her PhD candidature.

Funding

Funding from the Commonwealth of Australia and the New South Wales and Queensland government was received for this project.

Authors' contributions

JM designed the survey, with significant input from MT, CS, HF, KA and NL. JM jointly wrote the Human Research Ethics Committee application with MT. JM recruited the veterinary clinics, administered the survey, designed the

Facebook link, and collated all the data. KA provided significant guidance of design of the research project and was responsible for running the statistical analyses in consultation with MT and JM. NL and MT provided advice on the qualitative coding. JM wrote the manuscript with MT and NL. CS, HF and KA provided extensive editing advice and all authors gave approval of the final version of the manuscript.

Competing interests
Authors JM and MT received funding (sources listed below) to carry out the research and prepare the papers.

Consent for publication
Not Applicable.

Author details
[1]Centre for Health Research, Western Sydney University, Sydney, Australia. [2]School of Animal Biology, University of Western Australia, PO BOX 7178, Tathra, NSW, Australia. [3]EcoHealth Alliance, New York, NY, USA. [4]Centre for Science Communication, University of Otago, Dunedin, New Zealand. [5]School of Science and Health, Western Sydney University, Sydney, Australia. [6]Department of Agriculture and Fisheries, Queensland Centre for Emerging Infectious Diseases, Biosecurity Queensland, Coopers Plains, QLD, Australia. [7]Department of Psychology, Macquarie University, Sydney, Australia.

References
1. Joffe H. Risk and 'the other'. New York: Cambridge University Press; 1999.
2. Davis M, Stephenson N, Flowers P. Compliant, complacent or panicked? Investigating the problematisation of the Australian general public in pandemic influenza control. Soc Sci Med. 2011;72(6):912–8.
3. Plough A, Krimsky S. The emergence of risk communication studies: social and political context. Sci Technol Hum Values. 1987;12(3/4):4–10.
4. Wynne B. Misunderstood misunderstandings: Social identities and public uptake of science. In: Misunderstanding Science? The public reconstruction of science and technology. edn. Edited by Irwin A, Wynne B. Trowbridge, Wiltshire: Cambridge University Press; 1996: 19-46.
5. Sandman P. Responding to community outrage: Strategies for Effective Risk Communication. American Industrial hygiene Association; 2012. petersandman.com/media/RespondingtoCommunityOutrage.pdf.
6. Slovic P. The Psychology of risk. Saúde Sociedade. 2010, 19(4):731-47.
7. Slovic P. Trust, emotion, sex, politics, and science: surveying the risk-assessment battlefield. Risk Anal. 1999;19(4):689–701.
8. Engdahl E, Lidskog R. Risk, communication and trust: towards an emotional understanding of trust. Public Underst Sci. 2014;23(6):703–17.
9. Kahan D, Braman D, Gastil J, Slovic P, Mertz C. Culture and identity-protective cognition: explaining the white-male effect in risk perception. J Empir Leg Stud. 2007;4(3):465–505.
10. Joffe H. Risk: from perception to social representation. Br J Soc Psychol. 2003;42(1):55–73.
11. Slovic P. The 'value' of smoking. Health Risk Soc. 2012;14(5):409–14.
12. Douglas M. Risk acceptability according to the social sciences. London: Routledge & Kegan Paul; 1986.
13. Xue W, Hine DW, Loi NM, Thorsteinsson EB, Phillips WJ. Cultural worldviews and environmental risk perceptions: a meta-analysis. J Environ Psychol. 2014;40:249–58.
14. Shi J, Visschers VHM, Siegrist M. Public perception of climate change: the importance of knowledge and cultural worldviews. Risk Anal. 2015;35(12):2183–201.
15. Thompson M, Ellis R, Wildavsky A. Cultural theory. Boulder, Colorado: Westview Press; 1990.
16. Douglas M, Wildavsky A. Risk and culture: an essay on the selection of technical and environmental dangers. Berkeley: University of California Press; 1982.
17. Kahan DM, Braman D, Cohen GL, Gastil J, Slovic P. Who fears the HPV vaccine, Who Doesn't, and Why? An experimental study of the mechanisms of cultural cognition. Law Hum Behav. 2010;34(6):501–16.
18. Fischhoff B, Lichtenstein S, Slovic P, Keeney R, Derby S. Approaches to acceptable risk : a critical guide / Baruch Fischhoff ... [et al.]; prepared by Decision Research for Oak Ridge National Laboratory under ORNL subcontract no. 7656; this work performed for U.S. Nuclear Regulatory Commission under NRC interagency agreement 40-550-75. Washinton DC: Oak Ridge National Laboratory; 1980.
19. Smith C, Skelly C, Kung N, Roberts B, Field H. Flying-fox species density–a spatial risk factor for Hendra virus infection in horses in eastern Australia. PloS One U6. 2014;9(6):1–7.
20. Halpin K, Young P, Field HE, Mackenzie JS. Isolation of Hendra virus from pteropid bats: a natural reservoir of Hendra virus. J Gen Virol. 2000;81(8):1927–32.
21. Goldspink LK, Edson DW, Vidgen ME, Bingham J, Field HE, Smith CS. Natural Hendra virus infection in flying-foxes - tissue tropism and risk factors. PLoS One. 2015;10(6):1–10.
22. Edson D, Field H, McMichael L, Vidgen M, Goldspink L, Broos A, Melville D, Kristoffersen J, de Jong C, McLaughlin A, et al. Routes of hendra virus excretion in naturally-infected flying-foxes: implications for viral transmission and spillover risk. PLoS One. 2015;10(10):1–15.
23. Martin G, Plowright R, Chen C, Kault D, Selleck P, Skerratt LF. Hendra virus survival does not explain spillover patterns and implicates relatively direct transmission routes from flying foxes to horses. J Gen Virol. 2015;96(6):1229–37.
24. Field H, Smith CS, Jong CE, Melville D, Broos A, Kung N, Thompson J, Dechmann DKN. Landscape utilisation, animal behaviour and hendra virus risk. EcoHealth. 2015;13(1):26–38.
25. Middleton D, Pallister J, Klein R, Feng Y-R, Haining J, Arkinstall R, Frazer L, Huang J-A, Edwards N, Wareing M, et al. Hendra virus vaccine, a one health approach to protecting horse, human, and environmental health. Emerg Infect Dis. 2014;20(3):372–9.
26. Government Q: Hendra Virus Information for horse owners, handlers, competitors and event organisers. In. Edited by Department of Agriculture FaF. Brisbane: Queensland Government Department of Agriculture and Fisheries; 2013.
27. Field H, Jordan D, Edson D, Morris S, Melville D, Parry-Jones K, Broos A, Divljan A, McMichael L, Davis R, et al. Spatiotemporal aspects of Hendra virus infection in pteropid bats (Flying-Foxes) in Eastern Australia. PLoS One. 2015;10(12):1–14.
28. Taylor M, Dhand NK, Toribio J-A, Wiethoelter A, Schembri N, Sawford K, Kung N, Field H, Moloney B, Wright T. Longitudinal cohort study of horse owners. HHALTER: Horse owners and Hendra Virus: A longitudinal study to evaluate risk, Final report. In.: Rural Industries Research and Development Coporation (RIRDC); 2016.
29. Kung N, McLaughlin A, Taylor M, Moloney B, Wright T, Field H. Hendra virus and horse owners – risk perception and management. PLoS One. 2013;8(11):1–9.
30. Vaughan E. Contemporary perspectives on risk perceptions, health-protective behaviors, and control of emerging infectious diseases. Int J Behav Med. 2011;18(2):83–7.
31. Bangerter A, Green E, Gilles I. Editorial introduction. Public Underst Sci. 2011;20(4):442–5.
32. Wynne B. Redefining the issues of risk and public acceptance. Futures. 1983;15(1):13–32.
33. Abraham T. Lessons from the pandemic: the need for new tools for risk and outbreak communication. 2011.
34. Ellis-Iversen J, Cook AJC, Watson E, Nielen M, Larkin L, Wooldridge M, Hogeveen H. Perceptions, circumstances and motivators that influence implementation of zoonotic control programs on cattle farms. Prev Vet Med. 2010;93(4):276–85.
35. Ochieng BJ, Hobbs JE. Incentives for cattle producers to adopt an *E. coli* vaccine: An application of best–worst scaling. Food Policy. 2016;59:78–87.
36. Browne M, Thomson P, Rockloff MJ, Pennycook G. Going against the herd: psychological and cultural factors underlying the 'vaccination confidence gap'. PLoS One. 2015;10(9):1–14.
37. Kahan D. A Risky Science Communication Environment for Vaccines. Science. 2013;342(6154):53–4.
38. Larson HJ. Understanding vaccine hesitancy around vaccines and vaccination from a global perspective: a systematic review of published literature. Vaccine. 2007–2012;32(19):2150–9.

39. Eskola J. How to deal with vaccine hesitancy? Vaccine. 2015;33(34):4215–7.
40. Hendra Virus Research Program Commissioned Projects [https://www.daf.qld.gov.au/animal-industries/animal-health-and-diseases/a-z-list/hendra-virus/intergovernmental-hendra-virus-taskforce/national-hendra-virus-research-program/commissioned-projects].
41. Braun V, Clarke V. Successful Qualitative research: a practical guide for beginners. London: SAGE Publications Ltd; 2013.
42. Buckley P, Dunn T, More SJ. Owners' perceptions of the health and performance of Pony Club horses in Australia. Prev Vet Med. 2004;63(1–2):121–33.
43. Braun V, Clarke V. Using thematic anaylsis in psychology. Qual Res Psychol. 2006;3:77–101.
44. Lanska DJ. The mad cow problem in the UK: risk perceptions, risk management, and health policy development. J Public Health Policy. 1998;19(2):160–83.
45. Leiss W, Powell D. Mad cows and Mother's milk. Quebec, Canada: McGill-Queen's University Press; 2004.
46. Cairns G, de Andrade M, MacDonald L. Reputation, relationships, risk communication, and the role of trust in the prevention and control of communicable disease: a review. J Health Commun. 2013;18(12):1550–65.
47. Permit for Equivac Hev Hendra virus vaccine for horses. http://apvma.gov.au/node/12876.
48. Field H. Hendra virus ecology and transmission. Curr Opin Virol. 2016;16:120–5.
49. Summary of adverse experience reports made to the APVMA about Hendra virus vaccine [http://apvma.gov.au/node/15786].
50. Harambam J, Aupers S. Contesting epistemic authority: Conspiracy theories on the boundaries of science. Public Underst Sci. 2015;24(4):466–80.
51. Smallman S. Whom do you trust? Doubt and conspiracy theories in the 2009 influenza pandemic. J Int Glob Stud. 2015;6(2):1–24.
52. Chong M. A crisis of epidemic proportions: What communication lessons can practitioners learn from the Singapore SARS crisis? Public Relat Q. 2006;51(1):6–11.
53. Frewer LJ, Miles S, Brennan M, Kuznesof S, Ness M, Ritson C. Public preferences for informed choice under conditions of risk uncertainty. Public Underst Sci. 2002;11(4):363–72.
54. Tversky A, Kahneman D, Slovic P. Judgment under uncertainty : heuristics and biases. New York: Cambridge University Press; 1982.
55. Field H, Young P, Yob JM, Mills J, Hall L, Mackenzie J. The natural history of Hendra and Nipah viruses. Microbes Infect. 2001;3(4):307–14.
56. Frewer LJ, Miles S. Temporal stability of the psychological determinants of trust: implications for communication about food risks. Health Risk Soc. 2003;5(3):259–71.
57. Kahan D. Ideology, motivated reasoning, and cognitive reflection. Judgment Decis Mak. 2013;8(4):407–24.
58. Rush for Hendra vaccine after death [https://au.news.yahoo.com/video/watch/17759685/rush-for-hendra-vaccine-after-death/#page1].
59. Smith CS, McLaughlin A, Field HE, Edson D, Mayer D, Ossedryver S, Barrett J, Waltisbuhl D. Twenty years of Hendra virus: laboratory submission trends and risk factors for infection in horses. Epidemiol Infect. 2016:1–8.
60. Schemann K, Firestone SM, Taylor M, Toribio JALML, Ward MP, Dhand NK. From the horse's mouth: perceptions of the management of the 2007 equine influenza outbreak in Australia. Transbound Emerg Dis. 2012;59(6):503–16.
61. Schemann K, Taylor M, Toribio JALML, Dhand NK. Horse owners' biosecurity practices following the first equine influenza outbreak in Australia. Prev Vet Med. 2011;102(4):304.
62. Taylor M, Agho KE, Stevens GJ, Raphael B. Factors influencing psychological distress during a disease epidemic: data from Australia's first outbreak of equine influenza. BMC Public Health. 2008;8(1):347–61.

13

Systemic immune response and virus persistence after foot-and-mouth disease virus infection of naïve cattle and cattle vaccinated with a homologous adenovirus-vectored vaccine

Michael Eschbaumer[1,2], Carolina Stenfeldt[1,2], Steven I. Rekant[1,2], Juan M. Pacheco[1], Ethan J. Hartwig[1], George R. Smoliga[1], Mary A. Kenney[1], William T. Golde[1], Luis L. Rodriguez[1] and Jonathan Arzt[1*]

Abstract

Background: In order to investigate host factors associated with the establishment of persistent foot-and-mouth disease virus (FMDV) infection, the systemic response to vaccination and challenge was studied in 47 steers. Eighteen steers that had received a recombinant FMDV A vaccine 2 weeks earlier and 29 non-vaccinated steers were challenged by intra-nasopharyngeal deposition of FMDV A24. For up to 35 days after challenge, host factors including complete blood counts with T lymphocyte subsets, type I/III interferon (IFN) activity, neutralizing and total FMDV-specific antibody titers in serum, as well as antibody-secreting cells (in 6 non-vaccinated animals) were characterized in the context of viral infection dynamics.

Results: Vaccination generally induced a strong antibody response. There was a transient peak of FMDV-specific serum IgM in non-vaccinated animals after challenge, while IgM levels in vaccinated animals did not increase further. Both groups had a lasting increase of specific IgG and neutralizing antibody after challenge. Substantial systemic IFN activity in non-vaccinated animals coincided with viremia, and no IFN or viremia was detected in vaccinated animals. After challenge, circulating lymphocytes decreased in non-vaccinated animals, coincident with viremia, IFN activity, and clinical disease, whereas lymphocyte and monocyte counts in vaccinated animals were unaffected by vaccination but transiently increased after challenge. The $CD4^+/CD8^+$ T cell ratio in non-vaccinated animals increased during acute infection, driven by an absolute decrease of $CD8^+$ cells.

Conclusions: The incidence of FMDV persistence was 61.5 % in non-vaccinated and 54.5 % in vaccinated animals. Overall, the systemic factors examined were not associated with the FMDV carrier/non-carrier divergence; however, significant differences were identified between responses of non-vaccinated and vaccinated cattle.

Keywords: FMDV, Vaccination, Persistence, Carrier, Flow cytometry, Lymphopenia, Interferon, ELISA, ELISPOT

* Correspondence: jonathan.arzt@ars.usda.gov
[1]United States Department of Agriculture (USDA), Plum Island Animal Disease Center (PIADC), Foreign Animal Disease Research Unit (FADRU), Agricultural Research Service (ARS), P.O. Box 848, Greenport, NY 11944, USA
Full list of author information is available at the end of the article

Background

Foot-and-mouth disease virus (FMDV; family *Picornaviridae*; genus *Aphthovirus*) causes a highly contagious, acute disease of cloven-hoofed animals, with fever, lameness, and vesicular lesions of the feet, tongue, muzzle, and teats reviewed in [1–3]. Foot-and-mouth disease (FMD) is a difficult and expensive disease to control and eradicate due to its wide host range, low minimum infectious dose, rapid rate of replication, high level of viral shedding, and multiple modes of transmission [1, 3]. The situation is further complicated by an important subclinical divergence that occurs after acute infection of ruminants: some animals remain subclinically infected for up to 3 years ("FMDV carriers") ([2], reviewed in [4, 5]), while others completely clear the virus within 1 to 2 weeks ("non-carriers"). The definition of an FMDV carrier established by the World Organisation for Animal Health (OIE) is an animal from which infectious FMDV can be recovered at greater than 28 days after infection [6].

The bovine nasopharynx [7–12] and regional lymph nodes [13] have been identified as sites of this persistence, but it is poorly understood how FMDV evades clearance by the host immune response at these sites [14]. It is also unknown whether there are pre-existent factors or patterns in the virus-host interaction during and after acute infection that can be used to predict or influence the ultimate outcome of virus clearance versus persistence.

Type I and type III interferons (IFN) are important parts of the early innate immune response to viral infection and are often crucial in controlling or eliminating infection (reviewed in [15]). All cells in the body are responsive to type I IFNs, whereas the type III IFN receptor is mostly restricted to gastrointestinal and airway epithelia [16]. Several reports have demonstrated strong IFN activity during FMDV infection in cattle using an Mx/CAT reporter system which does not differentiate between IFN type I and type III [17–22]. Using this method, type I/III IFN activity has been found in circulating plasmacytoid dendritic cells (pDCs) [18, 23] and in tissues at sites of virus replication [22]. However, it is unclear how much of the systemically detected IFN originates within the vasculature as opposed to from sites of infection in tissues.

In pigs, FMDV infection leads to lymphopenia and immune suppression, manifested as a significant loss of circulating T cells [24, 25]. Significant lymphopenia during acute FMDV infection of cattle has been described [20, 26], but other studies have reported that no changes occur in total circulating leukocytes or relative lymphocyte subpopulations [27, 28]. One report concluded that the T-cell response to mitogen and non-FMDV antigens was not impaired during acute FMDV infection, but no FMDV-specific T-cell responses were detected [28].

In earlier experiments, the depletion of $CD4^+$ cells in vivo significantly reduced neutralizing antibody titers and delayed class switching in cattle vaccinated with inactivated FMDV [29]. However, in non-vaccinated cattle, $CD4^+$ depletion before FMDV infection had no effect on clinical signs, the induction of neutralizing antibodies, or the acute clearance of virus from the circulation [27]. These and other studies have concluded that the antigenic structure of the FMDV capsid, the high local antigen concentration, and the strong cytokine response during acute infection likely are key factors in the efficient induction of T cell-independent antibody responses [29, 30].

$CD8^+$ cytotoxic T lymphocytes (CTLs) from vaccinated pigs are capable of selectively killing FMDV-infected cells in vitro [31], and infection of pigs with FMDV also leads to a clear CTL response [32]. However, in cattle, partial depletion of $CD8^+$ cells did not affect the resolution of acute FMDV infection [27]. Given that the acute phase of an FMDV infection is concluded before a significant adaptive CTL response can be mounted [28], it is likely that the control of the infection is mediated by a T-cell-independent neutralizing antibody response and type I/III interferon signaling. Overall, the role of bovine antigen-specific T cells in FMDV infection remains unresolved, and it is unclear how FMDV evades the CTL response during persistent infection.

The kinetics of circulating FMDV-specific antibody-secreting cells in the context of antibody levels and neutralizing activity have not yet been examined. FMDV infection generally elicits a rapid, strong, and lasting antibody response. Coincident with the first detection of antibody there is a rapid clearance of virus from the circulation and a more gradual reduction of virus shedding. Although circulating antibodies are generally believed to be the primary mediators of immunity after infection or vaccination [3], it is well known that vaccines prevent viremia and generalized disease, but not primary local infection, e.g., in the pharynx. Several studies have reported shedding of infectious FMDV in nasal, oral, or oropharyngeal fluids of vaccinated animals following virus exposure [10, 33–37], which is consistent with primary infection of the upper respiratory or gastrointestinal tracts. Virus replication in the nasopharyngeal mucosa of vaccinated animals in the present study has been demonstrated in a separate publication [38]. The occurrence of persistent, asymptomatic FMDV infection in vaccinated cattle [9, 10, 34, 36, 37, 39, 40] provides further unequivocal evidence that vaccination does not prevent primary infection.

Similarly, antibodies are ineffective in clearing virus from the pharynx of carrier ruminants [4], and substantial antibody levels – in serum as well as in secretions-have been reported in animals that remained persistently infected with FMDV [21, 41–43]. In vaccinated animals, protection against challenge is correlated with neutralizing antibody in circulation, but low antibody levels can also be protective [35, 44, 45] and animals with high neutralizing titers can develop disease after challenge [37].

The overarching goal of the present study was to elucidate systemic host factors associated with the response to FMDV in cattle during early and late stages of infection and to categorize these responses in the context of vaccination status and carrier-state divergence. For this purpose, serological and hematological parameters as well as lymphocyte sub-populations were investigated in vaccinated and non-vaccinated cattle from the day of FMDV vaccination and/or infection to the persistent/recovered phase. Trends associated with acute disease, vaccination, and the development of the FMDV-carrier state were examined in the context of clinical, virological, and serological data collected from the same animals.

Methods

Animals

Forty-seven Holstein steers (6 to 8 months, ~200 kg) were obtained from an experimental livestock provider (Thomas D. Morris Inc., Reisterstown, MD, USA) accredited by the Association for Assessment and Accreditation of Laboratory Animal Care International and registered with the United States Department of Agriculture (USDA). The animals were housed together in a BSL-3-Ag animal facility from the time of arrival until euthanasia, and were given an acclimation period of 2 weeks before the start of the experiment. The health status of all animals was assessed daily throughout the study period. Based on daily clinical assessments, analgesics and anti-inflammatory drugs (flunixin meglumine, 1.1–2.2 mg/kg; butorphanol tartrate, 0.1 mg/kg) were administered to mitigate pain associated with severe clinical FMD as needed. Steers were sedated with xylazine (intramuscular, 0.22 mg/kg) for inoculations and clinical exams; after the procedure, the sedation was reversed with tolazoline (intravenous, 2 mg/kg).

Vaccination

Two weeks before infection, eighteen of the 47 steers were immunized using a recently licensed recombinant FMD serotype A vaccine (USDA product code 1FM.1R0; manufactured by Antelope Valley Bios, Lincoln, NE, USA). This vaccine contains the P1-2A and 3Cpro coding regions from FMDV A24 Cruzeiro within a replication deficient human adenovirus serotype 5 vector [46]. The steers were intramuscularly injected with the product release dose in a 2 mL total volume containing commercially available adjuvant (product #7010101, VaxLiant, Lincoln, NE, USA).

Challenge infection

All animals were clinically evaluated and sampled prior to inoculation, to ensure their FMDV-free status and the absence of elevated systemic type I/III IFN levels that could interfere with initial FMDV replication. On day 0 of the experiment, all animals were inoculated with 10^5 infectious doses (titrated in bovine tongue epithelium) [6] of FMDV A_{24} Cruzeiro [47] in 2 mL of minimum essential medium (MEM) with 25 mM HEPES by intranasopharyngeal (INP) deposition [38, 48]. The successful deposition of virus was confirmed in all animals by collection of nasal and oral fluids after removal of the inoculation catheter (data not shown).

Clinical evaluation

From the day of challenge until 10 days post inoculation (dpi), clinical scores were recorded on a scale from 0 to 5 accounting for presence of FMD vesicles on each foot or anywhere on the head (oral cavity or nasal epithelia) [12]. Clinical examinations with sedation were performed daily in non-vaccinated animals and every other day in vaccinated animals, either throughout the first 10 dpi, or until the animal had reached full clinical score. Rectal body temperatures were taken every day for the entire duration of the experiment.

Euthanasia and tissue collection

A subset of study animals were euthanized at predetermined time points during acute and post-acute phases of infection (0 to 14 dpi) for detailed tissue-based pathogenesis studies which have been presented in separate publications [12, 38]. All samples and data collected before necropsy, however, are included herein. Specifically, four non-vaccinated animals were euthanized on 1 dpi, and two each on 2, 3, 4, 7, 10, and 14 dpi. Among vaccinated animals, two animals were euthanized on each of 1, 2, and 3 dpi, and one on 14 dpi (see Fig. 1). Sodium pentobarbital (intravenous, 86 mg/kg) was used for all euthanasias.

The OIE defines FMDV carriers as animals in which the virus persists for more than 28 days after infection [6]. For the animals in this study, however, it was found that the persistence status could be reliably determined by 21 dpi (see Results section for details).

Since the FMDV carrier status was not determined for animals euthanized earlier than 21 dpi, these animals were excluded from graphical and statistical analyses that discriminated animals by persistence status; however, these animals were included in all analyses that did not require their persistence status to be defined. Twenty-four out of 47 animals (13 non-vaccinated and 11 vaccinated) were kept alive beyond 21 dpi, which was determined to be the threshold at which it was possible to consistently conclude from oropharyngeal fluid samples whether an animal had

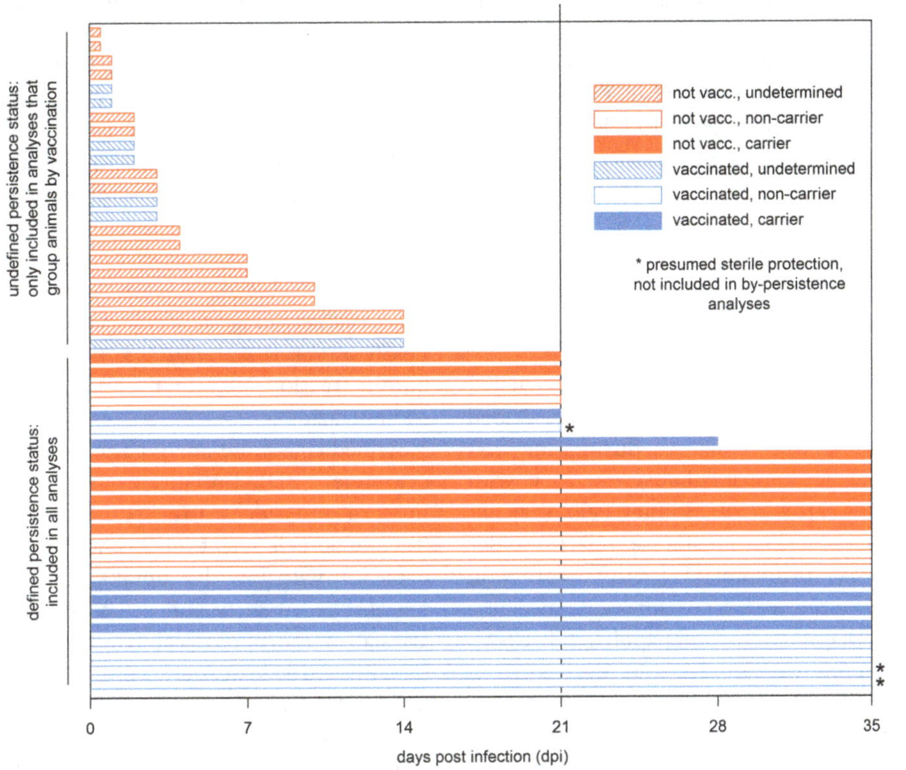

Fig. 1 Overview of the experimental timeline. Each bar represents one animal, with the length of the bar corresponding to the time the animal remained in the experiment after challenge infection (21 dpi, the revised cut-off by which FMDV persistence status could be determined, is marked by a *vertical line*). Non-vaccinated animals are shown in *red*, vaccinated animals in *blue*. *Solid-colored bars* are FMDV carriers, *unfilled bars* are non-carriers. *Striped bars* are used when the persistence status of an animal could not be determined because it was euthanized before 21 dpi. Asterisks mark the three animals without convincing evidence of infection (see Results section for details)

cleared the infection or entered the FMDV carrier state. With the exception of three vaccinated animals in which infection could not be confirmed (see Results section for details), all animals that were kept alive to 21 dpi or longer were included in all analyses.

Blood and probang samples

Blood was collected from the jugular vein on the day of vaccination (immediately before), on days 4 and 7 post-vaccination (dpv), on the day of challenge (immediately before), then daily for the first ten dpi and afterwards weekly until 35 dpi. Samples were collected in BD Vacutainer® tubes containing either K_2EDTA for hematology, heparin for PBMC separation, or serum-separator gel. Starting on 7 dpi (21 dpv) in vaccinated animals and 14 dpi in non-vaccinated animals, oropharyngeal fluids (OPF) were collected by probang cup [49] two times per week. Probang cup contents were mixed with an equal volume of cold MEM with 25 mM HEPES immediately after collection and then kept on ice. Upon arrival in the laboratory, serum tubes were centrifuged for harvesting (10 min at 1000 × g and 4 °C), and OPF samples were immediately processed as described previously [10], including treatment with 1,1,2-trichlorofluoroethane (TTE) to reactivate antibody-bound virus [50].

The PBMC preparation, surface marker staining, and flow cytometric data collection have been described previously [51]. Briefly, for separation of PBMCs, 18 mL of fresh heparinized blood were diluted in Dulbecco's phosphate-buffered saline (PBS; Life Technologies, Carlsbad, CA, USA), underlaid with Histopaque® 1083 (Sigma-Aldrich, St. Louis, MO, USA), and centrifuged. Harvested PBMCs were washed twice with PBS, counted, and resuspended at a concentration of 10^7 cells/mL in either fetal bovine serum (FBS; GE Healthcare Life Sciences, Logan, UT, USA) with 10 % (v/v) dimethyl sulfoxide (Sigma-Aldrich) for freezing (for flow cytometry) or in ELISPOT media (RPMI-1640 with antibiotics, 0.1 mM non-essential amino acids, 2 mM L-glutamine, 10 mM HEPES, 1 mM sodium pyruvate [all Life Technologies], and 10 % FBS) for immediate use. Frozen cells were stored at −70 °C for no longer than thirty days before flow cytometry analysis.

FMDV RNA detection and virus isolation

Real-time RT-PCR and virus isolation for FMDV detection in serum and OPF were performed as previously described

[52]. Briefly, FMDV viral RNA was quantified by real-time RT-PCR targeting the 3D region of the FMDV genome [53] with forward and reverse primers adapted from Rasmussen et al. [54]. Samples with cycle threshold (C_t) values lower than 45 were considered positive. Serial 10-fold dilutions of in vitro synthesized FMDV RNA of known concentration were used to convert C_t values to FMDV RNA genome copy numbers (GCN) per mL of sample. After the conversion, the cut-off C_t value corresponded to a detection limit of 1.57 $\log_{10}$ FMDV GCN/mL.

Type I/III IFN bioassay

Type I/III IFN activity in serum was quantified using the Mx/CAT reporter assay as previously described [22]. Briefly, serum samples collected during the first 10 days after challenge were incubated for 24 h with recombinant Madin-Darby bovine kidney cells that express chloramphenicol acetyltransferase (CAT) under the control of an Mx1 promoter [17]. CAT expression in the cells was measured with a commercially available ELISA kit (Roche Diagnostics, Indianapolis, IN, USA), and IFN levels in unknown samples were derived from a standard curve of serial dilutions of recombinant human interferon-α 2a with known potency (PBL Assay Science, Piscataway, NJ, USA) that was run in parallel. Results are reported as international units (IU) of IFN per mL of serum. The Mx/CAT assay does not distinguish between type I and type III interferon [20].

Hematology

For each whole blood sample from all animals, a complete blood count (CBC) was performed on the same day with a Hemavet 950FS veterinary hematology system (Drew Scientific, Waterbury, CT, USA), following the manufacturer's instructions. High and low values were flagged by the analyzer based on factory-set normal limits. Among the blood parameters reported by the analyzer, only the total white blood cell (WBC) count and its principal components are reported here (in 1000 s [K] of cells per μL of blood). The WBC count is the sum of five subpopulations, with neutrophils, lymphocytes, and monocytes together comprising over 90 % of all circulating white blood cells [55]. The bovine reference ranges are 600 to 4000 neutrophils, 2500 to 7500 lymphocytes, and 0 to 900 monocytes per μL of blood [56].

Flow cytometry

PBMCs from all animals were evaluated by flow cytometry. Cells were thawed in a water bath at 37 °C, slowly diluted in warm RPMI-1640 media with 10 % FBS, and washed twice with PBS [57]. All samples were stained in duplicate; first with an amine-reactive dye (LIVE/DEAD® Fixable Yellow; Life Technologies), then with monoclonal antibodies against bovine CD3 (MM1A, IgG_1, Washington State University, Pullman, WA, USA), the δ chain of the γδ T cell receptor (GB21A, IgG_{2b}, Washington State University), CD4 (CC8, IgG_{2a}, conjugated with FITC, Bio-Rad, Hercules, CA, USA), and CD8 (CC63, IgG_{2a}, Alexa Fluor® 647, Bio-Rad), and finally with polyclonal goat antibodies against murine IgG_1 (allophycocyanin-cyanine7; SouthernBiotech, Birmingham, AL, USA) and IgG_{2b} (R-phycoerythrin; SouthernBiotech). Compensation controls and fluorescence-minus-one controls were included for each antibody/dye combination. After each staining step, cells were washed twice in cold FACS buffer (PBS with 0.3 % [v/v] bovine serum albumin fraction V [Life Technologies] and 0.1 % [w/v] sodium azide).

Stained cells were analyzed in a three-laser LSR II flow cytometer (BD). Initially, events were gated based on forward and side scatter, equal pulse height/area ratio (for single-cell selection), as well as live/dead staining behavior, with low dye uptake considered indicative of membrane integrity and cell viability [58]. The boundaries of a morphological lymphocyte gate (defined by forward and side scatter) were established by backgating from CD3. Among all live cells in that gate, T lymphocytes were then identified by $CD3^+$ staining. At least 10000 $CD3^+$ cells were evaluated per sample. $CD3^+$ $\gamma\delta TCR^-$cells were presumed to be αβ T lymphocytes, and were examined for CD4 and CD8 expression. All surface marker gating was done automatically with "snap to" interval gates in single-parameter histograms in BD FACSDiva 8.

The flow cytometer only measures the relative quantities (percent abundance) of T lymphocyte subsets but does not provide absolute cell counts. Because percent abundance can be misleading when assessing the change in a population of cells over different experimental conditions [59], the flow cytometry and hematology data were combined [60] to obtain absolute counts of the $CD4^+$ and $CD8^+$ αβ T lymphocyte subpopulations. The absolute number of cells in each subpopulation was calculated based on the complete blood count obtained with the Hemavet analyzer as described by Riondato et al. [61]. Briefly, the total lymphocyte counts per mL of peripheral blood were assigned to the morphological lymphocyte gate on the flow cytometer. Absolute numbers for the subpopulations were then obtained by serially applying the percentage-of-parent values to this total count, beginning with the CD3 gate. Absolute counts are reported as number of cells per μL of blood.

Humoral immunity

All animals that survived for at least 21 days after challenge were included in the serological analyses; animals that were euthanized at earlier time points were not included.

Serum neutralization test (SNT)

FMDV-neutralizing antibody titers were determined for serum samples taken at − 14 and − 7 dpi (vaccinated animals only; 0 and 7 dpv, respectively), and at 0, 7, 14, 21, 28, and 35 dpi for all animals. Sera were heat inactivated for 30 min at 56 °C and used in a microtiter neutralization assay. Serial fourfold dilutions of serum (in MEM with 25 mM HEPES) on 96-well plates (from an initial dilution of 1/8 down to 1/32768) were incubated with 100 50 % tissue culture infective doses ($TCID_{50}$) of FMDV A24 Cruzeiro for 1 h at 37 °C and 5 % CO_2. Freshly trypsinized LFBK-αVβ6 cells [62, 63] were resuspended in MEM with 25 mM HEPES, 4×10^4 cells/well were added to the plates, and the plates were incubated for another 72 h at 37 °C and 5 % CO_2. After microscopic evaluation of cell monolayers, the plates were treated with crystal violet dissolved in tissue fixative (HistoChoice®; AMRESCO, Solon, OH, USA), then washed and air-dried before cytopathic effect was again evaluated visually. Titers were calculated as the reciprocal of the highest dilution of serum that fully neutralized the virus in 50 % of replicate wells.

FMDV-specific antibody ELISAs

Serum samples were collected on days − 14, −10, −7 (vaccinated animals only), 0 to 10, 14, and 21 after challenge infection and were used without prior heat inactivation. An indirect double antibody sandwich ELISA was developed for the detection of FMDV-specific IgM and IgG in serum. Optimal concentrations of reagents were determined by checkerboard titration. Each reagent was added at a volume of 100 µl per well, except where indicated. All incubations were at 37 °C for an hour, shaking, except where indicated. All washes were performed four times with PBST, 300 µl per well. All dilutions were performed in blocking buffer (BB, 10 % normal horse serum in PBST) except where indicated. Immulon 2HB plates (Thermo Scientific) were coated with anti-FMDV-A polyclonal rabbit serum (Pirbright Institute, Pirbright, United Kingdom) at a dilution of 1/1000 in fresh carbonate/bicarbonate buffer (0.05 M, pH 9.6, Sigma-Aldrich) by incubation overnight at 4 °C. After washing, plates were incubated with 200 µl per well of BB. After emptying plates, they were incubated with positive and negative (made by BEI inactivation of mock- and virus-infected cells) antigen preparations that were added to negative and positive columns, respectively. After washing, serum samples were added at a dilution of 1/100 for IgM detection, 100 µL each on negative- and positive-antigen coated wells. The same was true for IgG detection, but at a dilution of 1/500. In each plate, standard positive and negative sera were included. The standard negative serum was obtained from animals that were FMDV-antibody free. Standard positive sera were chosen during the initial phase of the development of the assays because of their high titer and high maximum absorbance value. After incubation and washing, the bound bovine antibodies were detected using sheep anti-bovine IgM or sheep anti-bovine IgG heavy chain directly conjugated to horseradish peroxidase (A10-101P or A10-118P, respectively; Bethyl Laboratories, Inc., Montgomery, Texas). After incubation and washing, ELISA was completed by addition of substrate solution (SureBlue peroxidase substrate, Kirkegaard & Perry Laboratories [KPL], Gaithersburg, MD, USA) and stopped after 10 min at room temperature by addition of 50 µl/well of stop solution (BlueStop; KPL). Absorbance was measured with an ELx808 microplate reader (BioTek, Winooski, VT, USA) using a 630-nm filter. For each sample, a net OD was calculated by subtracting the reading of the negative-antigen well from the positive-antigen well. For each plate, the net ODs of test samples were then divided by the net OD of the positive control sample on the same plate. Identical aliquots of the same positive control were used for all plates, and results are reported as fractions of the net OD of the positive control (nFPC). To further correct for non-specific reactivity, the nFPC value of the sample taken on the day of first exposure to FMDV (either vaccination or challenge) was subtracted from the nFPC values of all subsequent samples of the same animal.

FMDV-specific B-cell ELISPOT

FMDV-specific antibody-secreting-cell counts from six non-vaccinated animals that survived until 35 dpi were obtained by ELISPOT. Filter plates (EMD Millipore) were coated with monoclonal antibodies against bovine IgM (IL-A30; 1/1000), IgG_1 (IL-A60; 1/500) or IgG_2 (IL-A74; 1/25) (International Livestock Research Institute, Nairobi, Kenya) diluted in fresh carbonate/bicarbonate buffer (0.05 M, pH 9.6, Sigma-Aldrich), incubated overnight at 4 °C, and washed and blocked with ELISPOT media (supplemented RPMI-1640 with 12 % horse serum). Fresh PBMCs were serially diluted in ELISPOT media, and 5×10^5, 2.5×10^5 and 1.25×10^5 cells from each sample were seeded in duplicate wells on the same plate, together with a media-only control. After overnight incubation at 37 °C with 5 % CO_2 and thorough washing with PBS with 0.1 % polysorbate (TWEEN®) 20 (PBST) in an automated plate washer, biotinylated FMDV A24 Cruzeiro antigen (1/500 in PBST) was added to the plates. After a 1-h incubation at room temperature and further washing, HRP-conjugated neutravidin was added at a dilution of 1/1000 (in PBST), and the plates were incubated for 1 h at room temperature and washed again. Captured FMDV antigen was visualized with TrueBlue peroxidase substrate (KPL) and spots were counted with an ImmunoSpot Analyzer (Cellular Technology Limited, Shaker Heights, OH, USA). Spot counts were normalized to the total input of PBMCs, and the IgM count as well as the combined IgG_1 and IgG_2 counts were used for comparison with the FMDV antibody ELISA results.

Statistical analysis of hematology and flow cytometry data

For data analysis, animals were grouped by vaccination or persistence status. Twenty-four animals remained for at least 3 weeks after challenge and were classified as FMDV carriers or non-carriers based on virus isolation results from TTE-treated probang samples. Data were graphed and analyzed with Excel (Microsoft, Redmond, WA, USA) and the R statistical environment [64], particularly the *ggplot2* package [65]. Group means are generally annotated with their 95 % confidence intervals (CI95) to facilitate visual comparisons between groups. For group sizes of 3 or fewer, or where between-group comparisons are not meaningful, standard deviations are shown instead.

The hematology and flow cytometry data were analyzed in R with linear mixed-effects models as implemented in *lme4* [66], using the *car, phia,* and *lsmeans* packages for post-hoc analyses of specific linear combinations of factor levels. Two models were built for each outcome variable (white blood cells, neutrophils, lymphocytes, monocytes for hematology, and $CD3^+$, $CD3^+$ $\gamma\delta TCR^-CD4^+$, $CD3^+\gamma\delta TCR^-CD8^+$ for flow cytometry), one with only vaccination status, time, and their interaction term as fixed effects, and another that additionally included persistence status and all interactions between the main effects. This dual approach was chosen because information on persistence status was only available for half of the animals in the study. Animal ID was included as a random effect in all models. For flow cytometry outcome variables, intercepts and slopes were allowed to vary between animals (random intercept and slope), whereas hematology models only had random intercepts.

Where an initial ANOVA (Type II Wald chi-square tests) found significant interactions between status (by vaccination or persistence) and time after infection, pairwise contrasts for the levels of the status factor (vaccination or persistence) were evaluated for each level of the time factor – i.e., difference between vaccinated/non-vaccinated or persistent/non-persistent for each day. Changes in an outcome variable over time were evaluated with custom contrasts (e.g., dpi1 - dpi0) for each level of a status factor; similarly, the effect of time alone was evaluated by averaging across both levels of the status factor and applying the custom contrasts. *P*-values from linear hypothesis tests on the models are reported approximately; any p-value <0.05 was considered significant.

For the association between viremia and type I/III IFN activity in serum, the test statistic was calculated using Pearson's product moment correlation coefficient. The asymptotic 95 % confidence interval is based on Fisher's Z transform.

The difference between absolute $CD4^+$ and $CD8^+$ $\alpha\beta$ T cell counts in non-vaccinated animals before and after challenge (0 vs. 5 dpi) was evaluated with a paired t-test. The variance was estimated separately for both groups and the Satterthwaite approximation to the degrees of freedom was used. Exact p-values are reported for the t-test.

Results

FMDV carrier/non-carrier divergence

The overarching goal of this work was to investigate systemic trends associated with 2 categorical factors: vaccination status at the start of the experiment and FMDV carrier status determined at the end of the study. Animals are defined and stratified as "carrier", "non-carrier", or "undetermined" for the entire study based on their final status at the end of the experiment (Fig. 1).

The OIE defines FMDV carriers as animals in which the virus persists for more than 28 days after infection [6]. In the present study, however, all probang samples from non-carriers were virus-negative by 21 dpi and remained negative, whereas all animals that were virus-positive in their 21-dpi probangs remained virus-positive until 28 dpi and beyond; there was no change in viral shedding in probangs in any animal between 21 dpi and the end of the experiment. Thus, for the purposes of this study, FMDV persistence was defined by sustained detection of infectious FMDV in probang samples until at least 21 dpi, or until the day of necropsy, whichever was later. Using this definition, 8 out of 13 non-vaccinated animals (61.5 %) which had survived until or past 21 dpi were determined to be persistently infected carriers, whereas 5 out of 13 non-vaccinated animals (38.5 %) had successfully cleared the infection. Of 11 vaccinated animals, 6 were carriers (54.5 %) and 5 non-carriers (45.5 %). Animals that were euthanized before 21 dpi were assigned an "undetermined" persistence status.

The vaccinated non-carrier group was further segregated into two distinct categories based on the observation that three animals lacked convincing virological evidence of infection. All vaccinated non-carrier animals were similar in that there was no detectable viral RNA or infectious virus in OPF, nor was any infectious virus found in tissue samples taken at necropsy. However, two out of the five vaccinated non-carriers had FMDV RNA in nasopharyngeal tissues at 21 or 35 dpi, indicating previous infection, while the other three did not [12]. Additionally, the three tissue-RNA-negative cattle did not seroconvert against FMDV non-structural proteins, while all other vaccinated and non-vaccinated non-carriers did (not shown). Taken together, this was considered an indication of possible sterile protection, and on this basis, the animals were treated separately and not included with the other non-carriers except for the total count. Specifically, these animals were included in all analyses that stratify animals by vaccination status but were excluded from all analyses that stratify animals by persistence status.

Clinical disease, viremia, and type I/III IFN response

All non-vaccinated steers developed moderate to severe clinical FMD after virus exposure (Fig. 2a). Characteristic lesions were seen in and around the mouth, including vesicles on the tongue and dental pad as well as on the skin around nostrils and lips. Foot lesions, including vesicles in the interdigital clefts and on coronary bands were often accompanied by moderate lameness. Vesicular lesions first appeared between 2 and 6 dpi (generally on the first day after the onset of detectable viremia) and resolved within approximately 10 days. None of the vaccinated steers developed clinical FMD after challenge (Fig. 2b).

Viremia (defined by presence of viral RNA in serum) was detected in all non-vaccinated steers after virus challenge. The earliest detection of FMDV RNA occurred between 1 and 5 dpi (mean time to initial detection: 3 days), with levels again declining below assay detection limits after four to six days of detection. The peak of mean viremia (6.7 $\log_{10}$ FMDV GCN/mL) across all non-vaccinated animals occurred on 5 dpi. Viremia and type I/III IFN activity in serum were significantly correlated ($r = 0.53$ [0.37; 0.66], $p < 0.01$), and peak viremia coincided with peak type I/III IFN activity (Fig. 2a). No difference was seen in clinical disease, the magnitude of the IFN response, or the level of viremia between the groups of animals that subsequently diverged into carriers and non-carriers. FMDV RNA was not detected in sera of any of the vaccinated steers at any time, and there was no detectable type I/III IFN activity in the serum of

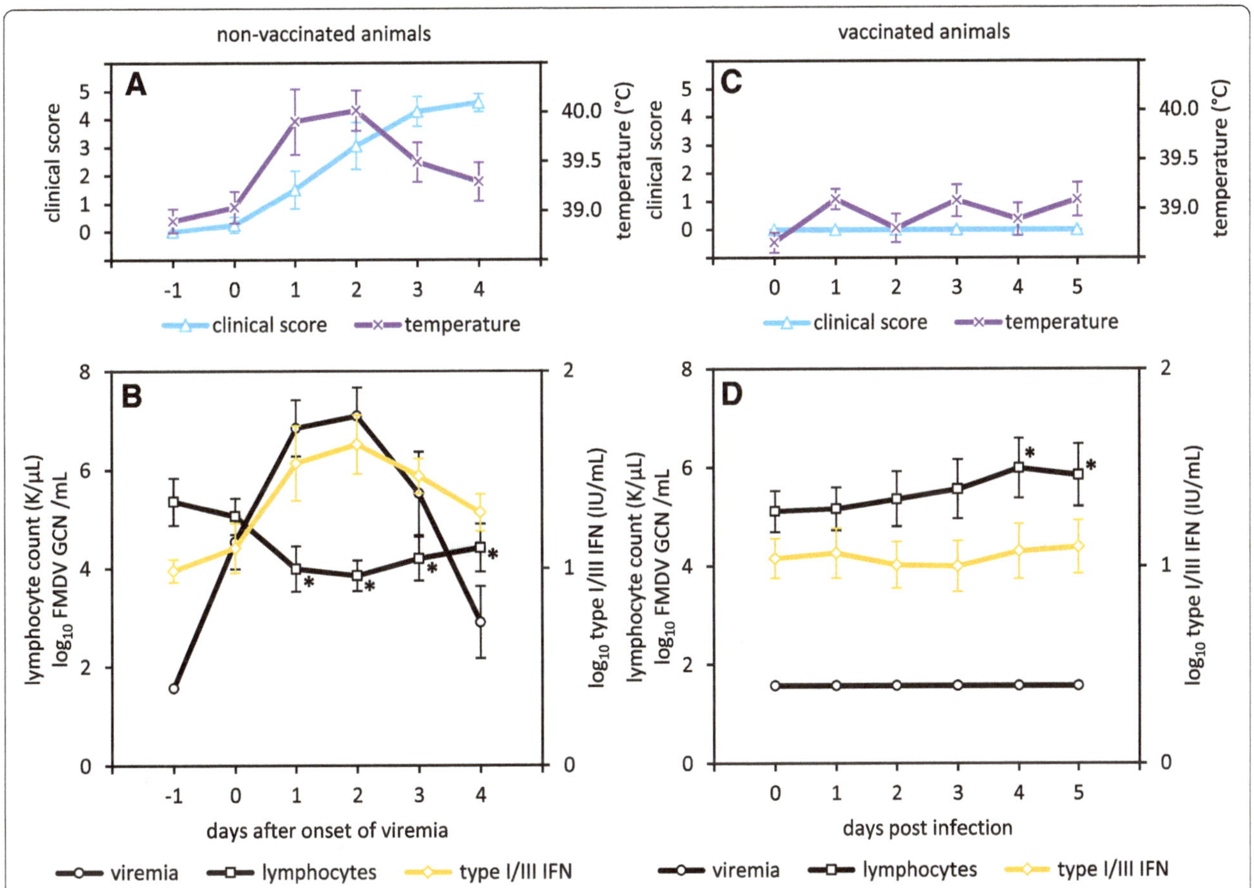

Fig. 2 Lymphopenia during acute FMDV infection. **a/b** non-vaccinated animals, **c/d** vaccinated animals. Mean lymphocyte counts (*black* squares), viral load (*red* circles), and type I/III IFN response (*gold* diamonds) in peripheral blood (**b/d**), as well as rectal temperature (*purple* crosses) and cumulative clinical score (*blue* triangles) (**a/c**) are shown with 95 % confidence intervals. The group means for non-vaccinated animals were calculated after individual timescales had been adjusted so that the onset of viremia coincided for all animals (0: first day of viremia). Asterisks mark days on which mean lymphocyte counts were significantly different from the initial value in the fitted model. The limit of detection for the FMDV real-time RT-PCR is 1.6 $\log_{10}$ FMDV GCN/mL

vaccinated animals after challenge (Fig. 2b). The Mx/CAT assay does not distinguish between type I and type III interferon [20]; hence it was not determined whether the observed interferon response was mediated by type I or type III interferon or both.

Hematology: vaccinated vs. non-vaccinated animals

No hematological changes were observed after vaccination, and the two groups (vaccinated and non-vaccinated) did not differ in any cell population in the complete blood count prior to challenge (Fig. 3). All further comparisons are made relative to the day of challenge. After challenge, the mean total WBC count decreased in non-vaccinated animals, while it increased in vaccinated animals. Neither change was significant within the groups, but the difference between non-vaccinated animals and vaccinated animals was significant between 4 and 10 dpi ($p < 0.05$) (Fig. 3a). Lymphocyte counts diverged starting at 4 dpi, with vaccinated steers having significantly higher counts than non-vaccinated steers ($p < 0.05$) (Fig. 3c). This separation was maintained throughout the early phase of the experiment (until 9 dpi). Within the vaccinated population, mean lymphocyte counts were significantly increased over pre-challenge levels (0 dpi) on 4 and 5 dpi and again from 7 to 9 dpi ($p < 0.05$). Lymphocyte counts were significantly decreased in non-vaccinated animals from 4 to 8 and on 10 dpi (Fig. 3c). The decrease in circulating lymphocytes closely followed the increase in viremia and type I/III IFN activity in serum detected in this group (Fig. 2). All group means were within established reference ranges for cattle; thus, the changes in lymphocyte quantities are indicative of relative lymphocytosis (in

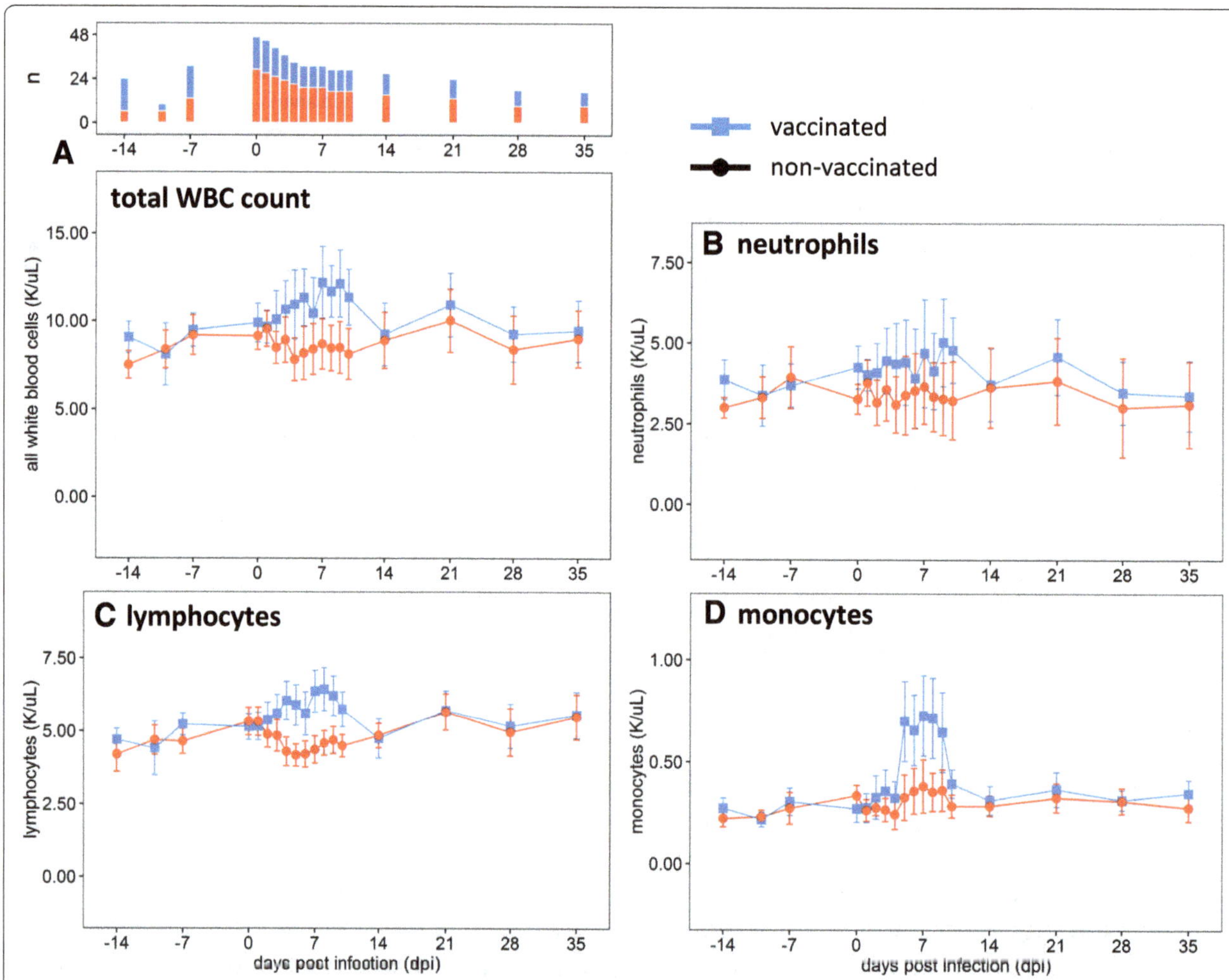

Fig. 3 White blood cell subpopulations in vaccinated and non-vaccinated steers. **a** Total WBC count. **b** Neutrophils. **c** Lymphocytes. **d** Monocytes. Animals were assigned to groups based on their FMDV vaccination status, without regard to their persistence status. Vaccinated animals have *blue lines* and *squares*, and non-vaccinated animals have *red lines* and *circles*. The plots show the group means with 95 % confidence intervals. The upper part of panel **a** shows the number of animals (n) that contributed data for each time point; this number is the same for all panels. All 47 animals contribute data to the 0-dpi group means; as animals are being euthanized beginning on 1 dpi, the size of each group decreases

vaccinated animals) and relative lymphopenia (in non-vaccinated animals) after challenge.

Similar to the mean lymphocyte counts, mean monocyte counts varied by vaccination status and time after infection. Mean monocyte counts in non-vaccinated steers were not significantly different over the course of the experiment. Vaccinated steers, however, had relative monocytosis from 5 to 9 dpi (p <0.05) (Fig. 3d). Six individual animals exceeded the threshold for absolute monocytosis at least once, but the group means did not. The three vaccinated animals (out of 18) that lacked definitive evidence of local virus replication did not have increased monocyte counts (not shown).

Mean neutrophil counts did not differ significantly between vaccinated and non-vaccinated steers, nor did they vary significantly over the course of infection (Fig. 3b).

Hematology: FMDV carriers vs. non-carriers

FMDV persistence status did not correlate with differences in total WBC count or any of its subpopulations. Carrier and non-carrier steers had similar mean hematological parameters over the course of infection (Fig. 4). Non-carrier steers had slightly higher mean lymphocyte counts from 3 to 10 dpi, but there was no statistically significant difference (p > 0.05). Overall, the observed hematological differences were more substantively associated with vaccination status than with persistence status.

In Fig. 3, animals are assigned to groups based on their FMDV vaccination status, without regard to their persistence status, whereas in Fig. 4, they are assigned to groups based on their FMDV persistence status, without regard to their vaccination status. A set of charts showing the hematology data stratified by vaccination and persistence

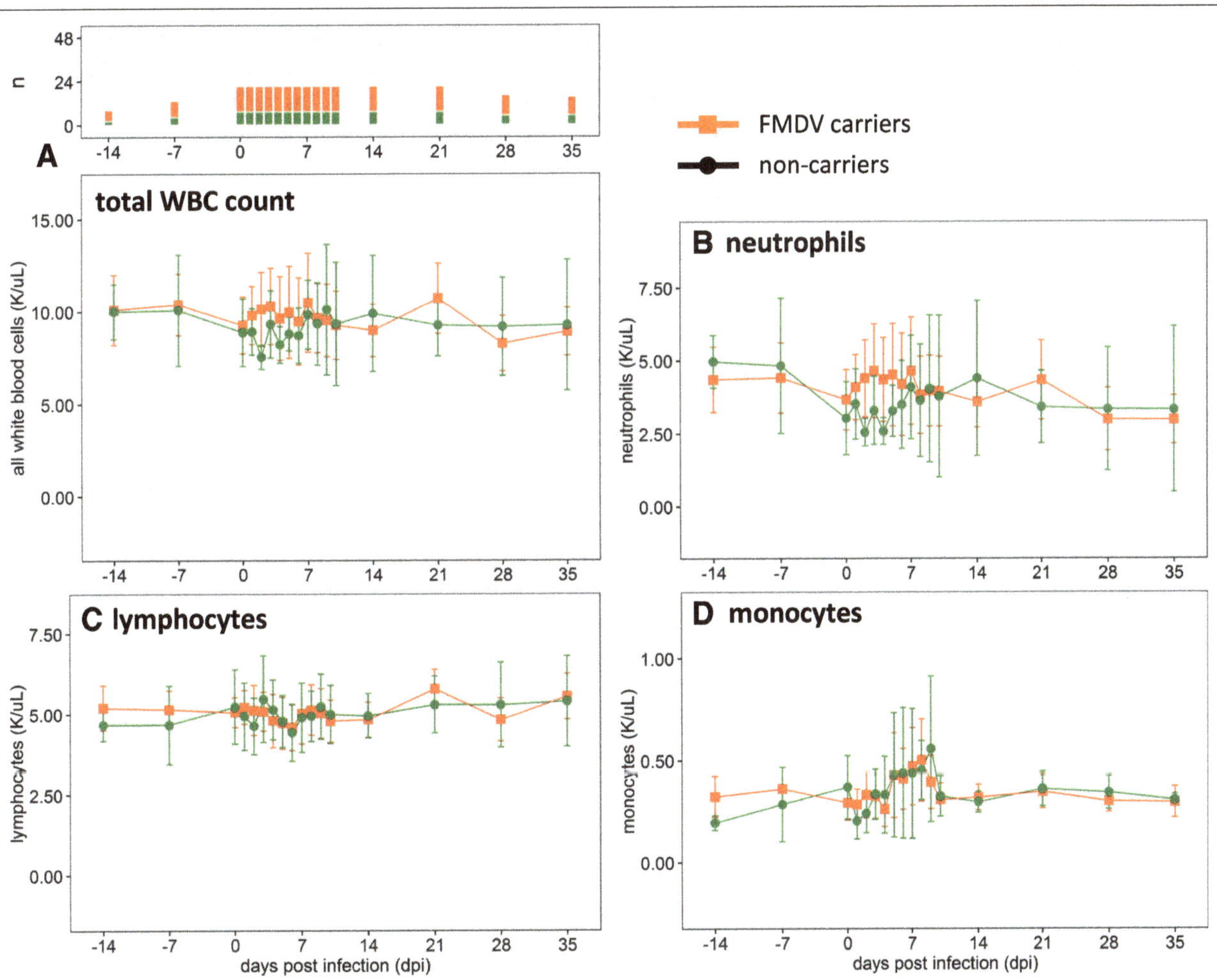

Fig. 4 White blood cell subpopulations in carriers and non-carriers. **a** Total WBC count. **b** Neutrophils. **c** Lymphocytes. **d** Monocytes. Animals were assigned to groups based on their FMDV persistence status, without regard to their vaccination status. Persistently infected FMDV carrier animals have *orange lines* and *squares*, and non-carriers have *green lines* and *circles*. The plots show the group means with 95 % confidence intervals. The upper part of panel **a** shows the number of animals (n) that contributed data for each time point; this number is consistent for all panels. The number of animals contributing data to each time point is stable between 0 and 21 dpi

status at the same time is included as Additional file 1: Figure S1 in the online version of this article.

Flow cytometry: Vaccinated vs. non-vaccinated animals

Serial examinations of phenotypic characteristics of PBMCs from forty-seven steers were performed on up to 22 samples per animal by staining in duplicate and evaluating by flow cytometry. The mean coefficent of variation between replicates of the same sample was less than 3 %.

The relative size of the $CD3^+$ population within the morphological lymphocyte gate (forward and side scatter) was variable over time, and trended lower in non-vaccinated animals after challenge. There was a significant difference between vaccinated and non-vaccinated animals on 4 and 5 dpi (p <0.05; not shown).

Based on relative percentage-of-parent values, the $CD4^+$ and $CD8^+$ αβ T cell subpopulations in vaccinated animals did not change significantly after challenge, but there was a significant increase of $CD4^+$ αβ T cells and a corresponding decrease of $CD8^+$ αβ T cells in non-vaccinated animals from 3 to 6 dpi (compared to day 0; p <0.05 for all 4 days, Fig. 5a, b). For each subpopulation, the difference between vaccinated and non-vaccinated animals was significant for the same time period (3 to 6 dpi, p <0.05). The $CD4^+/CD8^+$ ratio in non-vaccinated animals transiently increased from 3.2 at the day of challenge to 4.0 on 5 dpi, while it slightly decreased (from 3.3 to 3.1) in vaccinated animals.

In order to translate relative population measures obtained by flow cytometry to absolute counts, the percentage-of-parent values from the flow cytometry analysis were applied to the lymphocyte counts obtained with the hematology analyzer. When this conversion was performed, the increase in total circulating lymphocytes (compared to the day of challenge) of up to 25 % in vaccinated animals (Fig. 3c) had greater influence than the relative differences between vaccinated and non-vaccinated animals that have been described above. Thus, absolute quantities of both $CD4^+$ as well as $CD8^+$ αβ T cells were significantly higher in PBMCs of vaccinated steers than in non-vaccinated steers (p <0.05) from 2 to 10 dpi (Fig. 5c, d).

The absolute decrease (compared to the day of challenge) of the total lymphocyte count in non-vaccinated animals also influenced the counts of the $CD4^+$ and $CD8^+$ αβ T cell subpopulations. In relative terms, $CD4^+$ αβ T cells had been transiently increased in non-vaccinated

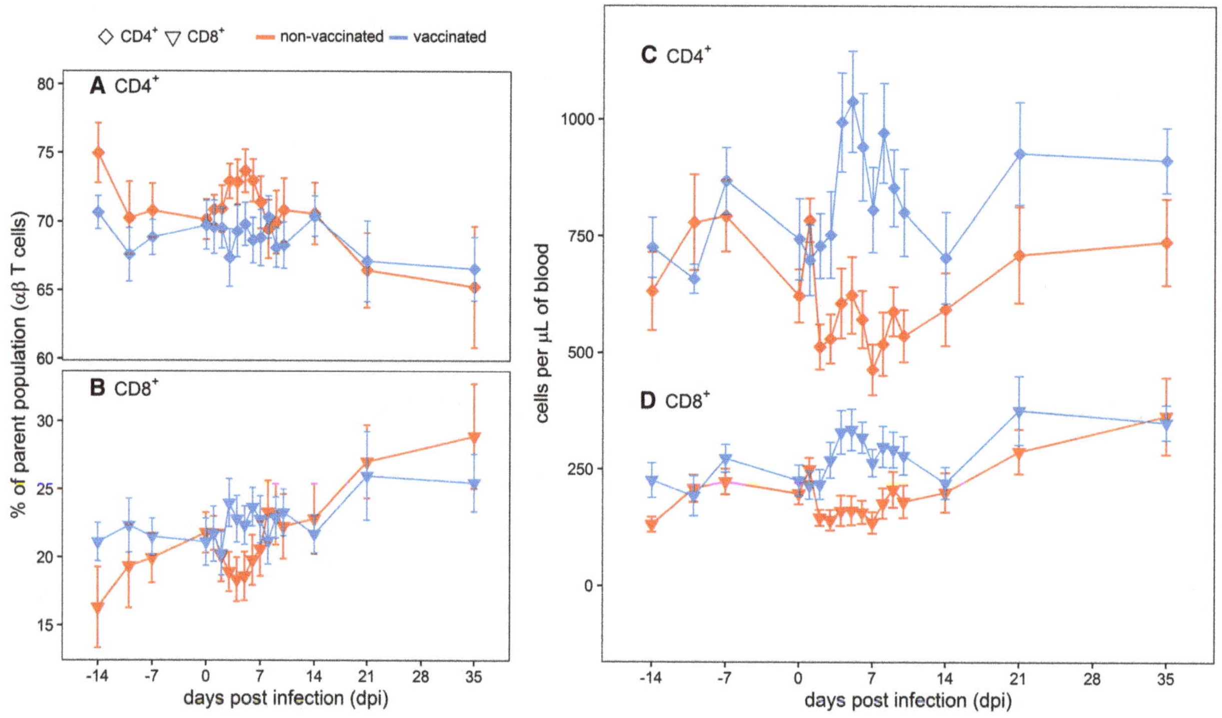

Fig. 5 $CD4^+$ and $CD8^+$ αβ T cells in vaccinated and non-vaccinated animals. Panels **a** and **b** show percentage values relative to the $CD3^+$ αβ T cell parent population, and panels C and D show absolute cell counts per μL of blood obtained by a dual-platform method. Group means ($CD4^+$: diamonds, $CD8^+$: triangles) are annotated with their 95 % confidence intervals, non-vaccinated animals are shown in *red* and vaccinated animals in *blue*. Based on relative percentage-of-parent values, there was a significant increase of $CD4^+$ αβ T cells (panel **a**) and a corresponding decrease of $CD8^+$ αβ T cells (**b**) in non-vaccinated animals. Translated to absolute counts, the increase in total circulating lymphocytes of up to 25 % in vaccinated animals had greater influence than the relative differences between vaccinated and non-vaccinated animals. Thus, absolute quantities of both $CD4^+$ (**c**) as well as $CD8^+$ αβ T cells (**d**) were significantly higher in PBMCs of vaccinated steers than in non-vaccinated steers

animals, while $CD8^+$ αβ T cells had shown a complementary decrease (Fig. 5a, b). The relative increase in $CD4^+$ cells partially counteracted the total decrease in lymphocytes, whereas the decrease in $CD8^+$ cells became more pronounced once absolute counts were taken into account (Fig. 5c, d). Absolute $CD4^+$ cell counts during acute infection fluctuated substantially more than $CD8^+$ counts (Fig. 5c, d). On day 5 after infection, the day with the largest $CD4^+/CD8^+$ ratio (4.0, see above) as well as the nadir of the lymphocyte count in non-vaccinated animals (Fig. 3c), the absolute $CD8^+$ cell count in non-vaccinated animals was reduced by approximately 20 % compared to day 0 (166 ± 34 vs. 202 ± 30 per μL of blood; means and CI95, $p = 0.03$), while the absolute $CD4^+$ count was similar to the initial level (624 ± 85 vs. 619 ± 66, $p = 0.91$).

Flow cytometry: FMDV carriers vs. non-carriers

There were no significant differences between carrier and non-carrier animals in the kinetics of any T cell population investigated herein, independent of whether vaccinated and non-vaccinated animals were analyzed together or separately, and independent of the measurement scale (relative or absolute).

FMDV-specific humoral immune response

In vaccinated animals, no FMDV-specific antibodies were detected at 4 dpv (by ELISA only; the 4-dpv sample was not tested in the SNT), but all vaccinated animals had developed FMDV-specific IgM and IgG by 7 dpv, and most had detectable neutralizing antibody at the day of challenge (14 dpv; Fig. 6).

All vaccinated animals had detectable FMDV-specific IgM on the day of challenge. Vaccinated animals that went on to become FMDV carriers maintained their pre-challenge FMDV IgM levels for the duration of the study, whereas FMDV-specific IgM in vaccinated animals that did not become persistently infected was markedly reduced by 7 dpi (see boxes in Fig. 6a, b). In contrast, FMDV-specific IgM in serum from non-vaccinated animals was first detected on day 5 after challenge. Levels increased quickly over the next few days and peaked on 9 dpi. In carriers and non-carriers IgM then declined steadily until the end of the experiment, but remained detectable throughout.

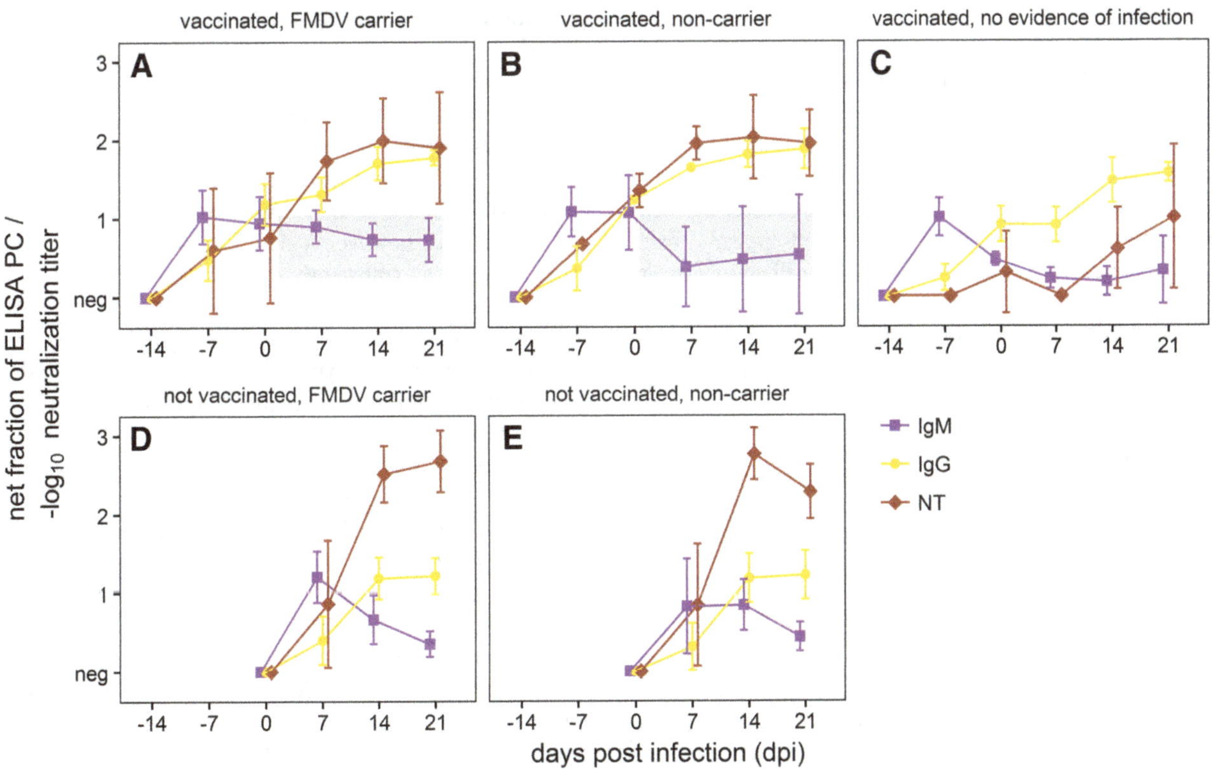

Fig. 6 Serological response to FMDV vaccination and challenge. Animals are grouped by vaccination status ("vaccinated", "not vaccinated") and FMDV persistence status ("carrier", "non-carrier", or "no evidence of infection" for vaccinated non-carriers without virological evidence of FMDV replication after challenge). Each panel shows group means with standard deviation for one combination of the two categories. In all five panels, *purple lines with square* markers show FMDV-specific IgM levels, *golden lines with round markers* show FMDV-specific IgG and *maroon lines with diamond markers* show FMDV A24 neutralization titers. The *gray boxes* highlight the potentially different post-challenge IgM kinetics in vaccinated carriers and non-carriers (see text). PC = positive control

After the first detection on 7 dpv, FMDV-specific IgG in vaccinated animals increased steadily until 14 dpi. All vaccinated animals had detectable FMDV-specific IgG on the day of challenge. In non-vaccinated animals, specific IgG was first detectable on 6 dpi and rose quickly until 14 dpi. After 14 dpi, the levels of specific IgG remained stable in vaccinated and non-vaccinated animals, but the final levels in vaccinated animals were higher than in non-vaccinated animals (Fig. 6a, b).

Neutralizing antibody levels in vaccinated and non-vaccinated animals generally correlated with FMDV-specific IgG rather than with IgM. However, in contrast to the ELISA data, final levels of neutralizing antibodies were higher in animals that had not been vaccinated before challenge and thus had developed fulminant FMD (Fig. 6d, e). The three vaccinated animals without virological evidence of local FMDV replication or dissemination had lower specific antibody levels than other vaccinated animals, both before and after challenge (Fig. 6c); however they did have increases in IgG and neutralization titers after challenge.

Apart from the slightly different IgM kinetics in vaccinated animals after challenge, there was no difference in FMDV-specific circulating antibody between carriers and non-carriers.

Isotype-specific characterization of anti-FMDV B cells

FMDV-specific circulating B cells of six non-vaccinated animals were evaluated using an antibody ELISPOT assay. Anti-FMDV antibody-secreting cells were first detected in non-vaccinated animals on 5 dpi. IgM-secreting cells peaked between 7 and 14 dpi, and had disappeared from peripheral blood by 14 dpi. IgG-secreting cell counts in circulation increased until 14 dpi, and then declined. Low levels of FMDV IgG-secreting cells remained detectable in peripheral blood until the end of the experiment (Fig. 7).

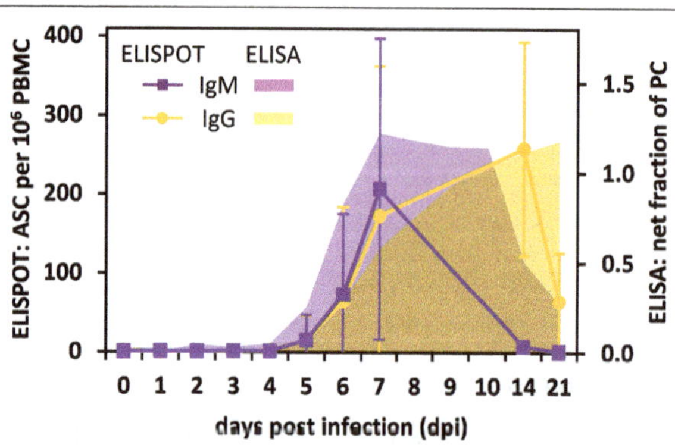

Fig. 7 FMDV-specific humoral immune response in 6 non-vaccinated animals. Antibody-secreting cells (ASC) in peripheral blood were counted with ELISPOT assays, and circulating antibody was measured by sandwich ELISAs. IgM is shown in *purple*, IgG in *gold*. Error bars show sample standard deviation. PC = positive control

Discussion

The present study examined the systemic response to FMDV infection in cohorts of non-vaccinated and vaccinated cattle with the purpose of investigating systemic immune system factors that may correlate with the divergence between FMDV carriers and non-carriers. Persistent infection can follow either a clinical or a subclinical FMDV infection and generally occurs at the same rate regardless of vaccination reviewed in [67]. The protective efficacy of Ad5-FMDV vaccination against disseminated disease has been demonstrated previously [46, 68, 69], but the incidence and characteristics of persistent infection after challenge of Ad5-FMDV-vaccinated cattle was studied here for the first time. Complete blood counts, T lymphocyte subpopulations, type I/III IFN response, as well as FMDV-specific antibody production and activity were compared between vaccinated and non-vaccinated animals and between carriers and non-carriers at an unprecedented level of detail. Before challenge, vaccinated cattle had detectable humoral immunity against FMDV. After challenge, all non-vaccinated steers became viremic and developed clinical disease, while the vaccinated steers did not. This divergence coincided with distinctive differences in several parameters. On the other hand, only slight differences were identified between animals that went on to become FMDV carriers compared to those which cleared the infection.

The present study confirmed earlier findings that summary WBC levels in non-vaccinated animals remain within the clinical reference range during acute FMDV infection and do not change significantly from the outset [28]. There was, however, a significant change in lymphocyte levels, which transiently decreased in non-vaccinated animals after FMDV challenge. This relative lymphopenia was significant compared to pre-infection levels; however, the animals were never lymphopenic relative to the established clinical reference range [56], which underscores the utility of reference change values over population-level standards in animal research [70].

Lymphopenia is a common feature of acute viral infections [71]. It is a well-described phenomenon in FMDV-infected pigs [24, 25, 72], and has previously been reported in FMDV-infected cattle in at least two studies [20, 26]. There are several mechanisms by which viruses can cause lymphopenia. Lymphocytes may be redistributed from the blood into infected tissues, e.g. through the action of type I IFNs. Alternatively, apoptosis of lymphocytes can be a direct result of viral infection or caused indirectly through cytokine induction [73]. In the present study, the decrease in circulating lymphocytes closely followed the increase in systemic type I/III IFN activity, which in turn was highly correlated with FMDV viremia. Thus, these findings are consistent with the observed lymphopenia being due to IFN-induced lymphocyte migration from the blood to sites of infection or lymphoid tissues [74]. The CBC only examines circulating cells; animals with a relative lymphopenia may have normal or even increased levels of total body lymphocytes and the reduction in circulating lymphocytes alone does not necessarily represent a decline in immune competence. It has been argued that transient virus-induced and IFN-mediated lymphopenia is, in fact, a physiological response and beneficial to the host reviewed in [74].

Similarly, increased lymphocyte counts, as were detected in the vaccinated animals in the present study, are often seen after antigenic stimulation [71]. The recall response after challenge of vaccinated animals is the result of an increased quantity of primed antigen-specific B and T cells, which can expand more quickly. Memory cells are activated more readily than naïve cells and can respond to lower doses of antigen [75].

As the bridge between innate and adaptive immunity, monocytes and macrophages are a key component in antigen presentation, phagocytosis, and viral clearance [76]. They usually form only a small part of the circulating leukocyte pool. In the present study, monocyte numbers did not change significantly after vaccination, or after FMDV infection of non-vaccinated animals, but there was a striking pattern in vaccinated steers after challenge. Four days after challenge, and two days after circulating lymphocyte counts had started to increase, monocyte counts rose sharply and remained high (approximately 50 % above baseline) for several days. Sigal et al. [77] have previously reported a similar increase of monocytes in FMDV-vaccinated animals 1 week after challenge.

Monocytes are released into circulation from the bone marrow and spleen in response to inflammation signals [78], and move quickly to sites of infection where they differentiate into macrophages or dendritic cells. Increased antigen presentation and lymphocyte activation stimulate additional monocyte recruitment through positive feedback loops [79]. Opsonization by specific antibody and phagocytosis are major factors in the immune defense against FMDV [80, 81]. Additionally, pDC activation by FMDV is also substantially enhanced in the presence of FMDV-specific antibodies [82]. In the vaccinated animals, protection from FMD occurred in the presence of abundant anti-FMDV immunoglobulin combined with elevated circulating monocyte counts, both of which were likely contributors to the effective immune response.

It has previously been shown that there is a strong systemic type I/III IFN response during acute FMDV infection of cattle [19, 21, 22], and this was again confirmed in the large cohort of unvaccinated cattle in the present study. High IFN activity is also detectable in tissues of FMDV-infected animals, but it is restricted to sites of virus replication [22]. It is unclear how much of the locally produced IFN enters the vasculature, and it has been suggested that the circulating type I/III IFN is instead produced by CD4$^+$ pDCs interacting with immune-complexed virus [18]. A flow cytometric analysis of ex vivo interferon production in pDCs from the FMDV-infected animals would have provided useful information in this regard, but this was beyond the scope of the present study.

No infectious virus or FMDV RNA was detected in serum of vaccinated animals in the present study; thus, the lack of a systemic type I/III IFN response could be explained by the absence of the crucial stimulus for its production. However, induction of transcription of IFN genes and IFN bioactivity was detected in pharyngeal tissues of vaccinated cattle from this study [38].

In addition to its critical role in innate immunity, type I IFN can act directly on both CD4$^+$ and CD8$^+$ T cells, positively or negatively influencing their function reviewed in [83]. T cells are the dominant lymphocyte population in peripheral blood of cattle [84]. For the first time, the present study identified significant changes in αβ T cells in non-vaccinated steers challenged with FMDV, complementing earlier work on γδ T cells [85]. After infection, non-vaccinated animals had a significant decrease in the relative quantity of CD8$^+$ αβ T cells for several days, while the same cell population in vaccinated animals remained stable. Conversely, the relative CD4$^+$ αβ T cell population in non-vaccinated animals was larger during that time, but did not change in vaccinated animals. In order to determine which subset was responsible for the change in the CD4$^+$/CD8$^+$ ratio, lymphocyte counts from the CBC were applied to the relative changes of lymphocyte subpopulations – commonly referred to as the dual-platform method of obtaining absolute counts [60]. The multicolor staining panel used in the present study also accounts for non-T lymphocytes and γδ T cells. Using this method, absolute CD4$^+$ counts in non-vaccinated animals were found to be stable during acute infection, while the absolute CD8$^+$ counts were significantly decreased. This indicates selective depletion (or redistribution) of circulating CD8$^+$ αβ T lymphocytes in FMDV-infected non-vaccinated cattle. A similar pattern has been previously described in swine [24, 25], compounded by evidence of functional impairment (e.g., mitogen unresponsiveness) of the residual circulating T cell population. A variety of explanations for these observations have been suggested [74], including FMDV infection of T lymphocytes or T-cell suppression by IL-10 overproduction [86]. Joshi et al. [87] reported a similarly inhibited response to mitogen in FMDV-infected bovine lymphocytes, but other studies found no evidence of changes in CD4$^+$ and CD8$^+$ populations, T-cell impairment or increased circulating IL-10 during acute FMDV infection in small cohorts of cattle [27, 28].

The time course of the FMDV-specific antibody response observed in the present study was similar to previously published results from other groups [27, 88–90]. Direct comparisons of the magnitude of the response, however, are impossible because of differences in the test format (endpoint dilution vs. optical density at a fixed dilution, use of monoclonal anti-isotype vs. polyclonal anti-isotype antibodies, etc.). In addition, neither system allows for a fully quantitative comparison of different immunoglobulin isotypes within a sample, only of relative levels of the same isotype between samples [89].

When comparing the antibody development after challenge between FMDV-vaccinated and non-vaccinated animals, Mulcahy et al. [89] saw a transient increase of specific IgM in non-vaccinated animals, followed by a sustained increase of specific IgG. This is the classical pattern of a primary immune response [91] that was also seen in non-vaccinated animals in the present study. Similar to what has been discussed for cellular adaptive responses, secondary or recall antibody responses differ from primary responses. They occur more rapidly, they consist of relatively more IgG than IgM, and they are of higher affinity [75]. Indeed, no rise in specific IgM was seen after challenge in the vaccinated animals in the present study, but FMDV-specific IgG levels in vaccinated animals did increase after challenge.

This increase was also seen in the three vaccinated animals that lacked evidence of local virus replication, possibly because antibody-bound FMDV was recognized by the immune system and induced an anamnestic response. Alternatively, there could have been low-level replication that was not directly detectable and which was insufficient to induce measurable antibodies against non-structural proteins. Overall, the data support these animals not having been infected. Strikingly, they only had low neutralizing antibody titers and no detectable type I/III interferon in serum before challenge; thus, the specific mechanisms that facilitated their apparent sterile protection remains undetermined. While the neutralizing antibody profiles between serum and nasal fluid of FMDV-vaccinated pigs are similar, this is not necessarily true for cattle [92], and the low serum titers are not indicative of a similarly low mucosal response.

Persisting serum IgM is used to diagnose chronic viral infections such as hepatitis B and C in humans. Contrary to the results presented here, Salt et al. [90] had not seen such a pattern for FMDV-specific IgM in carriers. In the present study, modestly elevated FMDV-specific IgM was detected in carriers. This may be because persistent FMDV infection is not highly productive, unlike the aforementioned chronic infections. It is interesting to note, too, that while IgM remains detectable, IgM-secreting cells disappear from circulation, possibly indicating a more localized production of the antibodies-similar to what has been described for the IgA response to persistent infection [42]. The magnitude of the difference in IgM kinetics between carriers and non-carriers, however, appears to be too small to be of diagnostic utility. As has been reported previously reviewed in [4], no component of the serum antibody response in the present study was significantly different between carriers and non-carriers.

Conclusions

This study corroborates the notion that vaccination and prevention of clinical disease offer no protection against either primary or persistent FMDV infection [12, 38, 90]. This is the first use of high-resolution hematology and multi-color flow cytometry data from a large cohort of animals, all exposed to the virus under simulated-natural conditions and closely monitored for the full course of infection. Lymphopenia and selective CTL depletion were found to be significant phenomena during the acute infection of naïve cattle, in contrast with a robust cellular immune response in vaccinated animals. However, none of the systemic parameters examined–type I/III interferon, FMDV-specific antibodies, circulating leukocyte populations and T-lymphocyte subsets–were associated with the FMDV carrier state divergence, emphasizing the highly localized nature of persistent FMDV infection. This suggests that tissue-level studies of sites of persistence may be required to elucidate the mechanisms associated with establishment and resolution of persistent FMD, and such studies are currently underway in our laboratory.

Additional files

Additional file 1: Figure S1. White blood cell subpopulations by vaccination and persistence status. A: Total WBC count. B: Neutrophils. C: Lymphocytes. D: Monocytes. Animals were assigned to one of four groups based on their FMDV vaccination and persistence status. Group means are shown with 95 % confidence intervals. Means are marked with orange circles for carrier animals and green circles for non-carriers; individual time points are connected with blue lines for vaccinated animals and with red lines for non-vaccinated animals. Small numbers at the bottom of each panel state the number of animals that contributed data to each time point. (PDF 595 kb)

Additional file 2: Table S1. Full dataset in tab-separated format. (TSV 70 kb)

Abbreviations

ANOVA: Analysis of variance; ARS: Agricultural Research Service; BB: Blocking buffer; CAT: Chloramphenicol acetyltransferase; CBC: Complete blood count; CD: Cluster of differentiation; CI95: 95 % confidence interval; CO_2: Carbon dioxide; C_t: Cycle threshold; CTL: Cytotoxic T lymphocyte(s); Dpi: Days post-infection; Dpv: Days post-vaccination; ELISA: Enzyme-linked immunosorbent assay; ELISPOT: Enzyme-linked immunospot; FACS: Fluorescence-activated cell sorting; FADRU: Foreign Animal Disease Research Unit; FBS: Fetal bovine serum; FMD: Foot-and-mouth disease; FMDV: Foot-and-mouth disease virus; GCN: Genome copy number; HEPES: 4-(2-hydroxyethyl)-1-piperazineethanesulfonic acid; HRP: Horseradish peroxidase; IFN: Interferon; IgG: Immunoglobulin gamma; IgM: Immunoglobulin mu; IL-10: Interleukin 10; INP: Intranasopharyngeal; K_2EDTA: Dipotassium ethylenediaminetetraacetic acid; LFBK: Lois' and Fran's bovine kidney cells; MEM: Minimum essential medium; Mx: Mx1, Myxovirus resistance protein 1; nFPC: Fraction of the net OD of the positive control; NSP: Non-structural protein; OD: Optical density; OPF: Oropharyngeal fluid(s); ORISE: Oak Ridge Institute for Science and Education; PBMC: Peripheral-blood mononuclear cell(s); PBS: Phosphate-buffered saline; PBST: Phosphate-buffered saline with TWEEN(R); PC: Positive control; pDC: Plasmacytoid dendritic cell; PIADC: Plum island animal disease center; RNA: Ribonucleic acid; RPMI: Roswell park memorial institute; RT-PCR: Reverse transcription polymerase chain reaction; SNT: serum neutralization test; $TCID_{50}$: 50 % tissue culture infective doses; TTE: 1,1,2-trichlorofluoroethane; USDA: United States Department of Agriculture; WBC: White blood cell(s)

Acknowledgments
Elizabeth Rieder and Michael LaRocco provided anti-NSP ELISA data for a subset of animal samples. The authors thank the Animal Resource Branch at PIADC for assistance with animal procedures.
This work is dedicated to the memory of Bernd Haas.

Funding
This work was funded in part by CRIS project 1940-32000-057-00D (USDA, Agricultural Research Service), as well as through an interagency agreement with the Science and Technology Directorate of the U.S. Department of Homeland Security under Award Number HSHQPM-13-X-00131. ME, CS, and SIR are recipients of PIADC Research Participation Program fellowships, administered by the Oak Ridge Institute for Science and Education (ORISE) through an interagency agreement with the U.S. Department of Energy. The sponsors had no involvement in the study design, in the collection, analysis and interpretation of data, in the writing of the manuscript, or in the decision to submit the manuscript for publication.

Authors' contributions
ME carried out the flow cytometry assays and the statistical analysis, participated in the development of the flow cytometry assays, in the animal experiments, sample processing and data analysis, the interferon bioassay, hematology, neutralization tests, and the ELISPOT, and wrote and revised the manuscript. CS coordinated and carried out the animal experiments, participated in the sample processing, data analysis and the conception, design, and coordination of the study, and co-wrote the manuscript. SIR carried out the antibody ELISA and hematology, and participated in the interferon bioassay, animal experiments, sample processing, data analysis and the editing of the manuscript. JMP developed the antibody ELISA, adapted the neutralization test, and participated in the coordination of the animal experiments, the conception, design and coordination of the study, data analysis and the revision of the manuscript. EJH and GRS participated in the sample processing, and carried out the virus isolation, real-time RT-PCR and the neutralization test. MAK performed the ELISPOT, and participated in the sample processing, the development of the ELISPOT and the flow cytometry assays and the data analysis. WTG participated in the development of the ELISPOT and flow cytometry assays, the data analysis, study design and coordination, and the revision of the manuscript. LLR participated in the conception and the design of the study and reviewed the manuscript. JA conceived, designed and coordinated the study, co-wrote the manuscript, and coordinated and participated in the animal experiments. All authors read and approved the final manuscript.

Competing interests
The authors declare that they have no competing interests. Mention of trade names or commercial products in this article is solely for the purpose of providing specific information and does not imply recommendation or endorsement by the USDA. The content is solely the responsibility of the authors and does not necessarily represent the official views of the USDA or any other U.S. federal entity.

Consent for publication
Not applicable.

Author details
[1]United States Department of Agriculture (USDA), Plum Island Animal Disease Center (PIADC), Foreign Animal Disease Research Unit (FADRU), Agricultural Research Service (ARS), P.O. Box 848, Greenport, NY 11944, USA. [2]Oak Ridge Institute for Science and Education, PIADC Research Participation Program, Oak Ridge, TN, USA.

References
1. Grubman MJ, Baxt B. Foot-and-mouth disease. Clin Microbiol Rev. 2004;17(2):465–93.
2. Arzt J, Juleff N, Zhang Z, Rodriguez LL. The pathogenesis of foot-and-mouth disease I: viral pathways in cattle. Transbound Emerg Dis. 2011;58(4):291–304.
3. Alexandersen S, Zhang Z, Donaldson AI, Garland AJM. The pathogenesis and diagnosis of foot-and-mouth disease. J Comp Pathol. 2003;129(1):1–36.
4. Alexandersen S, Zhang Z, Donaldson AI. Aspects of the persistence of foot-and-mouth disease virus in animals–the carrier problem. Microbes Infect. 2002;4(10):1099–110.
5. Salt JS. The carrier state in foot and mouth disease–an immunological review. Br Vet J. 1993;149(3):207–23.
6. OIE. Foot-and-Mouth Disease. In: Manual of Diagnostic Tests and Vaccines for Terrestrial Animals. 7th ed. 2012. p. 163.
7. Stenfeldt C, Belsham GJ. Detection of foot-and-mouth disease virus RNA in pharyngeal epithelium biopsy samples obtained from infected cattle: investigation of possible sites of virus replication and persistence. Vet Microbiol. 2012;154(3–4):230–9.
8. Zhang ZD, Kitching RP. The localization of persistent foot and mouth disease virus in the epithelial cells of the soft palate and pharynx. J Comp Pathol. 2001;124(2–3):89–94.
9. Burrows R. Studies on the carrier state of cattle exposed to foot-and-mouth disease virus. J Hyg (Lond). 1966;64(1):81–90.
10. Pacheco JM, Smoliga GR, O'Donnell V, Brito BP, Stenfeldt C, Rodriguez LL, Arzt J. Persistent Foot-and-Mouth Disease Virus Infection in the Nasopharynx of Cattle; Tissue-Specific Distribution and Local Cytokine Expression. PLoS ONE. 2015;10(5), e0125698.
11. Prato Murphy ML, Forsyth MA, Belsham GJ, Salt JS. Localization of foot-and-mouth disease virus RNA by in situ hybridization within bovine tissues. Virus Res. 1999;62(1):67–76.
12. Stenfeldt C, Eschbaumer M, Rekant SI, Pacheco J, Smoliga G, Hartwig E, Rodriguez L, Arzt J. The foot-and-mouth disease carrier state divergence in cattle. J Virol. 2016. in press.
13. Juleff N, Windsor M, Reid E, Seago J, Zhang Z, Monaghan P, Morrison IW, Charleston B. Foot-and-mouth disease virus persists in the light zone of germinal centres. PLoS ONE. 2008;3(10), e3434.
14. Zhang ZD, Hutching G, Kitching P, Alexandersen S. The effects of gamma interferon on replication of foot-and-mouth disease virus in persistently infected bovine cells. Arch Virol. 2002;147(11):2157–67.
15. Reid E, Charleston B. Type I and III interferon production in response to RNA viruses. J Interferon Cytokine Res. 2014;34(9):649–58.
16. Sommereyns C, Paul S, Staeheli P, Michiels T. IFN-lambda (IFN-lambda) is expressed in a tissue-dependent fashion and primarily acts on epithelial cells in vivo. PLoS Pathog. 2008;4(3), e1000017.
17. Fray MD, Mann GE, Charleston B. Validation of an Mx/CAT reporter gene assay for the quantification of bovine type-I interferon. J Immunol Methods. 2001;249(1–2):235–44.
18. Reid E, Juleff N, Gubbins S, Prentice H, Seago J, Charleston B. Bovine plasmacytoid dendritic cells are the major source of type I interferon in response to foot-and-mouth disease virus in vitro and in vivo. J Virol. 2011;85(9):4297–308.
19. Howey R, Bankowski B, Juleff N, Savill NJ, Gibson D, Fazakerley J, Charleston B, Woolhouse ME. Modelling the within-host dynamics of the foot-and-mouth disease virus in cattle. Epidemics. 2012;4(2):93–103.
20. Perez-Martin E, Weiss M, Diaz-San Segundo F, Pacheco JM, Arzt J, Grubman MJ, Delos Santos T. Bovine type III interferon significantly delays and reduces the severity of foot-and-mouth disease in cattle. J Virol. 2012;86(8):4477–87.
21. Stenfeldt C, Heegaard PM, Stockmarr A, Tjørnehøj K, Belsham GJ. Analysis of the acute phase responses of Serum Amyloid A, Haptoglobin and Type 1 Interferon in cattle experimentally infected with foot-and-mouth disease virus serotype O. Vet Res. 2011;42:66.

22. Arzt J, Pacheco JM, Smoliga GR, Tucker MT, Bishop E, Pauszek SJ, Hartwig EJ, Delos Santos T, Rodriguez LL. Foot-and-mouth disease virus virulence in cattle is co-determined by viral replication dynamics and route of infection. Virology. 2014;452–453:12–22.
23. Sei JJ, Ochoa AS, Bishop E, Barlow JW, Golde WT. Phenotypic, ultra-structural, and functional characterization of bovine peripheral blood dendritic cell subsets. PLoS ONE. 2014;9(10), e109273.
24. Bautista EM, Ferman GS, Golde WT. Induction of lymphopenia and inhibition of T cell function during acute infection of swine with foot and mouth disease virus (FMDV). Vet Immunol Immunopathol. 2003;92(1–2):61–73.
25. Diaz-San Segundo F, Salguero FJ, De Avila A, De Marco MM, Sanchez-Martin MA, Sevilla N. Selective lymphocyte depletion during the early stage of the immune response to foot-and-mouth disease virus infection in swine. J Virol. 2006;80(5):2369–79.
26. Maddur MS, Gajendragad MR, Gopalakrishna S, Singh N. Comparative study of experimental Foot-and-Mouth Disease in cattle (Bos indicus) and buffaloes (Bubalis bubalus). Vet Res Commun. 2008;32(6):481–9.
27. Juleff N, Windsor M, Lefevre EA, Gubbins S, Hamblin P, Reid E, McLaughlin K, Beverley PC, Morrison IW, Charleston B. Foot-and-mouth disease virus can induce a specific and rapid CD4+ T-cell-independent neutralizing and isotype class-switched antibody response in naive cattle. J Virol. 2009;83(8):3626–36.
28. Windsor MA, Carr BV, Bankowski B, Gibson D, Reid E, Hamblin P, Gubbins S, Juleff N, Charleston B. Cattle remain immunocompetent during the acute phase of foot-and-mouth disease virus infection. Vet Res. 2011;42:108.
29. Carr BV, Lefevre EA, Windsor MA, Inghese C, Gubbins S, Prentice H, Juleff ND, Charleston B. CD4+ T-cell responses to foot-and-mouth disease virus in vaccinated cattle. J Gen Virol. 2013;94(Pt 1):97–107.
30. Pega J, Bucafusco D, Di Giacomo S, Schammas JM, Malacari D, Capozzo AV, Arzt J, Pérez-Beascoechea C, Maradei E, Rodríguez LL, et al. Early adaptive immune responses in the respiratory tract of foot-and-mouth disease virus-infected cattle. J Virol. 2013;87(5):2489–95.
31. Patch JR, Pedersen LE, Toka FN, Moraes M, Grubman MJ, Nielsen M, Jungersen G, Buus S, Golde WT. Induction of foot-and-mouth disease virus-specific cytotoxic T cell killing by vaccination. Clin Vaccine Immunol. 2011;18(2):280–8.
32. Patch JR, Kenney M, Pacheco JM, Grubman MJ, Golde WT. Characterization of cytotoxic T lymphocyte function after foot-and-mouth disease virus infection and vaccination. Viral Immunol. 2013;26(4):239–49.
33. Cox SJ, Voyce C, Parida S, Reid SM, Hamblin PA, Paton DJ, Barnett PV. Protection against direct-contact challenge following emergency FMD vaccination of cattle and the effect on virus excretion from the oropharynx. Vaccine. 2005;23(9):1106–13.
34. McVicar JW, Sutmoller P. Growth of foot-and-mouth disease virus in the upper respiratory tract of non-immunized, vaccinated, and recovered cattle after intranasal inoculation. J Hyg (Lond). 1976;76(3):467–81.
35. Aggarwal N, Zhang Z, Cox S, Statham R, Alexandersen S, Kitching RP, Barnett PV. Experimental studies with foot-and-mouth disease virus, strain O, responsible for the 2001 epidemic in the United Kingdom. Vaccine. 2002;20(19–20):2508–15.
36. Cox SJ, Voyce C, Parida S, Reid SM, Hamblin PA, Hutchings G, Paton DJ, Barnett PV. Effect of emergency FMD vaccine antigen payload on protection, sub-clinical infection and persistence following direct contact challenge of cattle. Vaccine. 2006;24(16):3184–90.
37. Golde WT, Pacheco JM, Duque H, Doel T, Penfold B, Ferman GS, Gregg DR, Rodriguez LL. Vaccination against foot-and-mouth disease virus confers complete clinical protection in 7 days and partial protection in 4 days: Use in emergency outbreak response. Vaccine. 2005;23(50):5775–82.
38. Stenfeldt C, Eschbaumer M, Pacheco JM, Rekant SI, Rodriguez LL, Arzt J. Pathogenesis of Primary Foot-and-Mouth Disease Virus Infection in the Nasopharynx of Vaccinated and Non-Vaccinated Cattle. PLoS ONE. 2015;10(11), e0143666.
39. Doel TR, Williams L, Barnett PV. Emergency vaccination against foot-and-mouth disease: rate of development of immunity and its implications for the carrier state. Vaccine. 1994;12(7):592–600.
40. Hedger RS. Observations on the carrier state and related antibody titres during an outbreak of foot-and-mouth disease. J Hyg (Lond). 1970;68(1):53–60.
41. Parida S, Cox SJ, Reid SM, Hamblin P, Barnett PV, Inoue T, Anderson J, Paton DJ. The application of new techniques to the improved detection of persistently infected cattle after vaccination and contact exposure to foot-and-mouth disease. Vaccine. 2005;23(44):5186–95.
42. Parida S, Anderson J, Cox SJ, Barnett PV, Paton DJ. Secretory IgA as an indicator of oro-pharyngeal foot-and-mouth disease virus replication and as a tool for post vaccination surveillance. Vaccine. 2006;24(8):1107–16.
43. Maddur MS, Gajendragad MR, Kishore S, Chockalingam AK, Suryanarayana W, Gopalakrishna S, Singh N. Enhanced mucosal immune response in cattle persistently infected with foot-and-mouth disease virus. Vet Immunol Immunopathol. 2008;125(3–4):337–43.
44. McCullough KC, Bruckner L, Schaffner R, Fraefel W, Muller HK, Kihm U. Relationship between the anti-FMD virus antibody reaction as measured by different assays, and protection in vivo against challenge infection. Vet Microbiol. 1992;30(2–3):99–112.
45. Robiolo B, La Torre J, Maradei E, Beascoechea CP, Perez A, Seki C, Smitsaart E, Fondevila N, Palma E, Goris N, et al. Confidence in indirect assessment of foot-and-mouth disease vaccine potency and vaccine matching carried out by liquid phase ELISA and virus neutralization tests. Vaccine. 2010;28(38):6235–41.
46. Brake DA, McIlhaney M, Miller T, Christianson K, Keene A, Lohnas G, Purcell C, Neilan J, Schutta C, Barrera J, et al. Human adenovirus-vectored foot-and-mouth disease vaccines: establishment of a vaccine product profile through in vitro testing. Dev Biol (Basel). 2012;134:123–33.
47. Rieder E, Henry T, Duque H, Baxt B. Analysis of a foot-and-mouth disease virus type A24 isolate containing an SGD receptor recognition site in vitro and its pathogenesis in cattle. J Virol. 2005;79(20):12989–98.
48. Stenfeldt C, Pacheco JM, Singanallur NB, Ferreira HC, Vosloo W, Rodriguez LL, Arzt J. Clinical and virological dynamics of a serotype O 2010 South East Asia lineage foot-and-mouth disease virus in sheep using natural and simulated natural inoculation and exposure systems. Vet Microbiol. 2015;178:50–60.
49. Sutmoller P, Gaggero A. Foot-and mouth diseases carriers. Vet Rec. 1965;77(33):968–9.
50. Sutmoller P, Cottral GE. Improved techniques for the detection of foot-and-mouth disease virus in carrier cattle. Arch Gesamte Virusforsch. 1967;21(2):170–7.
51. Eschbaumer M, Stenfeldt C, Pacheco JM, Rekant SI, Arzt J. Effect of storage conditions on subpopulations of peripheral blood T lymphocytes isolated from naive cattle and cattle infected with foot-and-mouth disease virus. Vet Clin Pathol. 2016;45(1):110–5.
52. Stenfeldt C, Pacheco JM, Smoliga GR, Bishop E, Pauszek SJ, Hartwig EJ, Rodriguez LL, Arzt J. Detection of Foot-and-mouth Disease Virus RNA and Capsid Protein in Lymphoid Tissues of Convalescent Pigs Does Not Indicate Existence of a Carrier State. Transbound Emerg Dis. 2014.
53. Callahan JD, Brown F, Osorio FA, Sur JH, Kramer E, Long GW, Lubroth J, Ellis SJ, Shoulars KS, Gaffney KL, et al. Use of a portable real-time reverse transcriptase-polymerase chain reaction assay for rapid detection of foot-and-mouth disease virus. J Am Vet Med Assoc. 2002;220(11):1636–42.
54. Rasmussen TB, Uttenthal A, De Stricker K, Belak S, Storgaard T. Development of a novel quantitative real-time RT-PCR assay for the simultaneous detection of all serotypes of foot-and-mouth disease virus. Arch Virol. 2003;148(10):2005–21.
55. Weiss DJ, Wardrop KJ. Schalm's Veterinary Hematology. 6th ed. Hoboken: Wiley-Blackwell; 2010.
56. Merck Manual. Hematologic Reference Ranges. In: Aiello SE, editor. The Merck Veterinary Manual. 2012.
57. Ramachandran H, Laux J, Moldovan I, Caspell R, Lehmann PV, Subbramanian RA. Optimal thawing of cryopreserved peripheral blood mononuclear cells for use in high-throughput human immune monitoring studies. Cells. 2012;1(3):313–24.
58. Perfetto SP, Chattopadhyay PK, Lamoreaux L, Nguyen R, Ambrozak D, Koup RA, Roederer M. Amine reactive dyes: an effective tool to discriminate live and dead cells in polychromatic flow cytometry. J Immunol Methods. 2006;313(1–2):199–208.
59. Montes M, Jaensson EA, Orozco AF, Lewis DE, Corry DB. A general method for bead-enhanced quantitation by flow cytometry. J Immunol Methods. 2006;317(1–2):45–55.
60. Hultin LE, Chow M, Jamieson BD, O'Gorman MR, Menendez FA, Borowski L, Denny TN, Margolick JB. Comparison of interlaboratory variation in absolute T-cell counts by single-platform and optimized dual-platform methods. Cytometry B Clin Cytom. 2010;78(3):194–200.
61. Riondato F, D'Angelo A, Miniscalco B, Bellino C, Guglielmino R. Effects of road transportation on lymphocyte subsets in calves. Vet J. 2008;175(3):364–8.
62. LaRocco M, Krug PW, Kramer E, Ahmed Z, Pacheco JM, Duque H, Baxt B, Rodriguez LL. A continuous bovine kidney cell line constitutively expressing bovine alphavbeta6 integrin has increased susceptibility to foot-and-mouth disease virus. J Clin Microbiol. 2013;51(6):1714–20.

63. LaRocco M, Krug PW, Kramer E, Ahmed Z, Pacheco JM, Duque H, Baxt B, Rodriguez LL, Correction for LaRocco, et al. A Continuous Bovine Kidney Cell Line Constitutively Expressing Bovine alphaVbeta6 Integrin Has Increased Susceptibility to Foot-and-Mouth Disease Virus. J Clin Microbiol. 2015;53(2):755.
64. R: A Language and Environment for Statistical Computing [https://www.R-project.org/]
65. Wickham H. ggplot2: elegant graphics for data analysis. New York: Springer; 2009.
66. Bates D, Maechler M, Bolker BM, Walker S. lme4: Linear mixed-effects models using Eigen and S4. J Stat Softw. 2014.
67. Moonen P, Jacobs L, Crienen A, Dekker A. Detection of carriers of foot-and-mouth disease virus among vaccinated cattle. Vet Microbiol. 2004;103(3–4):151–60.
68. Grubman MJ, Moraes MP, Schutta C, Barrera J, Neilan J, Ettyreddy D, Butman BT, Brough DE, Brake DA. Adenovirus serotype 5-vectored foot-and-mouth disease subunit vaccines: the first decade. Future Virol. 2010;5(1):51–64.
69. Pacheco JM, Brum MC, Moraes MP, Golde WT, Grubman MJ. Rapid protection of cattle from direct challenge with foot-and-mouth disease virus (FMDV) by a single inoculation with an adenovirus-vectored FMDV subunit vaccine. Virology. 2005;337(2):205–9.
70. Walton RM. Subject-based reference values: biological variation, individuality, and reference change values. Vet Clin Pathol. 2012;41(2):175–81.
71. Roland L, Drillich M, Iwersen M. Hematology as a diagnostic tool in bovine medicine. J Vet Diagn Invest. 2014;26(5):592–8.
72. Nfon CK, Toka FN, Kenney M, Pacheco JM, Golde WT. Loss of plasmacytoid dendritic cell function coincides with lymphopenia and viremia during foot-and-mouth disease virus infection. Viral Immunol. 2010;23(1):29–41.
73. Cusick MF, Libbey JE, Fujinami RS. Picornavirus infection leading to immunosuppression. Future Virol. 2014;9(5):475–82.
74. Golde WT, De Los Santos T, Robinson L, Grubman MJ, Sevilla N, Summerfield A, Charleston B. Evidence of activation and suppression during the early immune response to foot-and-mouth disease virus. Transbound Emerg Dis. 2011;58(4):283–90.
75. Ahmed R, Gray D. Immunological memory and protective immunity: understanding their relation. Science. 1996;272(5258):54–60.
76. Janeway C. Basic concepts in immunology. In: Murphy K, Travers P, Walport M, editors. Janeway's Immunobiology. 7th ed. New York: Garland Science; 2008. p. 1–38.
77. Sigal LJ, Gomez G, Braun M. Changes in mononuclear peripheral blood cells in cattle with foot-and-mouth disease. Vet Immunol Immunopathol. 1992;30(4):431–8.
78. Shi C, Pamer EG. Monocyte recruitment during infection and inflammation. Nat Rev Immunol. 2011;11(11):762–74.
79. Deshmane SL, Kremlev S, Amini S, Sawaya BE. Monocyte chemoattractant protein-1 (MCP-1): an overview. J Interferon Cytokine Res. 2009;29(6):313–26.
80. McCullough KC, Parkinson D, Crowther JR. Opsonization-enhanced phagocytosis of foot-and-mouth disease virus. Immunology. 1988;65(2):187–91.
81. Quattrocchi V, Langellotti C, Pappalardo JS, Olivera V, Di Giacomo S, Van Rooijen N, Mongini C, Waldner C, Zamorano PI. Role of macrophages in early protective immune responses induced by two vaccines against foot and mouth disease. Antiviral Res. 2011;92(2):262–70.
82. Guzylack-Piriou L, Bergamin F, Gerber M, McCullough KC, Summerfield A. Plasmacytoid dendritic cell activation by foot-and-mouth disease virus requires immune complexes. Eur J Immunol. 2006;36(7):1674–83.
83. McNab F, Mayer-Barber K, Sher A, Wack A, O'Garra A. Type I interferons in infectious disease. Nat Rev Immunol. 2015;15(2):87–103.
84. Tizard IR. Veterinary Immunology. St. Louis: Elsevier Health Sciences; 2013.
85. Toka FN, Kenney MA, Golde WT. Rapid and transient activation of γδ T cells to IFN-γ production, NK cell-like killing, and antigen processing during acute virus infection. J Immunol. 2011;186(8):4853–61.
86. Diaz-San Segundo F, Rodriguez-Calvo T, De Avila A, Sevilla N. Immunosuppression during acute infection with foot-and-mouth disease virus in swine is mediated by IL-10. PLoS ONE. 2009;4(5), e5659.
87. Joshi G, Sharma R, Kakker NK. Phenotypic and functional characterization of T-cells and in vitro replication of FMDV serotypes in bovine lymphocytes. Vaccine. 2009;27(48):6656–61.
88. Abu Elzein EM, Crowther JR. Detection and quantification of IgM, IgA, IgG1 and IgG2 antibodies against foot-and-mouth disease virus from bovine sera using an enzyme-linked immunosorbent assay. J Hyg (Lond). 1981;86(1):79–85.
89. Mulcahy G, Gale C, Robertson P, Iyisan S, DiMarchi RD, Doel TR. Isotype responses of infected, virus-vaccinated and peptide-vaccinated cattle to foot-and-mouth disease virus. Vaccine. 1990;8(3):249–56.
90. Salt JS, Mulcahy G, Kitching RP. Isotype-specific antibody responses to foot-and-mouth disease virus in sera and secretions of "carrier" and "non-carrier" cattle. Epidemiol Infect. 1996;117(2):349–60.
91. Janeway C. Janeway's Immunobiology. 7th ed. New York: Garland Science; 2008.
92. Eble PL, Bouma A, Weerdmeester K, Stegeman JA, Dekker A. Serological and mucosal immune responses after vaccination and infection with FMDV in pigs. Vaccine. 2007;25(6):1043–54.

14

Protection of farm goats by combinations of recombinant peptides and formalin inactivated spores from a lethal *Bacillus anthracis* challenge under field conditions

Susanne M. Koehler[1,6], Fatih Buyuk[2], Ozgur Celebi[2], Hayati Demiraslan[3], Mehmet Doganay[3], Mitat Sahin[2], Jens Moehring[4], Okechukwu C. Ndumnego[5,7], Salih Otlu[2], Henriette van Heerden[5] and Wolfgang Beyer[1*]

Abstract

Background: *Bacillus* (*B.*) *anthracis,* the causal agent of anthrax, is effectively controlled by the Sterne live spore vaccine (34F2) in animals. However, live spore vaccines are not suitable for simultaneous vaccination and antibiotic treatment of animals being at risk of infection in an outbreak situation. Non-living vaccines could close this gap.

Results: In this study a combination of recombinant protective antigen and recombinant *Bacillus* collagen-like antigen (rBclA) with or without formalin inactivated spores (FIS), targeted at raising an immune response against both the toxins and the spore of *B. anthracis*, was tested for immunogenicity and protectiveness in goats. Two groups of goats received from local farmers of the Kars region of Turkey were immunized thrice in three weeks intervals and challenged together with non-vaccinated controls with virulent *B. anthracis,* four weeks after last immunization. In spite of low or none measurable toxin neutralizing antibodies and a surprisingly low immune response to the rBclA, 80% of the goats receiving the complete vaccine were protected against a lethal challenge. Moreover, the course of antibody responses indicates that a two-step vaccination schedule could be sufficient for protection.

Conclusion: The combination of recombinant protein antigens and FIS induces a protective immune response in goats. The non-living nature of this vaccine would allow for a concomitant antibiotic treatment and vaccination procedure. Further studies should clarify how this vaccine candidate performs in a post infection scenario controlled by antibiotics.

Keywords: Bacillus anthracis, Anthrax, Vaccination, Animal vaccine

Background

Anthrax was one of the first bacterial diseases to be controlled by vaccination. Starting with the famous vaccination of sheep conducted at Pouilly-le-Fort, France, by Louis Pasteur [1] his duplex vaccine became widely used for cattle and sheep in Europe and South America for about 50 years. It was, however, Max Sterne's live-spore vaccine [2] which in the long run became the world's most used live vaccine against anthrax in the veterinary field [3]. It remains the veterinary vaccine in use in most countries encountering anthrax [4].

Sterne's own trials with his vaccine [5, 6] had shown effectiveness in diminishing outbreaks in South Africa over the period 1925 to 1941. Nevertheless, while proving effective in controlling anthrax worldwide over the last 75 years, usage of the Sterne live spore vaccine poses a number of problems. These include problems related to the standardization of vaccine production and avoidance of batch to batch variation in content and immunogenicity, and the residual virulence known from several laboratory species and livestock [2, 7–9], in particular goats [3]. More importantly, especially for use

* Correspondence: wolfgang.beyer@uni-hohenheim.de
[1]Department of Infectiology and Animal Hygiene, University of Hohenheim, Institute of Animal Science, 70593 Stuttgart, Germany
Full list of author information is available at the end of the article

in livestock and endangered wild species, the live vaccine has been noted to prevent development of vaccine induced antibodies when administered concomitantly with an antibiotic in small laboratory rodents [10, 11]. The simultaneous antibiotic treatment and vaccination would be of great importance for control of an outbreak situation where the possible infection of livestock or wild animals needs to be prevented after the activity of the antibiotic has ceased. This concept has led to the approval of a human vaccine (AVA, (BioThrax[R]), Emergent BioSolutions) for a post-exposure scenario in humans where antibiotics may be administered for up to 60 days [12]. In animals, the risk for infections by spores originally present in or newly shed to the environment by early victims of an outbreak is even much higher, as one-shot treatments with long-lasting antibiotics generally do not protect for more than 14 days.

So far non-living alternatives are not available for veterinary use, contrary to the licensed acellular human vaccines AVA and AVP whose main immunological ingredient is the so-called protective antigen (PA; see reviews in [13–16]). However these are imposed with limitations of their own like an extensive immunization schedule, batch to batch variations in the content and concentration of the antigens [17], and species-specific variations in the protective capacity [18–22]. Thus the search for more defined recombinant protein antigens analogous to the licensed acellular human vaccines is still ongoing.

Varying results have been published in laboratory animal models (reviewed in 13) with purified PA preparations and recombinant PA (rPA). Results indicated that vaccines solely based on the toxin derived antigens, mainly PA, are less protective than live-spore vaccines against virulent isolates of *B. anthracis* [7, 23–29]. Spore vaccines constructed from toxigenic, non-encapsulated strains have repeatedly demonstrated the capacity to confer protection in mice and guinea pigs against challenge with virulent *B. anthracis* [7, 9, 23, 24, 30, 31]. Better protection by live spore vaccines compared to AVA or AVP has been attributed to improved stimulation of the cellular or cell mediated immune response by both spore and vegetative cell components [7, 8, 23, 32].

Brahmbhatt et al. [33] showed a protective effect of an exosporium derived antigen, *Bacillus* collagen-like antigen (BclA), when added to suboptimal amounts of PA in a combination vaccine. This supported the results of Hahn et al. [34] that showed the protection afforded by a combination of rPA and rBclA encoding plasmids was significantly better than protection provided by vaccination with the single components. More recently it was shown that other spore derived antigens [27, 29, 35–37], surface layer proteins [28, 38] or inactivated full spore preparation such as FIS [39–41] can add to the protective efficacy of PA-based vaccines.

The PA-induced immune response is highly dependent on the adjuvant used [19, 20]. In recent trials a lipopeptide adjuvant (LP), already validated in other contexts [42–47], was compared with alhydrogel (Ah) in mice and rabbits. Animals immunized with rPA and LP had significantly higher antibody (IgG2a) titers than those given rPA and Ah. When NMRI mice were challenged subcutaneously with *B. anthracis* Ames spores the rPA/LP immunized group survived significantly better than both the negative controls and the rPA/Ah immunized group, whereas rabbits were completely protected. None of the animals showed clinical side effects with this adjuvant [48].

As early as in 1946 Gladstone [49] recognized the potential of a non-cellular vaccine against anthrax and tested a culture filtrate of *B. anthracis* in several laboratory species and sheep. Experiments in the 1950s in cattle, sheep, and pigs demonstrated the potential protectiveness of such a cell-free vaccine [50, 51], though the interpretation of these trials was always hampered by the inability to find a fully lethal dose with the challenge strains used. To the best of our knowledge there have been no further studies aimed at protecting livestock animals from a virulent infection with *B. anthracis* by a non-living vaccine since these early experiments.

Our study investigated the protective immune response induced by a combination of recombinant proteins with or without FIS in goats. This species was selected given the extremely high susceptibility of goats and their economic and social importance in many arid or semi-arid areas of the world. A threefold vaccination with a non-living vaccine comprising of rPA, rBclA and FIS as the relevant antigens in combination with LP adjuvant revealed 80% survival after a parenteral lethal challenge with spores of *B. anthracis*. This indicates the high potential of such vaccines as either a supplement or even alternative to living spore vaccines when (i) vaccination is desirable to prevent the re-activation of an outbreak after the initial antibiotic treatment or (ii) when other non-living components are used in so-called combination vaccines to immunize simultaneously against both *B. anthracis* and a different pathogen. Such combination vaccines are often used concomitantly with antibiotics in the veterinary practice.

Methods

Animals

Goats were purchased from local farmers and comprised of a phenotypically heterogeneous group of both males and females of ages around 1 year, belonging to the breed of Caucasian goats. Animals were sourced from farms not affected by anthrax and with no anthrax vaccine history in the last 5 years. All animals were tested for anti-PA antibodies by ELISA and only animals considered negative were enrolled. Initially 25 goats were held in one flock on a fenced pasture throughout the vaccination. To allow for acclimatization the goats were held at the site of the experiment for approximately 1 month prior to the start of the vaccination. All animals were treated with Ivermectin (7 mg, s. c.) and mineral supplement (Depomin, 10 ml orally per day, for 3 days) and the health status was monitored by local veterinarians. Two vaccine groups of 10 goats each (groups A and B) and one unvaccinated negative control of 5 goats (group NegCTL) were selected at random from the flock to make up the experimental groups. During the challenge period groups of animals were held in separate concrete barns equipped with water basins and racks containing hay. Hay was provided ad libitum. At the end of the trials barns and any non-burnable materials were disinfected by spraying with 10% formaldehyde solution. Carcasses and contaminated materials were incinerated. Two animals of group A and one animal in group NegCTL were lost during the time of vaccination but before challenge (Table 1) due to reasons unrelated to the vaccination procedure (two predations and one unknown loss). The immunological data of these animals were part of the evaluation.

Recombinant proteins

Escherichia coli BL21-CodonPlus-RIL cells (Stratagene, La Jolla, CA) harboring the plasmid pREP 4 and pQE-30 (both Qiagen, Venlo, Netherland) encoding either rPA83 or rBclA coupled to a HIS-tag were grown and purified as described previously [34]. Briefly, bacterial inoccula were grown in antibiotic supplemented Standard medium I (Roth, Karlsruhe, Germany). Upon reaching OD_{600nm} of 0.6, protein production was induced with IPTG (Roth, Karlsruhe, Germany). After incubation for 3 h at 37 °C shaking cultures were lysed and proteins purified on a HiTrap Sepharose column loaded with nickel(II)sulfate (Sigma-Aldrich, Taufkirchen, Germany) via FPLC with Äktaprime plus (GE Healthcare, Freiburg, Germany). After dialysis onto 5 mM HEPES-buffer (Roth, Karlsruhe, Germany) and quality assessment via SDS-page, protein yield was established via Bicinchoninsäure test (Interchim, Montlucon, France). Proteins used for ELISA received no further treatment while proteins used for vaccination were tested for endotoxin (ET) yield using the Limulus Amoebocyte Lysate Endochrome-K test kit (Charles River, Wilmington, MA) according to the manufactures's instructions. Endotoxin removal was performed via EndoTrap blue endotoxin removal system (Hyglos, Bernried, Germany) for proteins with ET values more than 50 ng/kg body weight.

Formalin inactivated spores (FIS)

Sterne vaccine strain 34F2 spores (strain collection of the University of Hohenheim) suspended in 0.9% NaCl containing 0.1% gelatin were pelleted, then re-suspended in PBS with 4% formalin and incubated at 37 °C overnight. The suspension was centrifuged (4000 x g) four times and re-suspended in 0.9% NaCl and 0.1% gelatin with the last pellet re-suspended in endotoxin free PBS. Sterility of 1 aliquot of the preparation was confirmed on blood agar after neutralization of formalin with 1 volume of a solution containing 20 g/L histidine at room temperature for 30 min.

Lipopeptide adjuvant

A lipopeptide adjuvant comprising Pam3Cys-SKKKK, a TLR2/1 activator admixed with Pam3Cys conjugated to the promiscuitive T-helper-cell epitope of the sperm whale myoglobin SFISEAIIHVLHSRHPG [46, 47, 52] was purchased from EMC Microcollections GmbH, Germany.

Serology

All sera were tested individually for IgG antibodies against the respective antigens rPA83, rBclA, and FIS in the ELISA. IgM titers against rBclA and FIS were assessed with pooled group sera from each sampling point. The ELISA tests were performed as described earlier [53]. Briefly 96-well Maxisorp plates (Sigma-Aldrich, Taufkirchen, Germany) were coated with 0.5 µg antigen or respectively 10^8 cfu FIS per well in coating buffer (8.4 g/L $NaHCO_3$, 3.56 g/L Na_2CO_3) over night. Sera were titrated on the plate in duplicates using a serial $\log_2$ dilution with a starting concentration of 1:100. Controls included an equivalently titrated goat serum positive for all antigen tested, as well as point measurements (concentration 1:100) of unvaccinated goat sera as a negative control. The secondary antibody rabbit anti-goat IgG HRP (Thermo Fischer, Waltham, MA USA) was used at a dilution of 1:6000. Endpoint titers were developed with ABTS (Roche, Mannheim, Germany) and defined as the reciprocal of the highest serum dilution that resulted in an OD_{414nm} greater than 0.1.

Toxin-neutralizing assay (TNA) was performed as published earlier [53] to qualitatively assess the ability of antibodies generated to neutralize lethal toxin. Briefly, heat inactivated individual sera were serially diluted in 8 $\log_2$ steps with a starting dilution of 1:50 on sterile 96 well plates (BD Biosciences, Heidelberg, Germany) seeded with 10^5 J774 A.1 macrophages per well. Lethal toxin (LF) was added at concentration of 500 ng/mL PA and 100 ng/mL LF (List Biological Laboratories, Campbell, CA, USA) and survival of macrophages was visualized through MTT (5 mg/mL, Alfa Aesar, Karsruhe, Germany), which is degraded by living cells to a measurable ($OD540_{nm}$) colour compound. The neutralization titer (NT) corresponds to the inverse serum dilution at which the macrophage survival yielded 50% (NT_{50}). ELISA titers and NT_{50} were estimated using the Sigma Plot regression wizard (4-parameter sigmoid regression curve).

Bacillus anthracis challenge strain

The virulent *B. anthracis* strain was isolated from the spleen of a deceased bovine in the Kars region (strain K-136, collection of the Department of Microbiology, Faculty of Veterinary Medicine of the Kafkas University, Turkey) and identified as described earlier [54]. Spores were prepared as described in the WHO guidelines "Anthrax in humans and animals" [4]. The presence of both virulence plasmids pX01 and pX02 was tested by PCR [4] from 10 single colonies randomly picked from an overnight culture of the spore suspension on blood agar. The virulence of the challenge strain was confirmed in BALB/c mice at Erciyes University Hakan Cetinsaya Animal Experimentation Laboratory, Kayseri/Turkey. For this, two groups of 2 mice were challenged with 625 or respectively 1250 spores given s. c. in the back. Death occurred within 68 h after the lethal challenge and was verified through re-isolation of the challenge strain from heart and lung tissue.

Immunizations and challenge

Goats of group A received a vaccine formulation comprising of 500 µg LP adjuvant, 75 µg rPA83 and 75 µg rBclA per dose and group B goats received the same formulation as A with the addition of 10^8 FIS per dose. The 75 µg of recombinant proteins was a 25-fold increase in PA that is present in a single dose of the human vaccine AVA [55]. The spore dose was as published for studies with mice and guinea pigs [39]. Group NegCTL served as an unvaccinated negative control without any injections. The groups were vaccinated three times with 3 week intervals by subcutaneous injection into the upper thigh of the hind leg with 1 mL of vaccine (components diluted in 1 mL of endotoxin free PBS). Blood samples were collected before each immunization, right before and 14 days after challenge from survivors (Fig. 1). All animals were challenged with approximately 1000 spores at one time, except for two randomly chosen members of group NegCTL (96,163 and kesik kulak) that were challenged before the rest of the groups to establish the virulence of the spore suspension prepared. Re-counting colony forming units on blood agar plates revealed a number of 1027 spores for the two negative controls challenged first and 918 spores for the other goats.

To assess the health status of the challenged goats the general behaviour was checked and rectal temperature was measured at least twice daily for 2 weeks after the challenge. In cases of temperatures of ≥40 °C a blood smear to determine the presence of encapsulated bacilli in the blood was made [55]. Animals with negative blood smears were monitored more frequently. Positive animals were treated with 1 mL/25 kg body weight Dipenisol (penicillin/streptomycin formulation, Bayer, Leverkusen). The day of treatment was recorded as "time of death" for the analysis of protectiveness. The animal trials were approved by the Ethic Committee of Animal Experimentation of the Erciyes University, No. 13/01, decision date 09.01.2013.

Statistics

Titer values for all four traits were transformed using a logarithmic transformation, as residuals visually indicate clearly increasing variances for larger expected values. These data were then analyzed using a mixed model assuming fixed effects for groups and time points and their interactions. Furthermore, the model accounts for repeated measures taken from each goat. Repeated measures can be modelled by an unstructured variance covariance matrix for observations from one goat, but for all traits fitting a random goat effect and a week-specific error variance increased model fit measured by the Akaike information criterion (AIC). Values under the detection limit were replaced by the halved value of the detection level on the transformed scale. If all observations from one time point or one group were under the detection level, the variance for these observations is zero. To avoid underestimation of variances, we dropped these observations and present means for them as under detection level in the results section. A Tukey tests accounting for multiple testing were performed only after finding differences for a factor via F-Test. A letter display was used were means with identical letters were not significant different from each other. Additionally, in case of non-significant interactions between group and time point simple means were calculated, but not used for testing. Predicted means were back transformed for presentation only. Standard errors were back transformed using the delta method. As titer values could only be measured from surviving goats, means from the last time point depend on the surviving of goats. For those titers animal effects were correlated for the traits anti-rPA83 and NT_{50} using a bivariate model. To elaborate survival time the log rank test was employed using data from all treated goats. Multiple comparison was done using the adjustment by Tukey. For all statistical evaluation a *P*-value of 0.05 was considered significant. All analysis were done using the procedures PROC MIXED and PROC LIFETEST of the SAS system.

Results

Anti-rPA-IgG titer

Titers of NegCTL group remained below the detection threshold (< 100) throughout the study. The F-tests

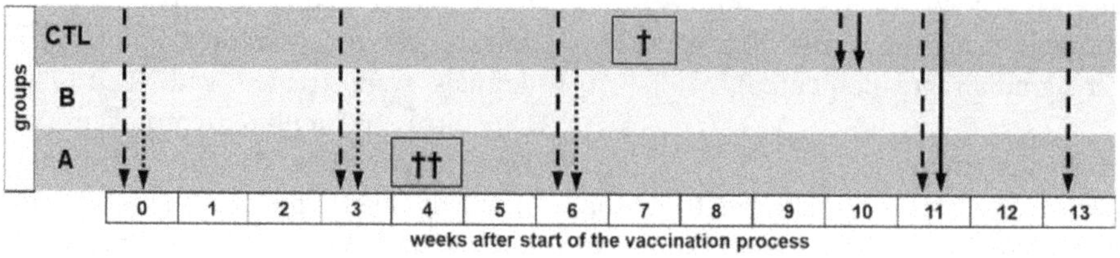

Fig. 1 Timeline of the vaccination and challenge schedule. Dashed arrows indicate blood sampling; dotted arrows indicate vaccination time points and continuous arrows indicate the application of the challenge dose; Arrow's lengths indicate schedule of the relevant groups (A-C); † indicates death of individual goats unrelated to the experimental set up within the indicated time frame; In week 10 only 2 individuals of group NegCTL (unvaccinated negative control) were bled and challenged to verify the functionality of the challenge set up, the remainder of group C was challenged and bled in week 11 together with group A (rBclA + rPA83), and B (rBclA + rPA83 + FIS). FIS: Formalin inactivated spores; rBcLA: Recombinant *Bacillus* collagen-like antigen; rPA: Recombinant protective antigen

indicated differences between time points, but titers of groups A and B show a similar development over time (P = 0.47) and means were not significantly different (P = 0.20). Mean anti-rPA83 titers increased significantly in both group A and B after the first and second vaccination (P = 0.0001) but decreased after the 3rd vaccination (P = 0.0051). Mean titers of goats surviving the challenge remained either nearly unchanged or raised strongly compared to values after second and third vaccination, leading to high variations within the groups (Fig. 2 and Additional file 1: Table S1).

Toxin neutralization titer (NT_{50})

Sera of group NegCTL as well as sera of all goats before the first immunization remained below the detection limit ($NT_{50} \leq 50$). The F-tests indicated differences between time points, but titers of groups A and B show a similar development over time (P = 0.81) and means were not significantly different (P = 0.25). After the first immunization only individual goats of groups A and B developed weak NT_{50} whereas the mean titers across groups A and B increased significantly (p = 0.0023) after the second immunization. In line with the tendency observed for anti-rPA83 IgG, the third immunization resulted in significant though lower mean titers (P = 0.0028) (Figs. 2 and 3, week 10/11). NT_{50} of goats surviving the challenge were highly variable (Fig. 3 and Additional file 1: Table S2). Animal showing high values for anti-rPA83 IgG also show high NT_{50} values (r = 0.956).

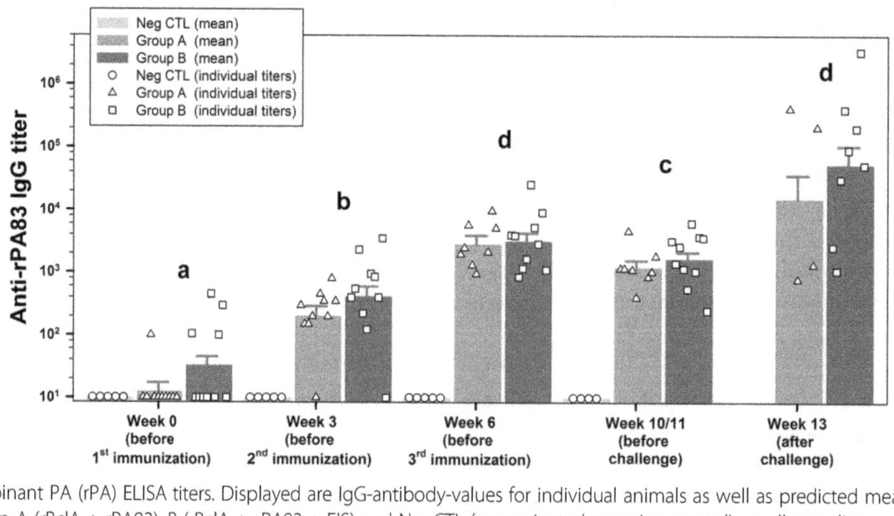

Fig. 2 Anti-recombinant PA (rPA) ELISA titers. Displayed are IgG-antibody-values for individual animals as well as predicted means and standard deviations for group A (rBclA + rPA83), B (rBclA + rPA83 + FIS) and NegCTL (unvaccinated negative control) on all sampling points measured via indirect ELISA against rPA83. Values below the detection limit (<100) were given an arbitrary value of 10. Individual values are given as symbols specific for each group (group A - triangle, group B - square and group NegCTL - circle). Mean values are given in the form of bar charts in the background and standard deviations as positive values above the bars. Mean values were analyzed for statistical differences with $P \leq 0.05$ as indicated by lower case letters for comparing time points above the respective bars. As there was no significant difference (P > 0.20) between group A and B for any sampling point concerning the anti-rPA83 IgG antibody titers, letters were displayed across both groups. Mean values with identical letters were not significant different from each other. Means from group NegCTL were always under the detection limit and therefore not included in the letter display. FIS: Formalin inactivated spores; rBcLA: Recombinant *Bacillus* collagen-like antigen; rPA: Recombinant protective antigen

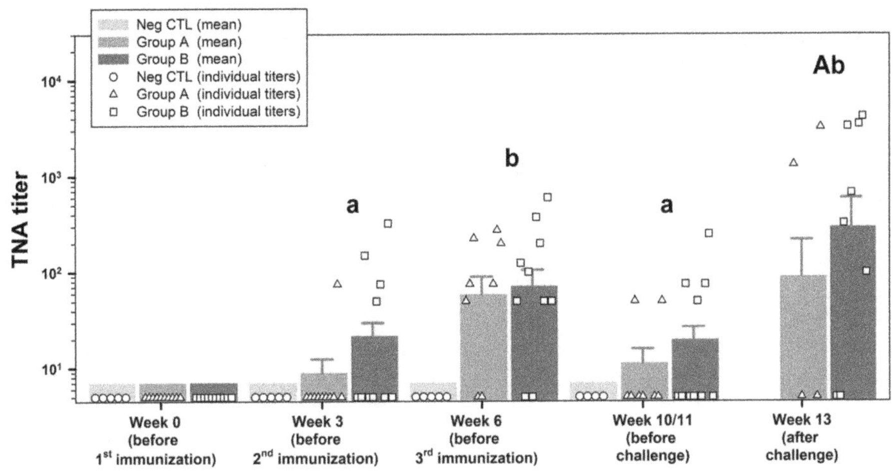

Fig. 3 Toxin neutralization assay (TNA)-titers. Displayed are toxin-neutralizing titers for individual animals as well as predicted means and standard deviations for group A (rBclA + rPA83), B (rBclA + rPA83 + FIS) and NegCTL (unvaccinated negative control) on all sampling points. Values below the detection limit (<50) were given an arbitrary value of . Individual values are given as symbols specific for each group (group A - triangle, group B - square and group NegCTL - circle). Means are given in the form of bar charts in the background and standard deviations as positive values above the bars. Results were analyzed for statistical differences with $P \leq 0.05$ indicated by lower case letters for comparing time points and upper case letters for comparing groups above the respective bars. Mean values of different time points with identical lower case letters were not significant different from each other. Mean values of different groups with identical upper case letters were not significant different from each other. As there was no significant difference ($P > 0.25$) between group A and B for any sampling point concerning the toxin-neutralizing titers, letters were displayed across both groups. Mean values with identical letters were not significant different from each other. Means from group NegCTL and before immunization were always under the detection limit and therefore not included in the letter display. FIS: Formalin inactivated spores; rBcLA: Recombinant *Bacillus* collagen-like antigen; rPA: Recombinant protective antigen

Anti-rBclA-IgG titer

The F-tests indicated a significant interaction term, thus different development of titers over time in different groups. The mean titers of group B slightly increased after the first and second immunization ($P = 0.0101$ and $P = 0.0078$) but differ significantly only in week 6 from the negative control group (Fig. 4 and Additional file 1: Table S3).

Anti-FIS-IgG titer

Again, F-tests indicated a significant interaction term, thus different development of titers over time in different groups. The mean titer of group B was significantly increased after the first ($P < 0.0001$) and second immunization ($P = 0.0027$) and stayed nearly constant after the third immunization and challenge ($P = 0.1573$, $P = 0.1273$). Titers from the NegCTL group were constant over time. Titers from group A, where FIS was not constituent of the vaccine formulation, remained nearly unchanged compared to serum before vaccination (Fig. 5 and Additional file 1: Table S4). Pooled group sera of every sampling point tested negative for IgM antibodies against rBclA and FIS (data not shown).

Challenge

In Fig. 6 the time to death curves are plotted, taking only full days into consideration. Two animals of group A got antibiotic treatment after a positive blood smear on days 3 and 9, respectively, according to the end point rules of this experiment. These animals were considered fatally infected and the day of intervention was taken for calculation of the death curve. Using the test for multiple comparisons group B shows a significant better survival than the negative control, with 8 out of 10 survivors ($P = 0.0015$) while group A with 4 out of 8 survivors did not ($P = 0.2895$). The difference in survival rate between group A and B is not significant ($P = 0.4614$) using the test approach described above. This test approach simultaneously used data from all goats. Note that using three two-sample log rank tests with a Bonferroni adjustment for multiple testing here showed significant increased survival rate for both groups A and B as compared to the unvaccinated negative group (NegCTL).

Discussion

Living spore vaccines, currently used as one of the most important measures for controlling anthrax in animals, are not suitable for simultaneous antibiotic treatment and vaccination. This scenario is relevant in veterinary practice when vaccination is desirable to prevent the re-activation of an outbreak after the initial antibiotic treatment or when other non-living components are used in so-called combination vaccines to immunize simultaneously against both *B. anthracis* and a different pathogen.

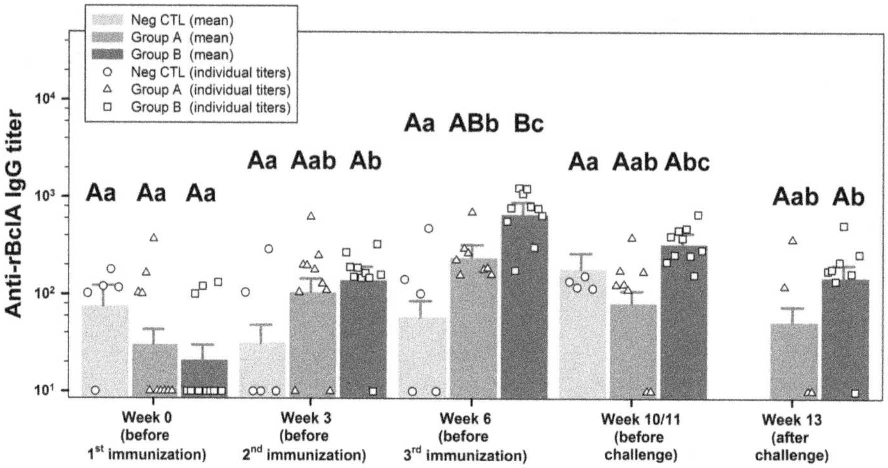

Fig. 4 Anti-rBclA ELISA titers. Displayed are IgG antibody-values for individual animals as well as predicted means and standard deviations for group A (rBclA + rPA83), B (rBclA + rPA83 + FIS) and NegCTL (unvaccinated negative control) on all sampling points measured via indirect ELISA against rBclA. Values below the detection limit (<100) were given an arbitrary value of 10. Individual values are given as symbols specific for each group (group A - triangle, group B - square and group NegCTL - circle). Means are given in the form of bar charts in the background and standard deviations as positive values above the bars. Results were analyzed for statistical differences with $P \leq 0.05$ indicated by lower case letters for comparing time points and upper case letters for comparing groups above the respective bars. Mean values of different time points with identical lower case letters were not significant different from each other. Mean values of different groups with identical upper case letters were not significant different from each other. Inter-group comparisons showed a significantly elevated mean IgG titer against rBclA for group B as compared to group NegCTL in week 6 only. FIS: Formalin inactivated spores; rBcLA: Recombinant *Bacillus* collagen-like antigen; rPA: Recombinant protective antigen

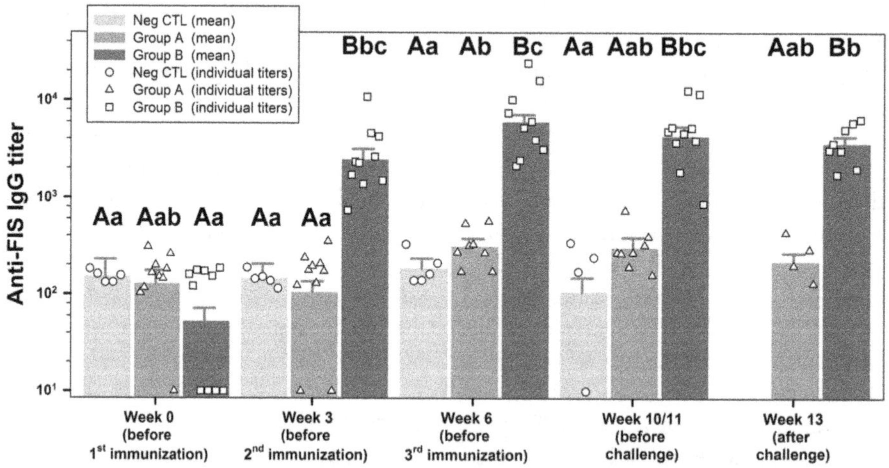

Fig. 5 Anti-FIS (formalin inactivated spores) ELISA titers. Displayed are IgG antibody-values for individual animals as well as predicted means and their standard deviations for group A (rBclA + rPA83), B (rBclA + rPA83 + FIS) and NegCTL (unvaccinated negative control) on all sampling points measured via indirect ELISA against FIS (formalin inactivated spores). Values below the detection limit (<100) were given an arbitrary value of 10 for better display. Individual values are given as symbols specific for each group (group A - triangle, group B - square and group NegCTL - circle). Means are given in the form of bar charts in the background and standard deviations as positive values above the bars. Results were analyzed for statistical differences with $P \leq 0.05$ indicated by lower case letters for comparing time points and upper case letters for comparing groups above the respective bars. Mean values of different time points with identical lower case letters were not significant different from each other. Mean values of different groups with identical upper case letters were not significant different from each other. Inter-group comparisons showed significantly elevated IgG titers for group B as compared to group A against FIS for all sampling points with the exception of week 0. FIS: Formalin inactivated spores; rBcLA: Recombinant *Bacillus* collagen-like antigen; rPA: Recombinant protective antigen

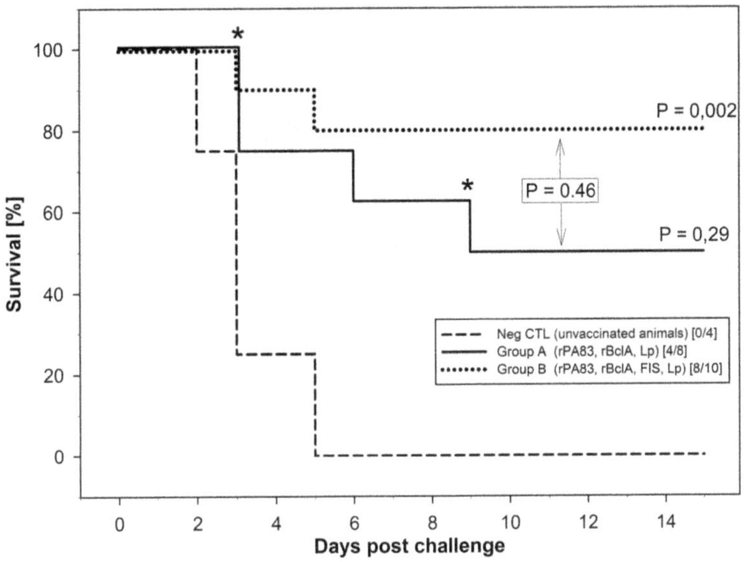

Fig. 6 Survival data. Displayed are survival data of goats immunized with protein component vaccines with or without FIS (formalin inactivated spores) and challenged with fully virulent wild type strain *Bacillus anthracis* K-136. Survival was monitored up to 15 days. Significance was tested via a log-rank test. *P*-values are as compared to the unvaccinated animals if not indicated otherwise. The time of death was either the day the animal was found dead or the day of antibiotic treatment, as was the case for 2 goats of group A. The time points of their antibiotic treatment are labelled with * in the figure

A growing body of data from vaccinations of laboratory animals show the superiority of vaccines supposed to elicit protective immune responses against both the action of the toxins and the replication of the bacterium. We sought to know whether an appropriate non-living combination vaccine could protect one of the most susceptible species of livestock, goats, against a lethal challenge with *B. anthracis*. This study demonstrated that goats were protected by a combination of recombinant peptides with or without FIS from a lethal *B. anthracis* challenge.

Based on promising results from earlier vaccination experiments in mice [56], goats were immunized three times at 3-week intervals with rPA and rBclA without (group A) or plus *B. anthracis* 34F2 strain derived FIS (group B) adjuvanted by a lipopeptide. This robust vaccination regimen was chosen in an "all or nothing" approach to ensure that in this pioneering experiment even a minimal protectiveness would be verifiable. The challenge with ~1000 spores of a fully virulent strain of *B. anthracis* revealed 50% (4/8) and 80% (8/10) survival for the 14 days monitoring period in group A and B, respectively, while all animals (4/4) of the negative control died within 5 days. According to the Tukey test for multiple comparisons only group B showed a significant protection in comparison to the negative control. This result falls in line with the observations made earlier where a combination of rPA83 and different concentrations of FIS in guinea pigs and several mice strains resulted in full protection [39, 40] whereas the components given in single did not. ELISA and TNA titers measured after each vaccination indicate that a two-step vaccination could be sufficient for protection as titers were higher after second vaccination than after third (Figs. 2, 3). This needs to be further investigated to determine if a two-step vaccination will protect target animals as well and to compare the protectiveness in different livestock animals to those of the current Sterne live spore vaccine (SLSV). In a previous trial on the long-term protectiveness of the SLSV in goats [57] a 100% survival from lethal challenge was only achieved when goats were freshly boostered. The single application of SLSV resulted in 60% (6 weeks post vaccination) and 80% (62 weeks post vaccination) survival. While the protectiveness of the threefold vaccination schedule conducted here with the non-living vaccine looks comparable to a single vaccination with SLSV anti-PA and TNA-titers were equal or higher with the latter at 4–6 weeks after vaccination compared to the peak titers (week 6) with the non-living vaccine. However, the titers of both anti-PA and TNA were fairly comparable right before challenge. Interestingly, anti-FIS titers were much lower after a single vaccination with SLSV (<1/10) compared to our group B titers but increased comparably after a second vaccination with living spores. Taken in mind the role of an anti-spore immune response the high anti-FIS titers may have contributed to the higher survival seen in group B.

Some animals showed measurable, but low ELISA titers against rPA83, rBclA and FIS before immunization. This has been observed in other trials before [57] and can be attributed to unspecific reactivity, as the animals utilized in this study had no historical vaccination background and were not connected to any anthrax outbreak. Furthermore, the background titers of unvaccinated animals did not change significantly over time and conveyed no protection. Because of this we focused our statistical evaluation on the progressive change in titers over time and between groups clearly showing a vaccine effect in terms of seroconversion and survival in the vaccinated animals. Of note, two animals in group A and B showed no increase in anti-rPA and TNA titers after the survival of the challenge as compared to before the challenge hinting at a sterile immunity [58].

As the exosporium is the outermost surface of a *B. anthracis* spore, it has been the focus of numerous novel vaccination approaches by several laboratories. BclA forms the hair-like extensions protruding from the exosporium membrane [59, 60]. It has been shown to be immunodominant [61] and adds to protectiveness of PA based vaccines [33, 34, 56]. Goats injected with a protein formulation of rPA83, rBclA and lipopeptide (group A) showed little to no increase in ELISA titers using either rBclA or FIS as the antigen. Goats supplementary injected with FIS (group B) showed a strong increase in anti-FIS IgG titers but still an only marginal increase in titers against rBclA. Given the previously described results from mouse experiments the low responsiveness of goats to either the recombinant or FIS-derived BclA was unexpected. Interestingly, these results are in line with serological data from a study in goats vaccinated with the commercial Sterne spore vaccine. Vaccinates also showed no change in anti-rBclA IgG titers over the course of a year as compared to titers before the vaccination while anti-FIS IgG titers increased strongly after the first and again after a booster immunization with the Sterne spore vaccine [57]. It has been stated that the main antibody response against BclA is directed against the proteinaceous parts of the native protein [62] and several reports have shown the immunogenic and protective capacity of a non-glycosylated rBclA [32–34, 56]. However, we cannot completely rule out that goats in group B may have elicited antibodies against the carbohydrate moieties of the glycosylated FIS-derived BclA which were not detectable using rBclA as the antigen in our ELISA. If so, such antibodies might have added to the better protection in group B and immunogenic oligosaccharide side chains of BclA may be considered part of future non-living vaccines, too. Taken together these results support the previously described notion [27, 29] that BclA, albeit highly immunogenic, might not be the only or even main relevant antigen from *B. anthracis* spores. Vergis et al. [29] observed an even better survival rate in mice challenged with Ames spores after immunization with a ΔBclA strain of the anthracis-like *B. cereus* G9241. The authors explained these surprising results with observations by Cybulski et al. [36] and Basu et al. [63], the latter demonstrating that the removal of the exosporium from a spore enhances the cytokine response in macrophages while the exosporium itself is inert in this regard. More recently, Wang et al. [64] implicated BclA in impairing antibody responses and protection against lethal infection of mice through inhibition of complement. The results of our study indicate that BclA might not only partially mask recognition of important antigens beneath the exosporium, but is in addition poorly immunogenic in goats as compared to mice and rabbits. If this has implications concerning the high susceptibility of goats against an infection with *B. anthracis*, needs further investigation.

Conclusions

The results of our study indicate the potential of an antigenic mixture eliciting an immune response against both the toxins and the spore components of *B. anthracis* to protect the extremely susceptible goat from a lethal infection with *B. anthracis*. The non-living nature of this vaccine would allow for a concomitant antibiotic treatment and vaccination procedure. Data from serological studies in goats support the robustness of immunogenicity of this vaccine also when administered in combination with long-term antibiotics (unpublished). Further studies will clarify how this vaccine candidate performs in a post infection scenario controlled by antibiotics.

Abbreviations

Ah: Alhydrogel; AVA: Anthrax Vaccine Adsorbed; AVP: Anthrax Vaccine Precipitated; B: *Bacillus*; BclA: *Bacillus* collagen-like antigen; ELISA: Enzyme Linked Immunosorbent Assay; ET: Endotoxin; FIS: Formalin Inactivated Spores; FPLC: Fast protein liquid chromatography; HRP: Horseredish Peroxidase; IgG: Immunoglobulin G; IgM: Immunoglobulin M; IPTG: Isopropyl-β-D-thiogalactopyranosid; LF: Lethal Factor; LP: Lipopeptide; NegCTL: Negative Control group; NT: Neutralization Titer; PA: Protective Antigen; PBS: Phosphate Buffered Saline; PCR: Polymerase Chain Reaction; RBclA: Recombinant BclA; rPA: Recombinant Protective Antigen; SDS: Sodium Dodecyl Sulfoxid; SLSV: Sterne's Live Spore Vaccine; TNA: Toxin Neutralization Assay

Acknowledgements

The authors would like to thank Peter Turnbull for his invaluable consultations during all phases of the work. We are very grateful for the technical assistance of Elisabeth Blaschke, Sabine Hoche and Mehmet Yetgin.

Funding

This work has been funded by Deutsche Forschungsgemeinschaft (BE 2157/4–1).

Authors' contributions

SMK was involved in every stage of planning, organizing and conducting the study and in manuscript writing, in partial fulfillment of her PhD studies. FB and OC characterized the challenge strain of *B. anthracis* at the Kars

University. HD and MD designed and carried out the mouse challenge study under BSL-3 conditions. MS and SO were responsible for planning, organizing and coordinating all the risk level 3 experiments at the Kars University, particularly the vaccination and challenge trials, and were involved in data collection and interpretation. FB, OC, and OCN were involved in the acquisition and analysis of data from the goat trials. OCN additionally carried out part of the immunoassays at the University of Pretoria. JM performed the statistical analysis. All authors have been involved in drafting the manuscript or revising it critically, have given final approval of the version to be published and agreed to be accountable for all aspects of the work in ensuring that questions related to the accuracy or integrity of any part of the work are appropriately investigated and resolved. HvH made substantial contributions to conception and study design. WB at University of Hohenheim has been the project leader and together with HvH from University of Pretoria was involved in every stage of the study and manuscript writing.

Authors' information
Not applicable.

Consent for publication
Not applicable.

Competing interests
The authors declare that they have no competing interests.

Author details
[1]Department of Infectiology and Animal Hygiene, University of Hohenheim, Institute of Animal Science, 70593 Stuttgart, Germany. [2]Faculty of Veterinary Medicine, Department of Microbiology, Kafkas University, 36300 Kars, Turkey. [3]Faculty of Medicine, Department of Infectious Diseases, Erciyes University, 38039 Kayseri, Turkey. [4]Institute for Crop Science, University of Hohenheim, Biostatistical Unit, 70593 Stuttgart, Germany. [5]Department of Veterinary Tropical Diseases, University of Pretoria, Onderstepoort 0110, South Africa. [6]Robert-Koch-Institut, 13353 Berlin, Germany. [7]Africa Health Research Institute, Durban 4013, South Africa.

References
1. Pasteur L. De l'atenuation des virus et de leur retour a la virulence. C Rend Acad Sci. 1881;92:429–35.
2. Sterne M. The immunization of laboratory animals against anthrax. Onderstepoort J Vet Sci Anim Indust. 1939;13:313–7.
3. Turnbull PCB. Anthrax vaccines: past, present and future. Vaccine. 1991;9:533–9.
4. Turnbull PCB. Anthrax in Humans and Animals. WHO Press, 4th ed Geneva; 2008.
5. Sterne M. The use of anthrax vaccines prepared from avirulent (uncapsulated) variants of bacillus anthracis. Onderstepoort J Vet Sci Anim Indust. 1939;13:307–12.
6. Sterne M, Nicol J, Lambrechts MC. The effect of large-scale active immunisation against anthrax. J S Afr Vet Med Assoc. 1942;13:53–63.
7. Little SF, Knudson GB. Comparative efficacy of *Bacillus anthracis* live spore vaccine and protective antigen vaccine against anthrax in the guinea pig. Infect Immun. 1986;52:509–12.
8. Turnbull PCB, Broster MG, Carman JA, Manchee RJ, Melling J. Development of antibodies to protective antigen and lethal factor components of anthrax toxin in humans and guinea pigs and their relevance to protective immunity. Infect Immun. 1986;52:356–63.
9. Ivins BE, Welkos SL, Knudson GB, Littl SF. Immunization against anthrax with aromatic compound-dependent (Aro-) mutants of *Bacillus anthracis* and with recombinant strains of *Bacillus subtilis* that produce anthrax protective antigen. Infect Immun. 1990;58:303–8.
10. Stepanov AV, Marinin LI, Pomerantsev AP, Staritsin NA. Development of novel vaccines against anthrax in man. J Biotechnol. 1996;44:155–60.
11. Webster A. Inhibiting effect of antibiotics on anthrax vaccination. Aust Vet J. 1973;49:545.
12. Ionin B, et al. Evaluation of Immunogenicity and Efficacy of Anthrax Vaccine Adsorbed for Postexposure Prophylaxis. Clin Vaccine Immunol. 2013;20:1016–26.
13. Cybulski RJ Jr, Sanz P, O'Brien AD. Anthrax vaccination strategies. JMAM. 2009;30:490–502.
14. Baillie LWJ. Past, imminent and future human medical countermeasures for anthrax. J Appl Microbiol. 2006;101:594–606.
15. Scorpio A, Blank TE, Day WA, Chabot DJ. Anthrax vaccines: Pasteur to the present. Cell Mol Life Sci. 2006;63:2237–48.
16. Little SF. Anthrax vaccines. BioDrugs. 2005;19:233–45.
17. Turnbull PCB. Anthrax vaccines. In: Artenstein AW, editor. Vaccines: a biography. Springer Verlag, London: Springer Verlag; 2010. p. 57–71.
18. Welkos SL, Friedlander AM. Comparative safety and efficacy against *Bacillus anthracis* of protective antigen and live vaccines in mice. Microb Pathog. 1988;5:127–39.
19. Ivins BE, Welkos SL, Little SF, Crumrine MH, Nelson GO. Immunization against anthrax with *Bacillus anthracis* protective antigen combined with adjuvants. Infect Immun. 1992;60:662–8.
20. Ivins B, Fellows PF, Pitt ML, Estep J, Farchaus JW, Friedlander AM, Gibbs PH. Experimental anthrax vaccines: efficacy of adjuvants combined with protective antigen against an aerosol *Bacillus anthracis* spore challenge in guinea pigs. Vaccine. 1995;13:1779–84.
21. Ivins BE, Pitt ML, Fellows PF, Farchaus JW, Benner GE, Waag DM, Little SF, Anderson GW Jr, Gibbs PH, Friedlander AM. Comparative efficacy of experimental anthrax vaccine candidates against inhalation anthrax in rhesus macaques. Vaccine. 1998;16:1141–8.
22. Fellows PF, Linscott MK, Ivins BE, Pitt ML, Rossi CA, Gibbs PH, Friedlander AM. Efficacy of a human anthrax vaccine in guinea pigs, rabbits, and rhesus macaques against challenge by *Bacillus anthracis* isolates of diverse geographical origin. Vaccine. 2001;19:3241–7.
23. Ivins BE, Ezzell JW, Jemski J, Hedlund KW, Ristroph JD, Leppla SH. Immunization studies with attenuated strains of bacillus anthracis. Infect Immun. 1986;52:454–8.
24. Welkos SL, Friedlander AM. Pathogenesis and genetic control of resistance to the Sterne strain of bacillus anthracis. Microb Pathog. 1988;4:53–69.
25. Cohen S, Mendelson I, Altboum Z, Kobiler D, Elhanany E, Bino T, Leitner M, Inbar I, Rosenberg H, Gozes Y, Barak R, Fisher M, Kronman C, Velan B, Shafferman A. Attenuated nontoxinogenic and nonencapsulated recombinant *Bacillus anthracis* spore vaccines protect against anthrax. Infect Immun. 2000;68:4549–58.
26. Rhie GE, Roehrl MH, Mourez M, Collier RJ, Mekalanos JJ, Wang JY. A dually active anthrax vaccine that confers protection against both bacilli and toxins. Proc Natl Acad Sci U S A. 2003;100:10925–30.
27. Cote CK, Kaatz L, Reinhardt J, Bozue J, Tobery SA, Bassett AD, Sanz P, Darnell SC, Alem F, O'Brien AD, Welkos SL. Characterization of a multi-component anthrax vaccine designed to target the initial stages of infections well as toxaemia. J Med Microbiol. 2012;61:1380–92.
28. Uchida M, Harada T, Enkhtuya J, Kusumoto A, Kobayashi Y, Chiba S, Shyaka A, Kawamoto K. Pro-tective effect of bacillus anthracis surface protein EA1 against anthrax in mice. Biochem Biophy Res Commun. 2012;421:323–8.
29. Vergis JM, Cote CK, Bozue J, Alem F, Ventura CL, Susan L, Welkos SL, O'Briena AD. Immunization of mice with formalin-inactivatedspores from avirulent Bacillus Cereus strains provides significant protection from challenge with bacillus anthracis Ames. Clin Vaccine Immunol. 2013;20:56–65.
30. Klein NF, DeArmon IA Jr, Lincoln RE, Mahlnadt BG, Fernelius AL. Immunological studies of anthrax. II. Levels of immunity against bacillus anthracis obtained with protective antigen and live vaccine. J Immunol. 1962;88:15–9.
31. Brossier F, Weber-Levy M, Mock M, Sirard JC. Role of toxin functional domains in anthrax pathogenesis. Infect Immun. 2000;68:1781–6.
32. Ivins BE, Welkos S. Recent advances in the development of an improved humen anthrax vaccine. Eur J Epidemiol. 1988;4:12–9.
33. Brahmbhatt TN, Darnell SC, Carvalho HM, Sanz P, Kang TJ, Bull RL, Rasmussen SB, Cross AS, O'Brien AD. Recombinant exosporium protein BclA of bacillus anthracis is effective as a booster for mice primed with suboptimal amounts of protective antigen. Infect Immun. 2007;75:5240–7.

34. Hahn UK, Böhm R, Beyer W. DNA vaccination against anthrax in mice – combination of anti-spore and anti-toxin components. Vaccine. 2006;24:4569–71.
35. Cote CK, Bozue J, Moody KL, DiMezzo TL, Chapman CE, Welkos SL. Analysis of a novel spore antigen in bacillus anthracis that contributes to spore opsonization. Microbiology. 2008;154:619–32.
36. Cybulski RJ Jr, Sanz P, McDaniel D, Darnell S, Bull RL, O'Brien AD. Recombinant bacillus anthracis spore proteins enhance protection of mice primed with suboptimal amounts of protective antigen. Vaccine. 2008;26:4927–39.
37. Enkhtuya J, Kawamoto K, Kobayashi Y, Uchida I, Rana N, Makino S. Significant passive protective effect against anthrax by antibody to bacillus anthracis inactivated spores that lack two virulence plasmids. Microbiology. 2006;152:3103–10.
38. Baillie LWJ, Hebdon R, Flick-Smith H, Williamson D. Characterisation of the immune response to the UK human anthrax vaccine. FEMS Immunol Med Microbiol. 2003;36:83–6.
39. Brossier F, Levy M, Mock M. Anthrax spores make an essential contribution to vaccine efficacy. Infect Immun. 2002;70:661–4.
40. Gauthier YP, Tournier JN, Paucod JC, Corre JP, Mock M, Goossens PL, Vidal DR. Efficacy of a vaccine based on protective antigen and killed spores against experimental inhalational anthrax. Infect Immun. 2009;77:1197–207.
41. Glomski IJ, Corre JP, Mock M, Goossens PL. Cutting edge: IFN-c-producing CD4 T lymphocytes mediate spore induced immunity to capsulated bacillus anthracis. J Immunol. 2007;178:2646–50.
42. Loleit M, Ihlenfeldt HG, Brünjes J, Jung G, Müller B, Hoffmann P, Bessler WG, Pierres M, Haas G. Synthetic peptides coupled to the lipotripeptide P3CSS induce in vivo B and T helper cell responses to HIV-1 reverse transcriptase. Immunobiology. 1996;195:61–76.
43. Schild H, Deres K, Wiesmüller KH, Jung G, Rammensee HG. Efficiency of peptides and lipopeptides for in vivo priming of virus-specific cytotoxic T cells. Eur J Immunol. 1991;21:2649–54.
44. Schlecht S, Wiesmüller K-H, Jung G, Bessler WG. Lipopeptide als natürliche Adjuvantien für Impfstoffe aus Gram-negativen Bakterien. Naturwissenschaften. 1993;80:9–17.
45. Wiesmüller KH, Jung G, Hess G. Novel low-molecular- weight synthetic vaccine against foot-and-mouth disease containing a potent B-cell and macrophage activator. Vaccine. 1989;7:29–33.
46. Wiesmüller KH, Fleckenstein B, Jung G. Peptide Vaccines and Peptide Libraries. Biol Chem. 2001;382:571–9.
47. Mittenbühler K, vdEsche U, Heinevetter L, Bessler WG, Huber M. Lipopeptides: adjuvanticity in conventional and genetic immunization. FEMS Immunol Med Microbiol. 2003;15:193–200.
48. Beyer W, Hahn UK, Boehm R. Lipopeptide adjuvant versus aluminium hydroxide in PA based vaccines. 5th International BACT-Conference. Abstract book. 2005;P14:49.
49. Gladstone GP. Immunity to anthrax: protective antigen present in cell-free culture filtrates. Br J Exp Pathol. 1946;27:394–418.
50. Schlingman AS, Devlin HB, Wright GG, Maine RJ, Manning MC. Immunizing activity of alum-precipitated protective antigen of bacillus anthracis in cattle, sheep, and swine. Am J Vet Res. 1956;4:256–61.
51. Jackson FC, Wright GG, Armstrong J. Immunization of cattle against experimental anthrax with alum-precipitated protective antigen or spore vaccine. Am J Vet Res. 1957;18:771–7.
52. Ghielmetti M, Reschner A, Zwicker M, Padovan E. Synthetic bacterial lipopeptide analogs: structural requirements for adjuvanticity. Immunbiol. 2005;210:211–5.
53. Hahn UK, Alex M, Czerny CP, Boehm R, Beyer W. Protection of mice against challenge with bacillus anthracis STI spores after DNA vaccination. Int J Med Microbiol. 2004;294:35–44.
54. Buyuk F, Sahin M, Cooper C, Celebi O, Saglam AG, Baillie L, Celik E, Akca D, Otluet S. The effect of prolonged storage on the virulence of isolates of Bacillus anthracis obtained from environmental and animal sources in the Kars Region of Turkey. FEMS Microbiol Lett. 2015;362:fnv102.
55. Joellenbeck LM, Zwanziger LL, Durch JS, Strom BL. The Anthrax Vaccine: Is it safe? Does it work? In: Committee to Assess the Safety and Efficacy of the Anthrax Vaccine. In: Medical Follow-Up Agency, Institute of Medicine; 2002. doi:10.17226/10310.
56. Köhler SM, Baillie LW, Beyer W. BclA and toxin antigens augment each other to protect NMRI mice from lethal bacillus anthracis challenge. Vaccine. 2015;33:2771–7.
57. Ndumnego OC, Köhler S, Crafford J, van Heerden H, Beyer W. Comparative analysis of the immunologic response and protective efficacy induced by the Sterne 34F2 live spore *Bacillus anthracis* vaccine in a ruminant model. Vet Immunol Immunop. 2016;178:14–21.
58. Hermanson G, et al. A cationic lipid-formulated plasmid DNA vaccine confers sustained antibody-mediated protection against aerosolized anthrax spores. Proc Natl Acad Sci U S A. 2004;101:13601–6.
59. Sylvestre P, Couture-Tosi E, Mock M. A collagen-like surface glycoprotein is a structural component of the bacillus anthracis exosporium. Mol Microbiol. 2002;45:169–78.
60. Sylvestre P, Couture-Tosi E, Mock M. Polymorphism in the collagen-like region of the bacillus anthracis BclA protein leads to variation in Exosporium filament length. J Bacteriol. 2003;185:1555–63.
61. Steichen CT, Kearney JF, Turnbough CL. Characterization of the exosporium basal layer protein BxpB of bacillus anthracis. J Bacteriol. 2005;187:5868–76.
62. Steichen C, Chen P, Kearney JF, Turnbough CL Jr. Identification of the immunodominant protein and other proteins of the bacillus anthracis exosporium. J Bacteriol. 2003;185:1903–10.
63. Basu S, Kang TJ, Chen WH, Fenton MJ, Baillie L, Hibbs S, Cross AS. Role of bacillus anthracis spore structures in macrophage cytokine responses. Infect Immun. 2007;75:2351–8.
64. Wang Y, Jenkins SA, Gu C, Shree A, Martinez-Moczygemba M, Herold J, Botto M, Wetsel RA, Xu Y. Bacillus anthracis spore surface protein BclA mediates complement factor H binding to spores and promotes spore persistence. PLoS Pathog. 2016;12:e1005678.

15

An inactivated gE-deleted pseudorabies vaccine provides complete clinical protection and reduces virus shedding against challenge by a Chinese pseudorabies variant

Jichun Wang[1,3], Rongli Guo[1,3], Yongfeng Qiao[1,3], Mengwei Xu[1,3], Zhisheng Wang[1,3], Yamei Liu[1,3], Yiqi Gu[1,2], Chang Liu[1,2] and Jibo Hou[1,3*]

Abstract

Background: Since the end of 2011 an outbreak of pseudorabies affected Chinese pig herds that had been vaccinated with the commercial vaccine made of Bartha K61 strain. It is now clear that the outbreak was caused by an emergent PRV variant. Even though vaccines made of PRV Bartha K61 strain can confer certain cross protection against PRV variants based on experimental data, less than optimal clinical protection and virus shedding reduction were observed, making the control or eradication of this disease difficult.

Results: An infectious clone of PRV AH02LA strain was constructed to generate a gE deletion mutant PRV(LA-A^B) strain. PRV(LA-A^B) strain can reach a titer of $10^{8.43}$ $TCID_{50}$ /mL (50% tissue culture infectious dose) on BHK-21 cells. To evaluate the efficiency of the inactivated vaccine made of PRV(LA-A^B) strain, thirty 3-week-old PRV-negative piglets were divided randomly into six groups for vaccination and challenge test. All five piglets in the challenge control showed typical clinical symptoms of pseudorabies post challenge. Sneezing and nasal discharge were observed in four and three piglets in groups C(vaccinated with inactivated PRV Bartha K61 strain vaccine) and D(vaccinated with live PRV Bartha K61 strain vaccine) respectively. In contrast, piglets in both groups A(vaccinated with inactivated PRV LA-AB strain vaccine) and B(vaccinated with inactivated PRV LA-A^B strain vaccine with adjuvant) presented mild or no clinical symptoms. Moreover, viral titers detected via nasal swabs were approximately 100 times lower in group B than in the challenge control, and the duration of virus shedding (3–4 days) was shorter than in either the challenge control (5–10 days) or groups C and D (5–6 days).

Conclusions: The infectious clone constructed in this study harbors the whole genome of the PRV variant AH02LA strain. The gE deletion mutant PRV(LA-A^B)strain generated from PRV AH02LA strain can reach a high titer on BHK-21 cells. An inactivated vaccine of PRV LA-A^B provides clinical protection and significantly reduces virus shedding post challenge, especially if accompanied by the adjuvant CVC1302. While Inactivated or live vaccines made of PRV Barth K61 strain can provide only partial protection in this test.

Keywords: Pseudorabies virus emerging variant, gE deletion, Inactivated vaccine, Adjuvant, Bacterial artificial chromosome, Challenge protection

* Correspondence: houjibo@jaas.ac.cn
[1]National Research Center of Engineering and Technology for Veterinary Biologicals/Institute of Veterinary Medicine, Jiangsu Academy of Agricultural Sciences, Nanjing, Jiangsu 210014, China
[3]Jiangsu Co-innovation Center for Prevention and Control of Important Animal Infectious Diseases and Zoonoses, Yangzhou, China
Full list of author information is available at the end of the article

Background

Pseudorabies, caused by pseudorabies virus(PRV), has leaded to significant economic losses to the pig industry in many countries. Pseudorabies is a porcine infectious disease that can be effectively controlled using gene deletion marked vaccines and serum monitoring, enabling differentiation of vaccinated from infected animals [1–3]. However, in 2011 an outbreak of pseudorabies affected Chinese pig herds that had been vaccinated with the standard PRV Bartha K61 strain [4–9]. It is now clear that the outbreak was caused by an emergent PRV variant [5–7, 9–13]. As a support for this finding, the widely used PRV Bartha K61 strain was shown to be incapable of providing complete protection against this new PRV variant in several experimental studies [4–8]. Thus, a more efficacious vaccine is perceived as a necessary tool to help affected herds revert to PRV virus negative status.

To develop an effective vaccine, gene deletion mutants were generated from the new PRV strain and evaluated for protection efficacy. Although live vaccine candidates based on gE, gE/gI, or TK/gE/gI gene deletion mutants are assumed to be highly protective, the safety issues of these preparations have to be demonstrated by lengthy testing [4, 14–18]. Alternatively, inactivated version of vaccine from the same mutants are promising to provide clinical protection as well based on relevant data about inactivated Bartha strain.

In this study, LA-A^B, a gE deleted mutant of the emerging PRV strain AH02LA, was constructed using a bacterial artificial chromosome clone. A vaccine utilizing this mutant was evaluated with and without adjuvant in regard to its ability to provide clinical protection and reduce virus shedding after lethal challenge.

Methods

Cells and viruses

BHK-21 cells (CVCC:CL5, from China Veterinary Culture Collection Center) and chicken embryo cells (CECs) (SPF chicken embryo eggs were from Beijing Merial Vital Laboratory Animal Technology Co., Ltd) were prepared using standard methods. The PRV Bartha K61 strain was kindly provided by Professor Ping Jiang of Nanjing Agricultural University. Virus cultures and stocks were prepared using CECs or BHK-21 cells before at -70 °C. Virus titers were determined by $TCID_{50}$ on BHK-21 cells following a standard protocol. Viral DNA extraction and transfection of plasmid, virus or bacterial artificial chromosome(BAC) DNAs were performed as described previously [19, 20].

Plasmid and BAC manipulation

The mini-F transfer vector pHA2-pUC19-H1-H2 was constructed as described [16]. Plasmid and BAC DNAs were isolated using commercial kits (Invitrogen PureLink® Quick Plasmid Miniprep and Qiagen Large-Construct Kit) following the manufacturer's instructions. Next, restriction fragment length polymorphism(RFLP) analyses of PRV BACs was conducted using the restriction endonucleases *BamH* I, *Kpn* I, *Pst* I and *Sph* I and digestion conditions recommended by the supplier (Takara). Electrocompetent *E.coli* cells (DH10B) were obtained commercially (Invitrogen). *E.coli* GS1783 was made electrocompetent using published protocols [21–23]. Electroporation was performed to transform viral or BAC DNA following established methods [23–25].

PCR and sequencing

A pair of primers (Table 1) was designed from reference sequence (GenBank:NC_006151.1) to amplify sequences

Table 1 Primers for PCR or sequencing

Primer	Sequence
PRV gD F	5′-AACACCTAATTTGCGTACGGC-3′
PRV gD R	5′-TCATCATCGACGCCGGTACT-3′
PRV gI F	5′-TGGGCGTGTGCGTCTACATCT-3′
PRV gI R	5′-CAACCCCGGTGTGTGTGAGA-3′
ΔgE T^V overlap1 F	5′-CCACGCCCAGCGGTCCATAAAATTGGGT-3′
ΔgE T^V overlap1 R	5′- TCATCACGAAGGAGCCCAGCAAAGGG CCGCATGG TCTCAACC-3′
ΔgE T^V overlap2 F	5′-GCTGGGCTCCTTCGTGATGA-3′
ΔgE T^V overlap2 R	5′-TCACGATCTGGGCATGCAGG-3′
SEQ-gI/gE F 1	5′-TTGCGTACGGCCTTGCTTAC-3′
SEQ-gI/gE F 2	5′-GACTACATGTTCCCCACGGA-3′
SEQ-gI/gE F 3	5′-ACGCCGTACGCCATCGACCC-3′
SEQ-gI/gE F 4	5′-ACGCTGCTGTTTCTGGAGGG-3′
SEQ-gI/gE F 5	5′-ACGAAGAGGAGGAGGACGAG-3′
SEQ-gI/gE F 6	5′-ACCATGCGGCCCTTTCTGCT-3′
SEQ-gI/gE F 7	5′-ACCACGGTGTGCTTCGAGAC-3′
SEQ-gI/gE F 8	5′-TGTACGAGCCCTGCATCTACCACCC-3′
SEQ-gI/gE F 9	5′-ACTACTACGACGGCGACGACGACGA-3′
SEQ-gI/gE F 10	5′-AACGAGACGCCCAGCGAGTT-3′
SEQ-gI/gE F 11	5′-AAGGTGCTCACCGAGTGGTGCTACG-3′
SEQ-gI/gE R 1	5′-TCTAGGAGATGGTACATCGCGGGGC-3′
SEQ-gI/gE R 2	5′-TGGTGATGTAGAACGGCGCC-3′
SEQ-gI/gE R 3	5′-ACAGCGAGCAGATGACCAGC-3′
SEQ-gI/gE R 4	5′-TCGCTGCTGAACTCGTCCTC-3′
SEQ-gI/gE R 5	5′-ATCACGAGCACGTACAGCCC-3′
SEQ-gI/gE R 6	5′-TGTAGAGGCCCGTGTCGTTG-3′
SEQ-gI/gE R 7	5′-AAAGGGCCGCATGGTCTCAACC-3′
SEQ-gI/gE R 8	5′-TCCTCCTCCTCTTCGTCGGA-3′
SEQ-gI/gE R 9	5′-AAAGAGGTCCGTGGTCCCGTTCAC-3′
SEQ-gI/gE R 10	5′-AGATGTAGACGCACACGCCCACCAG-3′
SEQ-gI/gE R 11	5′-GGGAACATGTAGTCCGCGGA-3′

of gI gene with isolated PRV AH02LA strain DNA as template. These primers were also used for sequencing gI gene (GeneScript, Nanjing China). To obtain the gE deletion, overlap PCR was conducted with two pairs of primers, ΔgE T^V overlap1 and ΔgE T^V overlap2 (Table 1). Briefly, with PRV AH02LA DNA as template, two PCR reactions were performed separately with the above two primer pairs. Next, the PCR products were gel purified to serve as templates in another PCR reaction with primers ΔgE T^V overlap1 F and ΔgE T^V overlap2 R to produce a fragment for gE deletion mutant generation. Thus the generated mutant, consists of upstream sequences, the intact gI gene, part of gE gene(1299 bp to 1735 bp of gE ORF), and downstream sequences (Fig. 1). Finally, the primers PRV Homo-1 F and PRV Homo-2R [16] were used to amplify the repairing viral DNA with the PRV AH02LA DNA as template.

Multistep growth kinetics

Multistep growth kinetics of parental AH02LA, gE deletion LA-A^B, and repair AH02LA^R viruses were tested on BHK-21 cells following methods as described [26] on monolayers (1×10^6 cells) of BHK-21 cells with a multiplicity of infection(MOI)of 0.01. Three independent experiments were conducted and one-way ANOVA (SPSS software package) was employed to identify significant differences.

LD_{50} determination for PRV AH02LA strain

To determine the LD_{50} of the virulent PRV AH02LA strain, the virus ($TCID_{50} = 10^{-8.25}$/mL) was serially diluted with DMEM to 10^{-1}, 10^{-2}, 10^{-3} and 10^{-4}. Twenty-five 77-day-old piglets were randomly divided into five groups. Piglets in each challenge group were inoculated intranasally(I.N.) with 1 mL diluted virus of different titers. Animals were observed for additional fourteen days. The number of piglets that died in each group was recorded to calculate LD_{50} using the Karber method.

Construction of PRV BAC and deletion mutants

The PRV BAC was constructed from an isolate of the emergent PRV variant following published methods (Fig. 1) [16, 26]. Briefly, After cotransfection of ~1.5 μg PRV AH02LA strain DNA and ~4 μg pHA2-pUC19-H1-H2 DNA, mini-F recombinant viruses with green fluorescence were purified to obtain a homogeneous population [27]. Next, mini-F containing PRV DNA was isolated and then transferred into *E. coli* cells DH10B and subsequently into *E.coli* strain GS1783 cells by electroporation for mutagenesis [23]. Finally, BAC DNA was isolated and RFLPs were identified as described [24] using *BamH* I, *Kpn* I, *Pst* I and

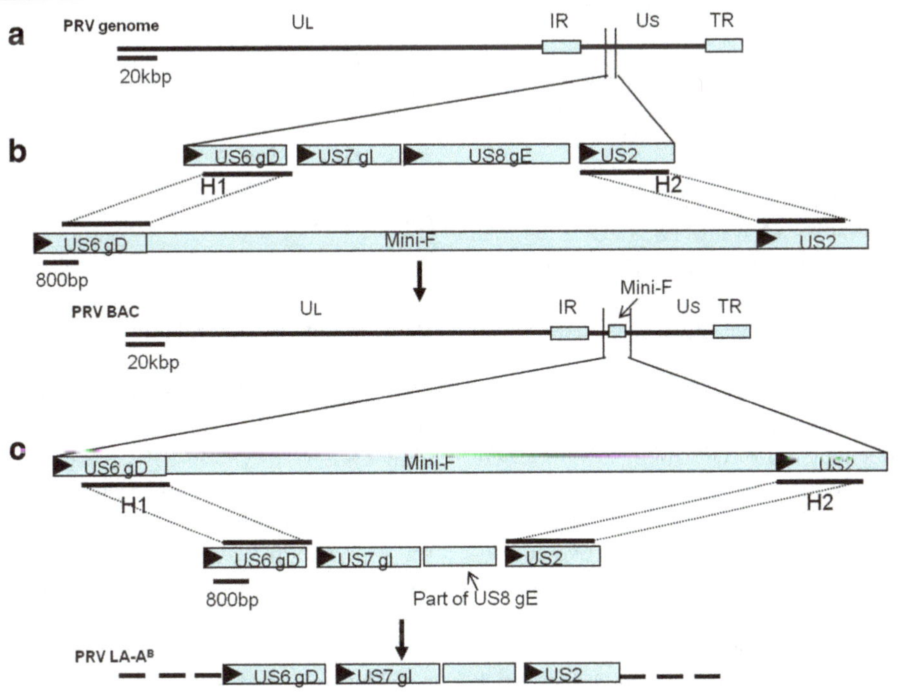

Fig. 1 Construction of mini-F recombinant PRV AH02LA strain and its gE deletion mutant virus (LA-A^B). **a** The whole genome of PRV. **b** Homologous recombination was conducted to insert mini-F in lieu of gI and gE to generate the mini-F recombinant PRV AH02LA strain for BAC construction. **c** Another recombination was performed to recover the whole gI gene and part of gE gene, the resulting $BAC^{PRV\text{-}G}$ was used to generate the gE deletion LA-A^B strain. Scales in bp or kbp are provided

Sph I, using the complete genome sequence of PRV ZJ01 strain (GenBank: KM061380.1) as a reference for *in silico* prediction.

To generate the gE deletion mutant of PRV AH02LA strain, another homologous recombination was performed to recover the gI gene and the undeleted sequences of gE as shown in Fig. 1. Briefly, PCR with primers ΔgE T^V overlap1 F and ΔgE T^V overlap2 R (Table 1) was performed with the PRV AH02LA DNA as template. And then CECs were co-transfected with approximately 5 μg PRV BAC DNA and 2 μg DNA of fragment from the second PCR reaction of overlap PCR with primersΔgE T^V overlap1 F andΔgE T^V overlap2 R by calcium phosphate precipitation. Using illumination at 488 nm, non-fluorescent virus isolates were selected and purified to homogeneity. Product structure was confirmed by sequencing with the same primers and other specific primers from the SEQ-gI/gE series (Table 1).

For generation of the gI/gE repair virus via homologous recombination, CECs were transfected with approximately 5 μg PRV BAC DNA and 2 μg PCR product generated using DNA of parental PRV as template and primers matching PRV Homo 1 F and PRV Homo 2R [16] (Fig. 1). Two to three days after transfection, non-fluorescent plaques (488 nm) were isolated and purified to obtain a homogeneous population. The structure of the recovered viruses was confirmed by PCR and sequencing with primers PRV Homo 1 F, PRV Homo 2R and sequencing primers of SEQ-gI/gE (Table 1).

Preparation of vaccine

PRV LA-A^B and Bartha K61 viruses were propagated in BHK-21 cells using a 5 liter bioreactor, each virus stock was diluted to $10^{8.5}$ $TCID_{50}$/mL. After inactivation with formalin (Sigma-Aldrich) as described [16], vaccines were prepared using mineral oil adjuvant (1:3 water in oil). All vaccines were confirmed to be free of bacteria and fungi, and had the expected physical properties according to standard protocols. Vaccines were stored at 4 °C until use.

Test of vaccine efficacy

Thirty piglets of 21-day-old (from Zhengzhuquan Pig Breeding Farm in Pukou district, Nanjing, China) were randomly divided into 6 groups (A-F) and housed in separated facilities. All piglets were antibody negative for PRV gB and gE, and free of porcine reproductive and respiratory syndrome virus, porcine parvovirus, porcine circovirus 2 and classical swine fever virus. All inoculations were given intramuscularly(I.M.) at 2 mL/pig. Group A piglets were inoculated with LA-A^B, group B piglets with LA-A^B plus adjuvant CVC1302 (Patent: CN103083663B, kindly provided by the group of Dr. Qisheng Zheng in our institute), group C piglets with inactivated Bartha K61, group D piglets with live Bartha K61 of $1 \times 10^{5.0}$ $TCID_{50}$ virus/dose, and groups E and F piglets were dosed with PBS only. Piglets in groups A, B, and C were inoculated at 28 days of age and again at 56 days. Group D piglets were inoculated once, at 28-day-old. Group E and F piglets were dosed once, at 28 days of age. Three weeks after the second inoculation (at which time the piglets were 11-week-old), groups A, B, C, D and E were challenged I.N. with $3 \times LD_{50}$ PRV AH02LA per piglet. Group F piglets were not challenged, serving as a negative control. Serum samples from all piglets were collected before inoculation, and at 7, 14, 21, 28, 35, 42 and 49 days post inoculation, and again at 14 days post challenge(P.C.). Serum was subjected to ELISA tests for PRV gB and gE antibodies, and cross-neutralizing (NA) antibodies against AH02LA or Bartha K61. Body temperature, clinical signs, and virus shedding were monitored and recorded daily until 14 days P.C.. The presence of lung lesions for died or survived piglets was noted at the end of the test.

Test for serological antibodies

ELISA tests were performed with the PRV gE or gB antibody detection kit (IDEXX, Maine, USA) following manufacturer's instructions. Cross neutralization tests were conducted according to the standard methods published by OIE (Veterinary Pharmacopoeia of the People's Republic of China (2010)) with slight modification. Briefly, serum samples were diluted two-fold with PBS, mixed with 100 $TCID_{50}$ PRV AH02LA or PRV Bartha K61 virus, and incubated for 1 h at 37 °C. The serum-virus mixture was used to inoculate BHK-21 cells which were then incubated at 37 °C, 5% CO_2 for 3–4 days to observe the development of CPE. Titers of neutralizing antibody were expressed as $n\log_2$ of highest dilution at which no CPE was observed, and mean titers of each group were calculated for comparison.

Detection of virus shedding

Nasal swab samples were collected from all piglets before challenge and daily to 14 days after challenge. After shaking at 5000–8000 RPM for 1–2 min, one freeze-thaw cycle (-70 °C and 37 °C) was conducted to release viruses from nasal swabs. Samples were centrifuged at 10,000 RPM for 15 min to pellet tissue and cell debris, the supernatants were collected to determine virus titers. Viruses titers were expressed as $TCID_{50}$ following the method of Karber.

All animal studies were conducted following guidelines provided by the Institutional Biosafety Committee and approved by the Institutional Animal Care and Use Committee at the Jiangsu Academy of Agriculture Sciences. Experiments involving virulent PRV were conducted under Biosafety Level 2+ containment.

Results

Isolation and identification of an emergent pseudorabies virus variant (AH02LA strain)

BHK-21 cells, inoculated with a sample of brain tissue from a stillborn piglet, exhibited cytopathogenic effects (CPE) after 3 days. After three rounds of plaque purification, a homogeneous population of virus was isolated and designated as the AH02LA strain. Using the viral DNA as template and the primers PRV gI F/ R (Table 1), PCR generated a product of 1250–1400 bp. Sequencing established that this fragment was homologous to the PRV gI gene. The AH02LA strain can be specifically neutralized with the standard antibodies against PRV (CIVDC, Beijing China) with a neutralizing index of 10,000. These results demonstrate that a variant PRV field isolate was identified.

Pathology of the PRV AH02LA strain

The LD_{50} of PRV AH02LA (Batch: JJ-R5) was determined using 77-day-old piglets free of antibodies against PRV. Three of five piglets in the 10^{-5} dosage group, and all of the piglets in the 10^{-4} dosage group, showed typical symptoms of PRV infection: sneezing, purulent nasal discharge, difficulty in breathing and ataxia, indicating the high virulence of this strain. The LD_{50} was $10^{-2.32}$/mL. The highly virulent character of AH02LA is shared by other emergent PRV strains isolated during the 2011 outbreaks [4–8]. The significant difference between these emerging strains and the conventional strain S (HWBD, Harbin China) is that the former cause mortalities in not only young piglets but also much older pigs, whereas the conventional strain S causes death only in young (less than 15-day-old) piglets (Veterinary Pharmacopoeia of the People's Republic of China (2005)).

Construction of a bacterial artificial chromosome containing the AH02LA genome

Green plaques of mini-F recombinant PRV AH02LA were observed under UV light (488 nm), and isolated after several rounds of plaque purification. The mini-F recombinant PRV AH02LA DNA was isolated and transfected into *Escherichia coli* DH10B competent cells, the resulting clone was designated $BAC^{PRV\text{-}AH02LA}$. $BAC^{PRV\text{-}AH02LA}$ DNA was electroporated into *E. coli* GS1783 competent cells, resulting in a clone designated $BAC^{PRV\text{-}G}$. This BAC was used for further gene manipulations using the *En Passant* protocol [20]. Restriction fragment length polymorphism (RFLP) analysis of $BAC^{PRV\text{-}G}$ with *BamH* I, *Kpn* I, *Pst* I and *Sph* I generated patterns similar to those predicted from the PRV ZJ01 strain sequence (GenBank: KM061380.1) with minor differences (Fig. 2). Virus was rescued successfully by transfection of the $BAC^{PRV\text{-}G}$ DNA into primary CECs, designated PRV $AH02LA^{R}$. In summary, an infectious clone containing the complete genome of the PRV emerging variant AH02LA strain was constructed successfully.

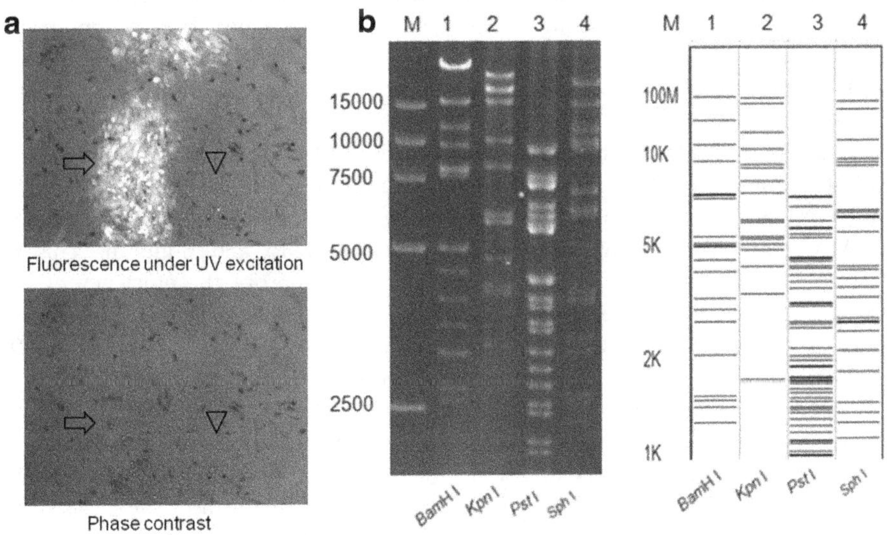

Fig. 2 Plaques of mini-F recombinant PRV AH02LA strain and RFLP of $BAC^{PRV\text{-}G}$. **a** Images of mini-F recombinant PRV AH02LA and the parental AH02LA plaques under UV excitation (upper) and phase contrast (lower) are shown. Arrowhead shows a plaque of parental PRV AH02LA virus and arrow shows a plaque formed by mini-F recombinant PRV AH02LA. Each panel represents a view of 200 × 200 μm in size. **b** RFLP of $BAC^{PRV\text{-}G}$, DNA from PRV AH02LA BAC clone $BAC^{PRV\text{-}G}$ was prepared by mini-prep and digested with *BamH* I, *Kpn* I, *Pst* I and *Sph* I (lanes 1–4). The digests were separated by 0.8% agarose gel electrophoresis for 16 h under 40 V (Left). Predicted RFLP patterns of $BAC^{PRV\text{-}G}$ with *BamH* I, *Kpn* I, *Pst* I and *Sph* I digestion respectively. Predictions of these digestions were performed with the whole genome sequence of PRV ZJ01 strain (GenBank: KM061380.1) as reference. M: DL 15,000 DNA Marker (Takara)

Construction of a gE deletion mutant virus

After co-transfection of $BAC^{PRV\text{-}G}$ DNA with a DNA fragment containing the gE deletion (obtained through PCR), several white plaques were observed under UV illumination at 488 nm. One was isolated after several rounds of plaque purification and designated PRV LA-A^B. The deletion was verified by PCR using primers of ΔgE TV overlap1 F andΔgE TV overlap2 R, followed by sequencing with the appropriate primers (Table 1).

Growth kinetics of the PRV LA-A^B virus

Multistep growth kinetics for the PRV LA-A^B, AH02LA, and $AH02LA^R$ viruses were determined. Peak supernatant titers for LA-A^B, AH02LA, and $AH02LA^R$ were $10^{8.18}$, $10^{9.01}$, and $10^{8.19}$ $TCID_{50}$ /mL respectively. At 48 hpi the titers for LA-A^B and $AH02LA^R$ were not significantly different from AH02LA ($p = 0.414$ and 0.362). For cell-associated virus titers LA-A^B, AH02LA, and $AH02LA^R$ were $10^{8.43}$, $10^{8.86}$, and $10^{8.13}$ $TCID_{50}$ /mL at 48 hpi, respectively. The titers of LA-A^B and $AH02LA^R$ are not significant different from the parental virus AH02LA at 48 hpi ($p = 0.126$ and 0.088).

Immunogenicity of the LA-A^B vaccine

In challenge control group, all piglets had typical clinical syndromes of pseudorabies infection including sneezing, coughing, difficulty breathing and nasal discharge P.C.. Two piglets died at 7 days and two at 8 days P.C. (Table 2). Body temperatures of these piglets reached over 41 °C and lasted for 4–5 days (Fig. 3(a)). All the piglets shed virus with titers of $10^{0.25} \sim 10^{5.25}$ $TCID_{50}$ /0.1 mL lasting for 5–7 days till death or 10 days for the surviving piglet (Fig. 3(b)). All piglets showed severe lung lesions from hemorrhaging and congestion (Table 2).

gB antibodies were detected in all piglets vaccinated with live Bartha K61 strain or the LA-A^B strain plus adjuvant at 7 days post vaccination(P.V.), while two of five piglets vaccinated LA-A^B strain alone or the inactivated Bartha K61 strain were anti-gB positive at 7 days P.V.. All samples collected at 14 days P.V. were positive for gB antibodies (Table 2). This result indicates the adjuvant CVC1302 helps the LA-A^B vaccine stimulate immunity against PRV more quickly. At 14 days P.C. all piglets were positive for gE antibodies (Table 2).

No neutralizing antibodies (NA) against the AH02LA or Bartha K61 strain, were detected in any of the piglets at 7 days P.V.. At 14 days P.V. neutralizing antibodies were detected in one piglet from group B (LA-A^B plus adjuvant) at a titer of 2. In groups A, B, and C, NA titers began increasing quickly seven days after the boost and continued to increase over the next two weeks. The LA-A^B vaccines induced higher titers of NA against the AH02LA and Bartha K61 strain, than vaccines made of Bartha K61. One dose of live Bartha K61 vaccine stimulated a weak NA titer of less than 4 against the AH02LA strain or the Bartha K61 strain. These results indicate that optimizing the prime-boost regimen is necessary for live Bartha K61 vaccine to stimulate strong humoral immunity. NA titers in group B piglets were higher than other groups, indicating that adjuvant CVC1302 helped stimulate higher specific immunity for LA-A^B vaccine (Table 2).

All piglets in the vaccinated groups (A, B, C and D) were protected against lethal challenge. Fevers in group A and B piglets were transient, and other clinical symptoms were mild or absent respectively. Titers of shed virus in LA-A^B vaccinated group A piglets were $10^{0.25} \sim 10^{3.75}$ $TCID_{50}$/0.1 mL lasting 3–4 days; in LA-A^B plus adjuvant group B piglets, titers were $10^{0.125} \sim 10^{2.875}$ $TCID_{50}$/0.1 mL lasting 3–4 days. Piglets in groups C and D (vaccinated with inactivated Bartha K61 and live Bartha K61 respectively) presented fevers of more than 41 °C lasting for 4–6 days (Fig. 3(a)), four and three piglets respectively, presented sneezing lasting for 2–4 days and nasal discharge lasting 2–3 days (Table 2). The titers of shed virus in these piglets were $10^{0.125} \sim 10^{4.125}$ $TCID_{50}$ /0.1 mL lasting for 5–6 days (Fig. 3(b)). No Lung lesions were observed in any group A or B piglets, while 2/5 group C piglets and in 1/5 group D piglets presented lesions from hemorrhage and congestion (Table 2).

Discussion

The results of vaccination test demonstrate that vaccines made of PRV LA-A^B elicit a more effective immune response against the emergent PRV AH02LA than the Bartha K61 vaccines. The immune response is even more pronounced when PRV LA-A^B is administered with adjuvant. Pigs vaccinated with LA-A^B produced lower titers of virus shedding over a shorter duration than pigs with Bartha K61. This is a clear advantage in the terms of controlling the spread of infection. Adjuvant CVC1302 is a mixture of monophosphoryl lipid A (MPLA), muramyl dipeptide (MDP) and β-glucan. This mixture has been shown to improve the efficiency of the inactivated vaccines of porcine epidemic diarrhea virus and foot and mouth disease virus (Patent:CN103083663B). MPLA, MDP and β-glucan can serve as delivery systems or stimulators for the immune system [28–31].

Bacterial artificial chromosome(BAC) of herpesvirus is a useful tool for generation of gene modified mutants to study the mechanism of the viruses. After the construction of the first BAC of mouse cytomegalovirus (MCMV) [32], a few of herpesvirus genomes have been maintained in BACs as infectious clones, which have provided great help for discovery of pathology of these viruses [27, 33] and construction of vectored vaccines [26, 34, 35], especially following the protocol of En Passant protocol [23]. The parental PRV AH02LA strain of

Table 2 Antibodies, clinical signs and lung lesions in animals

Groups			A	B	C	D	E	F
ELISA antibodies against PRV gB or gE	B.V.	gB+	0[a]/5[b]	0/5	0/5	0/5	0/5	0/5
		gE+	0/5	0/5	0/5	0/5	0/5	0/5
	7d P.V.	gB+	2/5	5/5	2/5	5/5	0/5	0/5
		gE+	0/5	0/5	0/5	0/5	0/5	0/5
	14d P.V.	gB+	5/5	5/5	5/5	5/5	0/5	0/5
		gE+	0/5	0/5	0/5	0/5	0/5	0/5
	21d P.V.	gB+	5/5	5/5	5/5	5/5	0/5	0/5
		gE+	0/5	0/5	0/5	0/5	0/5	0/5
	14d P.C.	gB+	5/5	5/5	5/5	5/5	2/2	0/5
		gE+	5/5	5/5	5/5	5/5	2/2	0/5
Mean titers of neutralizing antibodies	AH02LA	B.V.	<2[c]	<2	<2	<2	<2	<2
		7d P.V.	<2	<2	<2	<2	<2	<2
		14d P.V.	<2	0.4	<2	<2	<2	<2
		21d P.V.	2.00	2.80	<2	1.20	<2	<2
		28d P.V.	2.60	3.40	2.40	2.60	<2	<2
		35d P.V.	4.60	5.20	3.60	3.20	<2	<2
		42d P.V.	4.60	5.60	3.80	3.20	<2	<2
		49d P.V.	5.20	6.20	4.20	3.00	<2	<2
	Bartha K61	B.V.	<2	<2	<2	<2	<2	<2
		7d P.V.	<2	<2	<2	<2	<2	<2
		14d P.V.	<2	0.4	<2	<2	<2	<2
		21d P.V.	1.20	2.24	1.2	1.60	<2	<2
		28d P.V.	2.40	3.08	2.60	3.20	<2	<2
		35d P.V.	4.60	4.80	4.60	3.20	<2	<2
		42d P.V.	4.80	5.20	4.80	3.60	<2	<2
		49d P.V.	5.40	5.60	5.20	3.40	<2	<2
Clinical signs and lung lesions post challenge	Morbidity		1/5	0/5	4/5	3/5	5/5	0/5
	Duration of clinical signs(days)		1	-	2–4	2–3	4–7	-
	Mortality		0/5	0/5	0/5	0/5	4/5	0/5
	Lung lesions		0/5	0/5	2/5	1/5	5/5	0/5

B.V means before vaccination, *P.V* means post vaccination, *P.C* means post challenge. "a" indicates the number of piglets positive;"b" indicates the number of piglets in the group. "c" indicates mean titers of neutralizing antibody of each group expressed as $nlog_2$ of highest dilution at which no CPE was observed

the BAC constructed in this study is a virulent variant strain that caused severe losses in many porcine farms in China. So even though En Passant protocol was not performed in the generation of the gE deleted LA-A^B strain in this study, it will be used for further analysis of the mechanism of the high virulence of this variant.

The latent infection of PRV is always a potential threat to porcine herds [36]. So the eradication of PRV has been a direct aim of many farms for control of this disease. This aim has been achieved in a few countries [1] and the infection of wild PRV has been controlled to very low levels in some individual farms in China before 2011 [37, 38]. DIVA vaccine(vaccine allowing differentiating infected from vaccinated animals) has played an important role towards this aim [1]. In the project of eradication of PRV, the efficient reduction of virus shedding post infection with virulent strain is crucial [2]. In this study, the inactivated vaccine of LA-A^B strain with adjuvant CVC1302 reduced virus shedding significantly, despite that all vaccinated animals did not stop virus shedding post challenge.

We did find a difference in the profile of clinical symptoms between animals challenged through I.M. or I.N. route. During the challenge test in this study, we also tried the challenge route of I.M. injection for 11-week-old piglets (data not shown). We found that even though it caused high fever and obvious clinical syndromes of PR through this way, the virulence was significantly

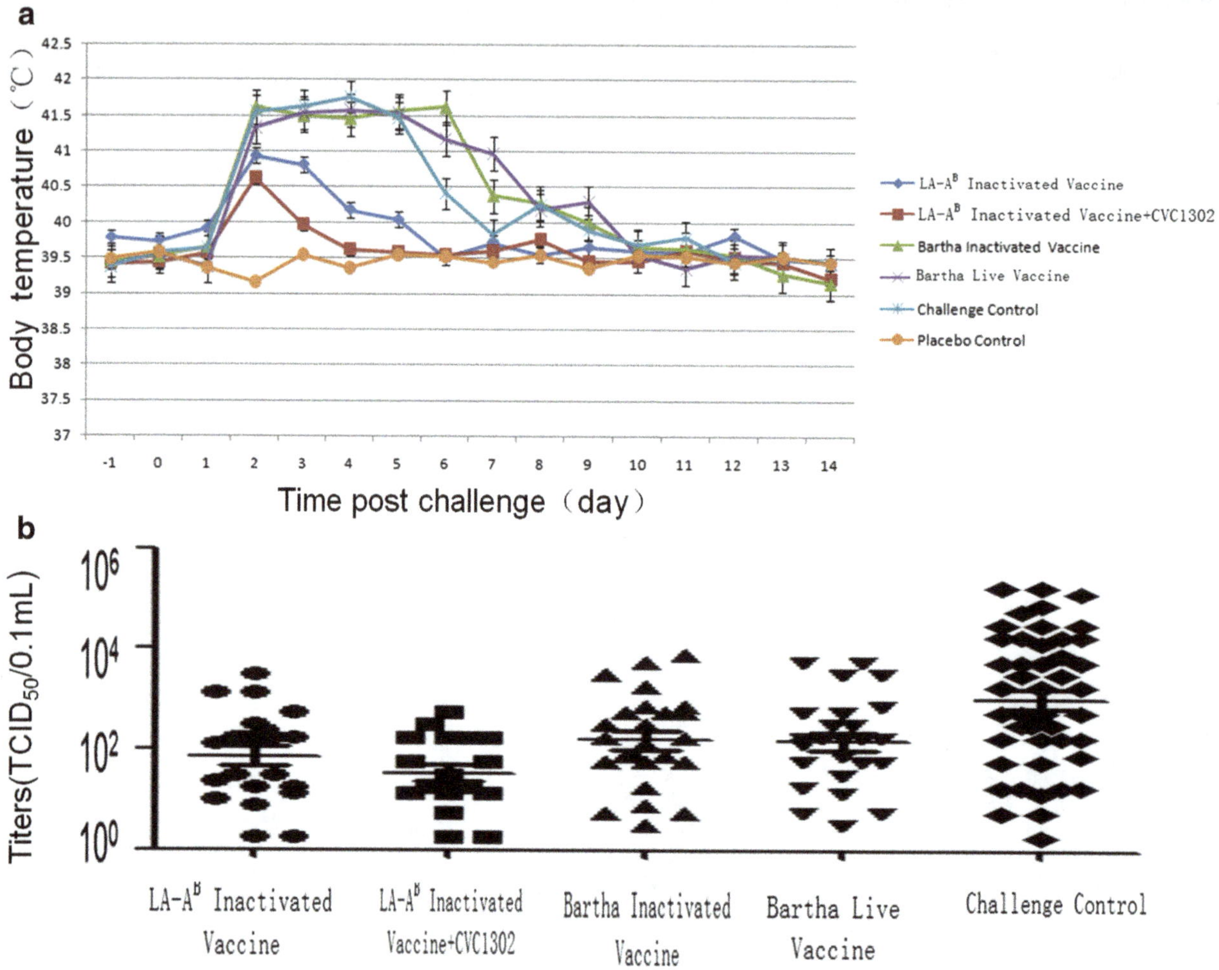

Fig. 3 Body temperatures and virus shedding post challenge with PRV AH02LA strain. **a** Body temperatures of piglets in vaccinated groups were detected together with challenge control and placebo control from one day before challenge to 14 days post challenge. Average temperatures of five piglets of each group were taken for comparison. Error bars represent the standard deviations. **b** Nasal swab samples of all piglets of vaccinated groups together with challenge control and placebo control groups were collected before challenge and daily up to 14 days after challenge for virus isolation and titer determination. The titers of viruses were expressed as $TCID_{50}$ on BHK-21 cells following the method of Karber. Average titers were determined with the samples that virus exceeding were detected

lower than through I.N. way. This difference is presumed to be associated with the increased titers of virus after replication on epithelial cells of respiratory tract. To mimick the nature infection of domestic pigs genuinely, we did the challenge protection test through I.N. way for evaluation of the vaccines in this study.

Conclusion

The infectious clone consists of the whole genome of PRV emerging variant AH02LA strain. Inactivated vaccine made of PRV LA-A^B strain can provide better clinical protection than vaccines made of Bartha K61. In addition, significant decrease of virus shedding was observed post lethal challenge when LA-A^B inactivated vaccine were adjuvanted with CVC1302.

Abbreviations

BAC: Bacterial artificial chromosome; CEC: Chicken embryo cell; CPE: Cytopathogenic effects; *E.coli*: Escherichia coli; ELISA: Enzyme-linked immunosorbent assay; gB: glycoprotein B; gE: glycoprotein E; gI: glycoprotein I; Hpi: Hour post infection; I.M: Intramuscularly; I.N: Intranasally; LD_{50}: 50% lethal dose; MCMV: Mouse cytomegalovirus; MDP: Muramyl dipeptide; MOI: Multiplicity of infection; MPLA: Monophosphoryl lipid; NA: Neutralizing antibodies; ORF: Open reading frame; PC: Post challenge; PV: Post vaccination; PBS: Phosphate buffer saline; PCR: Polymerase chain reaction; PRV: Pseudorabies virus; RFLP: Restriction fragment length polymorphism; $TCID_{50}$: 50% tissue culture infectious dose; TK: Thymidine kinase; VN: Virus neutralization

Acknowledgements

We thanks professor Nikolaus Osterrieder at the Free University of Berlin for kindly providing *E.coli* GS1783. We thanks Dr Qisheng Zheng for kindly providing adjuvant CVC1302.

Funding

This study was supported by the Special Fund for Agro-Scientific Research in the Public Interest (201303046), Program for Independence and Innovation in Agricultural Sciences of Jiangsu Province (CX(12)3061 and CX(14)2084), and the Natural Science Foundation of Jiangsu Province (BK20131334).

Availability of supporting data
The data set(s) supporting the results of this article is included within the article. And all row data are available in National Research Center of Engineering and Technology for Veterinary Biologicals/Institute of Veterinary Medicine, Jiangsu Academy of Agricultural Sciences, Nanjing Jiangsu, China upon official request via mail (jcwang@263.net).

Authors' contributions
JW and JH designed the generation of BAC and related mutants. JW, YQ, YG and CL contributed to the design and performance of animal tests. RG, YG, CL, YL and MX constructed the bacterial artificial chromosome of PRV and the related studies. JW ZW and RG constructed the gE deleted vaccine. ZW, JW, YQ and RG investigated the related properties of the vaccine and performed the animal experiments and related tests. All authors approved the final manuscript.

Competing interests
The authors declare that they have no conflicts of interest.

Consent for publication
Not applicable.

Author details
[1]National Research Center of Engineering and Technology for Veterinary Biologicals/Institute of Veterinary Medicine, Jiangsu Academy of Agricultural Sciences, Nanjing, Jiangsu 210014, China. [2]College of Veterinary Medicine, Nanjing Agricultural University, Nanjing 210095, China. [3]Jiangsu Co-innovation Center for Prevention and Control of Important Animal Infectious Diseases and Zoonoses, Yangzhou, China.

References
1. Zimmerman JJ, Karriker LA, Ramirez A, Schwartz KJ, Stevenson GW. Diseases of Swine. 10th Edition. Ames: Iowa State University Press, Wiley-Blackwell. 2014;1541-73.
2. Van Nes A, Stegeman JA, De Jong MC, Loeffen WL, Kimman TG JH. No massive spread of pseudorabies virus in vaccinated sow herds. Vet Microbiol. 1997;55(1-4):147–51.
3. Lyman M, Demmin G, Banfield B. The attenuated pseudorabies virus strain Bartha fails to package the tegument proteins Us3 and VP22. J Virol. 2003; 77(2):1403–14.
4. Wang C, Yuan J, Qin H, Luo Y, Cong X, Chen J, Li S, Sun Y, Qiu H. A novel gE-deleted pseudorabies virus (PRV) provides rapid and complete protection from lethal challenge with the PRV variant emerging in Bartha-K61-vaccinated swine population in China. Vaccine. 2014;32(27):3379–85.
5. Ye C, Zhang Q, Tian Z, Zheng H, Zhao K, Liu F, Guo J, Tong W, Jiang C, Wang S, et al. Genomic characterization of emergent pseudorabies virus in China reveals marked sequence divergence: Evidence for the existence of two major genotypes. Virology. 2015;483:32–43.
6. Yu X, Zhou Z, Hu D, Zhang Q, Han T, Li X, Gu X, Yuan L, Zhang S, Wang B, et al. Pathogenic pseudorabies virus, China, 2012. Emerg Infect Dis. 2014;20(1):102–4.
7. Wang Y, Qiao S, Li X, Xie W, Guo J, Li Q, Liu X, Hou J, Xu Y, Wang L, et al. Molecular epidemiology of outbreak-associated pseudorabies virus (PRV) strains in central China. Virus Genes. 2015;50(3):401–9.
8. An T, Peng J, Tian Z, Zhao H, Li N, Liu Y, Chen J, Leng C, Sun Y, Chang D, et al. Pseudorabies virus variant in bartha-k61-vaccinated pigs, china, 2012. Emerg Infect Dis. 2013;19(11):1749–55.
9. Sun Y, Luo Y, Wang C, Yuan J, Li N, Song K, Qiu H. Control of swine pseudorabies in China: Opportunities and limitations. Vet Microbiol. 2016; 183:119–24.
10. Peng JM, An TQ, Zhao HY, Liu YM, Chen JZ, Leng CL, Sun Y, Chang D, Tian ZJ, Tong GZ. Identification and antigenic variation of new epidemiology of pseudorabies virus from swine. Chin J Prev Vet Med. 2013;01:1–4.
11. Serena M, Geisler C, Metz G, Mórtola E, Echeverría M. Production of pseudorabies virus recombinant glycoprotein B and its use in an agar gel immunodiffusion (AGID) test for detection of antibodies with sensitivity and specificity equal to the virus neutralization assay. J Virol Methods. 2016;230:9–12.
12. Yang Q, Sun Z, Tan F, Guo L, Wang Y, Wang J, Wang Z, Wang L, Li X, Xiao Y, et al. Pathogenicity of a currently circulating Chinese variant pseudorabies virus in pigs. World J Virol. 2016;5(1):23–30.
13. Xiang S, Zhou Z, Hu X, Li Y, Zhang C, Wang J, Li X, Tan F, Tian K. Complete Genome Sequence of a Variant Pseudorabies Virus Strain Isolated in Central China. Genome Announc. 2016;4(2). doi: 10.1128/genomeA.00149-16
14. Papageorgiou K, Suárez N, Wilkie G, Filioussis G, Papaioannou N, Nauwynck H, Davison A, SK K. Genome sequences of two pseudorabies virus strains isolated in Greece. Genome Announc. 2016;4(1). doi: 10.1128/genomeA.01624-15.
15. Zhang C, Guo L, Jia X, Wang T, Wang J, Sun Z, Wang L, Li X, Tan F. Construction of a triple gene-deleted Chinese Pseudorabies virus variant and its efficacy study as a vaccine candidate on suckling piglets. Vaccine. 2015;33(21):2432–7.
16. Gu Z, Dong J, Wang J, Hou C, Sun H, Yang W, Bai J, Jiang P. A novel inactivated gE/gI deleted pseudorabies virus (PRV) vaccine completely protects pigs from an emerged variant PRV challenge. Virus Res. 2014; 195(14):57–63.
17. Miller L, Bayles D, Zanella E, Lager K. Effects of Pseudorabies Virus Infection on the Tracheobronchial Lymph Node Transcriptome. Bioinform Biol Insights. 2016;9 Suppl 2:25–36.
18. Wu C, Liao C, Chi J, Chien M, Huang C. Growth properties and vaccine efficacy of recombinant pseudorabies virus defective in glycoprotein E and thymidine kinase genes. J Biotechnol. 2016;229:58–64.
19. Morgan R, Cantello J, McDermott C. Transfection of chicken embryo fibroblasts with Marek's disease virus DNA. Avian Dis. 1990;34:345–51.
20. Boussif O, Lezoualc'h F, Zanta M, Mergny M, Scherman D, Demeneix B, Behr J. A versatile vector for gene and oligonucleotide transfer into cells in culture and in vivo: polyethylenimine. Proc Natl Acad Sci U S A. 1995;92:7297–301.
21. Muyrers J, Zhang Y, Testa G, Stewart A. Rapid modification of bacterial artificial chromosomes by ET-recombination. Nucleic Acids Res. 1999;27.
22. Narayanan K, Williamson R, Zhang Y, Stewart A, Ioannou P. Efficient and precise engineering of a 200 kb beta-globin human/bacterial artificial chromosome in E. coli DH10B using an inducible homologous recombination system. Gene Ther. 1999;6:442–7.
23. Tischer B, Smith G, Osterrieder N. En passant mutagenesis: a two step markerless red recombination system. Methods Mol Biol. 2010;634:421–30.
24. Schumacher D, Tischer B, Fuchs W, Osterrieder N. Reconstitution of Marek's disease virus serotype 1 (MDV-1) from DNA cloned as a bacterial artificial chromosome and characterization of a glycoprotein B-negative MDV-1 mutant. J Virol. 2000;74:11088–98.
25. Shizuya H, Birren B, Kim U, Mancino V, Slepak T, Tachiiri Y, Simon M. Cloning and stable maintenance of 300-kilobase-pair fragments of human DNA in Escherichia coli using an F-factor-based vector. Proc Natl Acad Sci U S A. 1992;89:8794–7.
26. Wang J, Osterrieder N. Generation of an infectious clone of duck enteritis virus and generation of a vectored DEV expressing hemagglutinin of H5N1 avian influenza virus. Virus Res. 2011;159(1):23–31.
27. Rudolph J, O'Callaghan D, Osterrieder N. Cloning of the genomes of equine herpesvirus type1 (EHV-1) strains KyA and racL11 as bacterial artificial chromosomes (BAC). J Vet Med B Infect Dis Vet Public Health. 2002;49:31–6.
28. Lerma L, Muñoz A, Wagner S, Dinu M, Martín B, Tabarés E. Construction of recombinant pseudorabies viruses by using PRV BACs deficient in IE180 or pac sequences: Application of vBAC90D recombinant virus to production of PRV amplicons. Virus Res. 2016;213:274–82.
29. Fan J, Zeng X, Zhang G, Wu Q, Niu J, Sun B, Xie Q, Ma J. Molecular characterization and phylogenetic analysis of pseudorabies virus variants isolated from Guangdong Province of Southern China during 2013-2014. J Vet Sci. 2015;[Epub ahead of print].
30. Le Luduec J, Debeer S, Piras F, Andréoni C, Boudet F, Laurent P, Kaiserlian D, Dubois B. Intradermal vaccination with un-adjuvanted sub-unit vaccines

triggers skin innate immunity and confers protective respiratory immunity in domestic swine. Vaccine. 2016;34(7):914–22.

31. Liang X, Sun L, Yu T, Pan Y, Wang D, Hu X, Fu Z, He Q, Cao G. A CRISPR/Cas9 and Cre/Lox system-based express vaccine development strategy against re-emerging Pseudorabies virus. Sci Rep. 2016;6:19176.
32. Messerle M, Crnkovic I, Hammerschmidt W, Ziegler H, Koszinowski U. Cloning and mutagenesis of a herpesvirus genome as an infectious bacterial artificial chromosome. Proc Natl Acad Sci U S A. 1997;94:14759–63.
33. Osterrieder N, Schumacher D, Trapp S, Beer M, von Einem J, Tischer K. Establishment and use of infectious bacterial artificial chromosome (BAC) DNA clones of animal herpesviruses. Berl Munch Tierarztl Wochenschr. 2003; 116:373–80.
34. Rosas C, Van de Walle G, Metzger S, Hoelzer K, Dubovi E, Kim S, Parrish C, Osterrieder N. Evaluation of a vectored equine herpesvirus type 1 (EHV-1) vaccine expressing H3 haemagglutinin in the protection of dogs against canine influenza. Vaccine. 2008;26:2335–43.
35. Wang J, Ge A, Xu M, Wang Z, Qiao Y, Gu Y, Liu C, Liu Y, Hou J. Construction of a recombinant duck enteritis virus (DEV) expressing hemagglutinin of H5N1 avian influenza virus based on an infectious clone of DEV vaccine strain and evaluation of its efficacy in ducks and chickens. Virol J. 2015;12:126.
36. Yoon H, Eo S, Aleyas A, Cha S, Lee J, Chae J, Jang H, Cho E, Song H. Investigation of pseudorabies virus latency in nervous tissues of seropositive pigs exposed to field strain. J Vet Med Sci. 2006;68(2):143–8.
37. Wang D, Huang R. Effect of eradication of pseudorabies virus in breeding pig farms. Anhui Agri Sci Bull. 2009;15(24):30–1.
38. Li G. Control and eradication of pseudorabies in large-scale pig farms. Hubei J Anim Vet Sci. 2009;11:39–40.

16

A rapid minor groove binder PCR method for distinguishing the vaccine strain *Brucella abortus* 104M

Wenlong Nan[1], Lide Qin[1], Yong Wang[1,2], Yueyong Zhang[1], Pengfei Tan[1,2], Yuqi Chen[4], Kairong Mao[3] and Yiping Chen[1*]

Abstract

Background: Brucellosis is a widespread zoonotic disease caused by Gram-negative *Brucella* bacteria. Immunisation with attenuated vaccine is an effective method of prevention, but it can interfere with diagnosis. Live, attenuated *Brucella abortus* strain 104M has been used for the prevention of human brucellosis in China since 1965. However, at present, no fast and reliable method exists that can distinguish this strain from field strains. Single nucleotide polymorphism (SNP)-based assays offer a new approach for such discrimination. SNP-based minor groove binder (MGB) and Cycleave assays have been used for rapid identification of four *Brucella* vaccine strains (*B. abortus* strains S19, A19 and RB51, and *B. melitensis* Rev1). The main objective of this study was to develop a PCR assay for rapid and specific detection of strain 104M.

Results: We developed a SNP-based MGB PCR assay that could successfully distinguish strain 104M from 18 representative strains of *Brucella* (*B. abortus* biovars 1, 2, 3, 4, 5, 6, 7 and 9, *B. melitensis* biovars 1, 2 and 3, *B. suis* biovars 1, 2, 3 and 4, *B. canis*, *B. neotomae*, and *B. ovis*), four *Brucella* vaccine strains (A19, S19, S2, M5), and 55 *Brucella* clinical field strains. The assay gave a negative reaction with four non-*Brucella* species (*Escherichia coli*, *Pasteurella multocida*, *Streptococcus suis* and *Pseudomonas aeruginosa*). The minimum sensitivity of the assay, evaluated using 10-fold dilutions of chromosomal DNA, was 220 fg for the 104M strain and 76 fg for the single non-104M *Brucella* strain tested (*B. abortus* A19). The assay was also reproducible (intra- and inter-assay coefficients of variation = 0.006–0.022 and 0.012–0.044, respectively).

Conclusions: A SNP-based MGB PCR assay was developed that could straightforwardly and unambiguously distinguish *B. abortus* vaccine strain 104M from non-104M *Brucella* strains. Compared to the classical isolation and identification approaches of bacteriology, this real-time PCR assay has substantial advantages in terms of simplicity and speed, and also reduces potential exposure to live *Brucella*. The assay developed is therefore a simple, rapid, sensitive, and specific tool for brucellosis diagnosis and control.

Keywords: Brucellosis, *Brucella abortus*, Minor groove binder, SNP-based assay

Background

Brucellosis is a widespread zoonotic disease caused by various Gram-negative *Brucella* bacterial species that damages human health and results in considerable economic losses. Annually, more than 500,000 new human brucellosis cases are reported worldwide [1], and cases have increased rapidly over the last decade in all provinces in China [2]. Human brucellosis is transmitted by eating contaminated food products of animal origin and via direct animal contact [2], and although rarely fatal, it can be severely debilitating and disabling [3].

For over a century, vaccination and the culling of animals has been performed to control this disease [4–6]. In China, live attenuated *Brucella* strains are widely used for the prevention and control of brucellosis, including *Brucella abortus* strain A19 in cattle, *B. suis* S2 used in

* Correspondence: cyp777@163.com
[1]Laboratory of Diagnositics Development, China Animal Health and Epidemiology Center, 369 Nanjing Road, Qingdao, Shandong 266032, China
Full list of author information is available at the end of the article

swine, and *B. melitensis* M5 in sheep and goat. In addition, live, attenuated *B. abortus* 104M has been adopted as a vaccine for use in humans since 1965. This strain, which was first isolated from the foetus of an aborted cow in the former Soviet republic in 1950, exhibits low virulence, high stability and high immuno-antigenicity [7].

However, since it is a live attenuated strain, vaccination with 104M may cause vaccine-related cases of brucellosis, and it may be difficult to differentiate between a vaccine response and a natural infection, which complicates diagnosis. At present, a rapid and reliable method for distinguishing 104M from field strains is not available. The main objective of this study was to develop a PCR assay for rapid and specific detection of 104M.

Methods

Strains and DNA extraction

Brucella strains used in the present study are listed in Table 1. These comprised 18 representative strains of *Brucella* species and biovars, five *Brucella* vaccine strains, and 55 *Brucella* field strains. In addition, four non-target organisms (*Escherichia coli* K99, *Pasteurella multocida* C48–1, *Pseudomonas aeruginosa* DI-1, and *Streptococcus suis* ST171) were included. *Brucella* strains were cultured on tryptose agar at 37 °C with 5–10% CO_2 when required for 48–72 h in a biosafety level 3-equipped laboratory. Bacteria were then washed with normal saline containing 0.5% formaldehyde, and inactivated at 37 °C for 24 h. The four non-*Brucella* species were cultivated as described previously [8], and harvested and inactivated as described above. Unless specified, genomic DNA was extracted with the QIAamp DNA mini kit according to the manufacturer's instructions (Qiagen GmbH., D40724 Hilden).

Minor groove binder (MGB) PCR

In this real-time PCR assay, a pair of short TaqMan 5′-labelled, 3′- MGB probes defining the single nucleotide polymorphism (SNP) were used to interrogate the 104M strain and non-104 M *Brucella* strains. Use of the MGB protein raises the melting temperature of probes meaning that a single base mismatch causes more destabilisation than would be the case with a longer probe [9]. This facilitates accurate SNP detection. For distinguishing *B. abortus* 104M, the SNP C_{228}–T_{228} in NL70_10085 was selected. This SNP was identified by comparison of the *B. abortus* 104M draft genomic sequence with the sequences of *B. abortus* 9–941, *B. melitensis* M28, *B. suis* S1330, *B. canis* ATCC 23365, and *B. ovis* ATCC 25840, *B. pinnipedialis* B2/94, *B. microti* CCM 4915. One set of primers and probes was designed based on this SNP (Table 2).

The assay was performed using the TransStart Green qPCR SuperMix kit (TransGen Biotech Co., Beijing, China) in a reaction volume of 25 μL containing a reaction mixture volume of 12.5 μL with the working concentrations of primers and probes listed in Table 2, together with the DNA template (2 μL). For detection of the 104M strain, the VAC probe was labelled with 6-carboxyfluorescein (FAM) at the 5′-end and MGB eclipse at the 3′-end. For detection of non-104 M *Brucella* strains, the NON probe was labelled with the fluorophore 4,7,2′-trichloro-7′-phenyl-6-carboxyfluorescein (VIC) at the 5′-end and MGB eclipse at the 3′-end.

PCR cycling parameters were as follows: 95 °C for 3 min, followed by 40 cycles of 95 °C for 5 s, 56 °C for 10 s, and 72 °C for 10 s. Amplification was performed using the Bio-Rad MiniOpticon system (Bio-Rad Laboratories, Inc., Hercules, CA).

Sensitivity, specificity, and reproducibility

For assay sensitivity tests, the minimum detection limit of MGB PCR was evaluated using 10-fold serial dilutions of genomic DNA from *B. abortus* 104M for FAM fluorescence, and *B. abortus* A19 for VIC fluorescence. Each dilution was included in the assay to determine the minimum discriminatory amount of genomic DNA detected in the assay.

For assay specificity tests, we evaluated whether MGB PCR could distinguish the 104M strain from common species and other vaccine strains of *Brucella* using the representative and vaccine *Brucella* strains listed in Table 1. These strains included almost all common species and biovars of *Brucella* and the vaccine strains currently used in China. The four non-*Brucella* spp. (*Escherichia coli* K99, *Pasteurella multocida* C48–1, *Streptococcus suis* ST171, and *Pseudomonas aeruginosa* DI-1) were also tested.

Assay reproducibility was determined by calculating the intra- and inter-assay coefficients of variation (CV), using at least three replicates of each of the 10-fold serial dilutions of genomic DNA to generate a standard curve. The efficiency of the assay was determined using the following calculation: Efficiency = 10 (− 1/slope) − 1.

Detection of clinical field strains

A further 55 *Brucella spp.* field isolates (see Table 1) that were isolated from different animal species and areas, identified and provided by China Veterinary Culture Collection Centre were also tested.

Results

Assay sensitivity

Using 10-fold serial dilutions of *B. abortus* 104M genomic DNA ranging from 1.1 ng/μL to 0.11 fg/μL, the minimum discriminatory sensitivity for detection of

Table 1 *Brucella spp.* strains used in the present study

Species (biovar)	Strain	Type	Host	Region
B. abortus (1)	A544 (CVCC790, ATCC23448)	Reference strain	Bovine	United Kingdom
B. abortus (2)	86/8/59 (CVCC12, ATCC23449)	Reference strain	Bovine	United Kingdom
B. abortus (3)	Tulya (CVCC13, ATCC23450)	Reference strain	Bovine	United Kingdom
B. abortus (4)	292 (CVCC16, ATCC23451)	Reference strain	Bovine	United Kingdom
B. abortus (5)	B3196 (CVCC14, ATCC23452)	Reference strain	Bovine	United Kingdom
B. abortus (6)	870 (CVCC17, ATCC23453)	Reference strain	Bovine	United Kingdom
B. abortus (7)	63/75 (CVCC15, ATCC23454)	Reference strain	Bovine	United Kingdom
B. abortus (9)	C68 (CVCC11, ATCC23455)	Reference strain	Bovine	United Kingdom
B. abortus (4)	C72–62 (CVCC887)	Field strain	Bovine	Inner Mongolia
B. abortus (4)	C72–63 (CVCC888)	Field strain	Bovine	Inner Mongolia
B. abortus (4)	C72–61 (CVCC886)	Field strain	Bovine	Inner Mongolia
B. abortus (Unknown)	SHDeer-74 (CVCC780)	Field strain	Cervine	Shanghai
B. abortus (Unknown)	C72–387 (CVCC785)	Field strain	Bovine	Heilongjiang
B. abortus (Unknown)	C72–10 (CVCC786)	Field strain	Bovine	Heilongjiang
B. abortus (Unknown)	2308 (CVCC788)	Field strain	Bovine	Heilongjiang
B. abortus (Unknown)	HBCow-1 (CVCC2408)	Field strain	Bovine	Hubei
B. abortus (Unknown)	HBCow-2 (CVCC2409)	Field strain	Bovine	Hubei
B. abortus (Unknown)	C72–12 (CVCC3621)	Field strain	Bovine	Heilongjiang
B. abortus (Unknown)	C72–8401 (CVCC3622)	Field strain	Bovine	Inner Mongolia
B. abortus (Unknown)	C72–8403 (CVCC3623)	Field strain	Bovine	Inner Mongolia
B. abortus (Unknown)	NMCow-2 (CVCC3635)	Field strain	Bovine	Inner Mongolia
B. melitensis (1)	16 M (CVCC70002, ATCC23456)	Reference strain	Caprine	United Kingdom
B. melitensis (2)	63/9 (CVCC21, ATCC23457)	Reference strain	Caprine	United Kingdom
B. melitensis (3)	Ether (CVCC20, ATCC23458)	Reference strain	Caprine	United Kingdom
B. melitensis (1)	Goat-901 (CVCC3627)	Field strain	Caprine	Inner Mongolia
B. melitensis (Unknown)	CVCC3620	Field strain	Unknown	Inner Mongolia
B. melitensis (Unknown)	C71–1257 (CVCC928)	Field strain	Caprine	Inner Mongolia
B. melitensis (Unknown)	C71–13 (CVCC929)	Field strain	Caprine	Inner Mongolia
B. melitensis (Unknown)	C71–35 (CVCC936)	Field strain	Ovine	Qinghai
B. melitensis (Unknown)	C71–44 (CVCC938)	Field strain	Caprine	Xinjiang
B. melitensis (Unknown)	Goat-963 (CVCC952)	Field strain	Caprine	Inner Mongolia
B. melitensis (Unknown)	M54–8 (CVCC3624)	Field strain	Ovine	Qinghai
B. melitensis (Unknown)	Goat-866 (CVCC3625)	Field strain	Caprine	Inner Mongolia
B. melitensis (Unknown)	Goat-872 (CVCC3626)	Field strain	Caprine	Inner Mongolia
B. melitensis (Unknown)	Goat-865 (CVCC3628)	Field strain	Caprine	Inner Mongolia
B. suis (1)	S1330 (CVCC70524, ATCC23444)	Reference strain	Porcine	United Kingdom
B. suis (2)	Thomsen (CVCC22, ATCC23445)	Reference strain	Porcine	United Kingdom
B. suis (3)	686 (CVCC23, ATCC23446)	Reference strain	Porcine	United Kingdom
B. suis (4)	40 (CVCC24, ATCC23447)	Reference strain	Porcine	United Kingdom
B. suis (3)	KP6 (CVCC3651)	Field strain	Porcine	Guangdong
B. suis (3)	ZC5 (CVCC3653)	Field strain	Porcine	Guangdong
B. suis (3)	ZC1 (CVCC3655)	Field strain	Porcine	Guangdong
B. suis (3)	ZC6 (CVCC3649)	Field strain	Porcine	Guangdong
B. suis (3)	KP1 (CVCC3658)	Field strain	Porcine	Guangdong
B. suis (3)	KP2 (CVCC3659)	Field strain	Porcine	Guangdong
B. suis (3)	KP3 (CVCC3660)	Field strain	Porcine	Guangdong

Table 1 *Brucella spp.* strains used in the present study *(Continued)*

Species (biovar)	Strain	Type	Host	Region
B. suis (3)	KP5 (CVCC3661)	Field strain	Porcine	Guangdong
B. suis (3)	HNPig-1 (CVCC3662)	Field strain	Porcine	Hainan
B. suis (3)	HNPig-2 (CVCC3663)	Field strain	Porcine	Hainan
B. suis (Unknown)	BS4 (CVCC1072)	Field strain	Porcine	Russian
B. suis (Unknown)	C73-5 (CVCC1080)	Field strain	Porcine	Guangxi
B. suis (Unknown)	C73-10 (CVCC1083)	Field strain	Porcine	Guangxi
B. suis (Unknown)	C73-11 (CVCC1084)	Field strain	Porcine	Guangxi
B. suis (Unknown)	C73-13 (CVCC1085)	Field strain	Porcine	Guangxi
B. suis (Unknown)	C73-23 (CVCC1089)	Field strain	Porcine	Guangxi
B. suis (Unknown)	C73-25 (CVCC1091)	Field strain	Porcine	Guangxi
B. suis (Unknown)	C73-26 (CVCC1092)	Field strain	Porcine	Guangxi
B. suis (Unknown)	Br.63/3 (CVCC3639)	Field strain	Unknown	United Kingdom
B. suis (Unknown)	Br.63/142 (CVCC3640)	Field strain	Unknown	United Kingdom
B. suis (Unknown)	Br.86/27 (CVCC3641)	Field strain	Unknown	United Kingdom
B. suis (Unknown)	Br.63/62 (CVCC3642)	Field strain	Unknown	United Kingdom
B. suis (Unknown)	Br.79/224 (CVCC3643)	Field strain	Unknown	United Kingdom
B. suis (Unknown)	Br.Thomsen1720 (CVCC3644)	Field strain	Unknown	United Kingdom
B. suis (Unknown)	Br.Thomsen5 (CVCC3645)	Field strain	Unknown	United Kingdom
B. suis (Unknown)	Br.63/225 (CVCC3646)	Field strain	Unknown	United Kingdom
B. suis (Unknown)	Br.63/32 (CVCC3647)	Field strain	Unknown	United Kingdom
B. suis (Unknown)	Br.64/24 (CVCC3648)	Field strain	Unknown	United Kingdom
B. suis (Unknown)	ZC2 (CVCC3656)	Field strain	Porcine	Guangdong
B. suis (Unknown)	ZC3 (CVCC3657)	Field strain	Porcine	Guangdong
B. suis (Unknown)	DF1 (CVCC3654)	Field strain	Porcine	Guangdong
B. suis (Unknown)	SD1 (CVCC3652)	Field strain	Porcine	Guangdong
B. suis (Unknown)	ZC4 (CVCC3650)	Field strain	Porcine	Guangdong
B. ovis	63/290 (CVCC70015, ATCC25840)	Reference strain	Ovine	United Kingdom
B. canis	RM6/66 (CVCC70701, ATCC23365)	Reference strain	Canine	United Kingdom
B. canis	KP4 (CVCC3664)	Field strain	Canine	Guangdong
B. neotomae	5 K33 (CVCC70721, ATCC23459)	Reference strain	Unknown	United Kingdom
B. abortus (1)	A19	Vaccine	–	–
B. melitensis (1)	M5	Vaccine	–	–
B. abortus (Unknown)	104 M	Vaccine	–	–
B. abortus (1)	S19	Vaccine	–	–
B. suis (1)	S2	Vaccine	–	–

Strains were identified and provided by the China Veterinary Culture Collection Centre (CVCC)
Unknown = unknown biovar or host

Table 2 Targets, primers and probes used for the MGB PCR assay with the associated working concentrations

Target (positon)	Gene description	Working concentration (nM)	
		Probe	Primer
NL70_10085 (228)	molecular chaperone DnaK	VAC: CCGTCG**T**TATGACGAT (160)	F: CCGGAAGGCACCCTTTTT (600)
		NON: CCGTCG**C**TATGACGA (400)	R: GATCCTTGTCCTTGGTGACCAT (600)

The position of the SNP within each target is shown in parentheses. The target SNP is shown in bold underlined font in both vaccine (VAC) and nonspecific (NON) probes

104M–specific strains was ~220 fg per reaction for MGB PCR (Table 3). Similarly, using 10-fold serial dilutions of *B. abortus* A19 genomic DNA ranging from 3.8 ng/μL to 0.38 fg/μL, the minimum discriminatory sensitivity for detection of non-104 M *Brucella* strains was ~76 fg per reaction for MGB PCR (Table 3). These results indicated that the assays were highly sensitive for the detection of 104M and non-104 M *Brucella* genomic DNA in a single reaction.

Assay specificity

For evaluating specificity, the representative and vaccine *Brucella* strains listed in Table 1 were tested using the MGB PCR method described. The results showed that 18 representative strains of *Brucella* (*B. abortus* biovars 1, 2, 3, 4, 5, 6, 7 and 9, *B. melitensis* biovars 1, 2 and 3, *B. suis* biovars 1, 2, 3 and 4, *B. canis, B. neotomae* and *B. ovis*), and four *Brucella* vaccine strains (A19, S19, S2, M5) gave strong VIC fluorescence and weak FAM fluorescence below the threshold detection level (Fig. 1a and b).

Only the *B. abortus* 104M vaccine strain gave strong FAM fluorescence and weak VIC fluorescence below the threshold detection level (Fig. 1a and b), indicating that the assay was 104M–specific. All four non-*Brucella* species (*Escherichia coli* K99, *Pasteurella multocida* C48–1, *Streptococcus suis* ST171 and *Pseudomonas aeruginosa* DI-1) were negative for both FAM and VIC fluorescence. These results suggest the MGB PCR assay was highly capable of differentiating 104M from non-104 M *Brucella* isolates and non-*Brucella* strains.

Assay reproducibility

The standard curve generated using genomic DNA was linear over a wide range of dilutions ($R^2 = 0.997$ and slope = – 3.645 for FAM fluorescence; R2 = 0.982 and slope = – 4.342 for VIC fluorescence). The assay was reproducible, with intra-assay CVs ranging from 0.006 to 0.022, and inter-assay CVs of 0.012 to 0.044. The efficiency of the assay was 88.1% for FAM fluorescence and 69.9% for VIC fluorescence. These figures were used to determine the threshold for detection.

Detection of clinical field strains

The results demonstrated strong VIC fluorescence and weak FAM fluorescence for all 55 *Brucella spp.* field isolates tested (Table 1), indicating that none were the 104M strain.

Discussion

The *B. abortus* vaccine strain 104M is a stable antigenic structure with low virulence and high immunogenicity, hence it has been used in China since 1965 to vaccinate cattle and humans against brucellosis. Because using a live vaccine may lead to severe pathogenic injury associated with allergy, the 104M strain was only recommended for high-risk populations in China [7], such as those at high risk due to their occupation [10]. The scratch vaccination method was used to introduce five billion bacteria, which achieved 90% protection for a 12 month duration [7]. In some areas in China, vaccination intervention in humans had an obvious effect; the reported cases of brucellosis in the Arong Banner declined sharply by 84.17% from 2005 to 2006 following vaccination, and the morbidity rate of brucellosis declined from 34,732 per 100,000 to 5454 per 100,000 [11].

However, due to lack of serological differentiation, it is difficult to distinguish 104M by serological assay alone. The recent development of SNP-based real-time assays offers a new approach for overcoming this hurdle. SNP-based MGB and Cycleave assays have been used for rapid identification of four *Brucella* vaccine strains (*B. abortus* strains S19, A19 and RB51, and *B. melitensis* Rev1) [12, 13].

In the present study, we developed a new MBG PCR assay that can successfully distinguish 104M strains from other bacterial strains, with a sensitivity of 220 fg, equating to around 60 cells. Furthermore, our MGB PCR assay can detect non-104 M *Brucella* strains in a single

Table 3 Mean quantification cycle (Cq) values resulting from MGB PCR[a]

Detection of 104M genomic DNA			Detection of A19 genomic DNA		
Concentration	Cq of FAM	Cq of VIC	Concentration	Cq of FAM	Cq of VIC
1.1 ng/μL	24.06	NA	3.8 ng/μL	NA	17.49
110 pg/μL	27.20	NA	380 pg/μL	NA	20.89
11 pg/μL	30.92	NA	38 pg/μL	NA	24.39
1.1 pg/μL	35.27	NA	3.8 pg/μL	NA	31.90
110 fg/μL	38.25	NA	380 fg/μL	NA	34.69
11 fg/μL	NA	NA	38 fg/μL	NA	38.11
1.1 fg/μL	NA	NA	3.8 fg/μL	NA	NA
0.11 fg/μL	NA	NA	0.38 fg/μL	NA	NA

[a]FAM = 6-carboxyfluorescein; VIC = 4,7,2′-trichloro-7′-phenyl-6-carboxyfluorescein; NA = not applicable

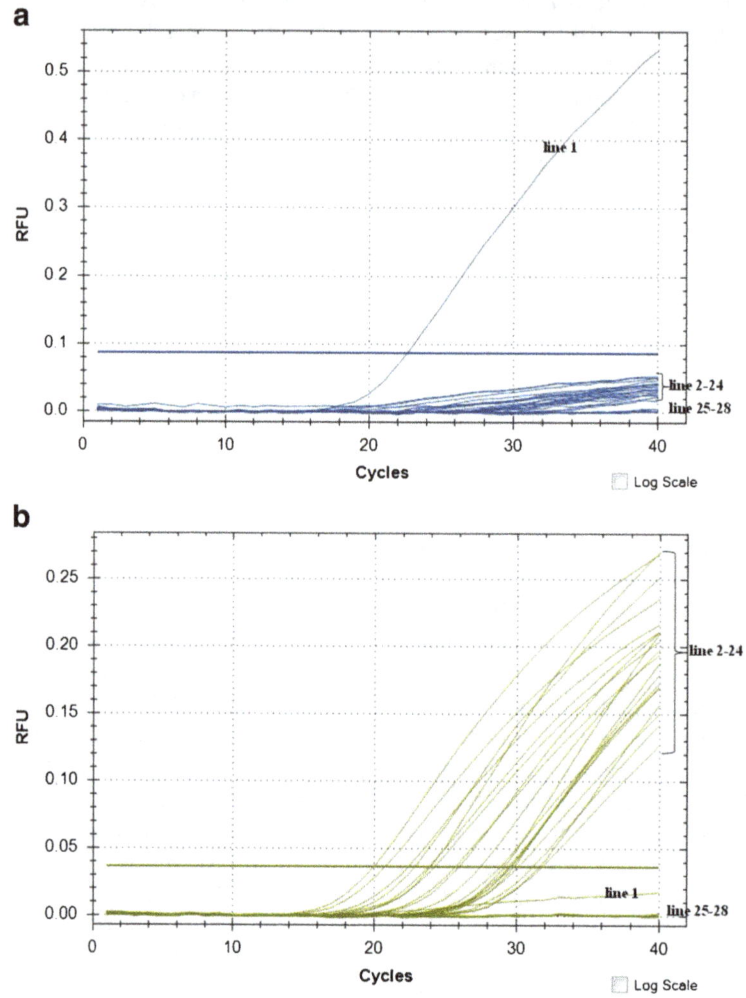

Fig. 1 Specificity of the MGB PCR assay using representative experiments for the detection of (**a**) FAM fluorescence and (**b**) VIC fluorescence. The following strains were subjected to amplification assays: Line 1, 104 M; Line 2 *Brucella suis* biovar 1 S1330; Line 3, *B. suis* biovar 2 Thomsen; Line 4, *B. suis* biovar 3686; Line 5, *B. suis* biovar 4 40; Line 6, *B. abortus* biovar 1 A544; Line 7, *B. abortus* biovar 2 86/8/59; Line 8, *B. abortus* biovar 3 Tulya; Line 9, *B. abortus* biovar 4292; Line 10, *B. abortus* biovar 5 B3196; Line 11, *B. abortus* biovar 6870; Line 12, *B. abortus* biovar 7 63/75; Line 13, *B. abortus* biovar 9 C68; Line 14, *B. melitensis* biovar 1 16 M; Line 15, *B. melitensis* biovar 2 63/9; Line 16, *B. melitensis* biovar 3442; Line 17, *B. ovis* 63/290; Line 18, *B. canis* RM6/66; Line 19, *B. neotomae* 5 K33; Line 20, S2; Line 21, S19; Line 22, A19; Line 23, M5; Line 24, S2; Line 25, *Escherichia coli* K99; Line 26, *Pasteurella multocida* C48–1; Line 27, *Streptococcus suis* ST171; Line 28, *Pseudomonas aeruginosa* DI-1

reaction with a sensitivity of 76 fg, equating to around 30 cells. This assay allows accurate and reliable discrimination of 104M and non-104 M *Brucella* strains from common species and biovars of *Brucella*, *Brucella* vaccines, and other bacterial strains. Our assay therefore provides a simple, rapid, sensitive, and specific tool for use in the control of brucellosis.

Conclusions

A SNP-based MGB PCR assay was developed that could straightforwardly and unambiguously distinguish *B. abortus* vaccine strain 104M. Results of our study indicate the assay allows accurate and reliable discrimination of 104M and non-104 M *Brucella* strains from common species and biovars of *Brucella*, *Brucella* vaccines, and other bacterial strains. The minimum detection limit of the assay was 220 fg for strain 104M and 76 fg for the single non-104 M *Brucella* strain tested. Compared to the classical isolation and identification approaches of bacteriology, this real-time PCR assay has substantial advantages in terms of simplicity and speed, and also reduces the potential for exposure to live *Brucella*. As real-time PCR instruments become more widely used in China, the approach will become widely applicable in routine diagnostics. The assay developed is therefore a simple, rapid, sensitive, and specific tool for brucellosis diagnosis and control.

Abbreviations
B. abortus: *Brucella abortus*; *B. canis*: *Brucella canis*; *B. melitensis*: *Brucella melitensis*; *B. neotomae*: *Brucella neotomae*; *B. ovis*: *Brucella ovis*; *B. suis*: *Brucella suis*; FAM: 6-carboxyfluorescein; MGB: Minor groove binder; SNP: Single nucleotide polymorphism-based; VIC: 4,7,2′-trichloro-7′-phenyl-6-carboxyfluorescein

Acknowledgements
Not applicable

Funding
This work was financially supported by the National Key Research and Development Program of China (No.2017YFF0208600).

Authors' contributions
YPC and WN conceived and designed the experiment. WN and YW designed the set of primers and probes. PT cultured all the *Brucella* and non-*Brucella* species. WN, LQ, YW and YZ carried out the experiment, including preparation of the bacterial genomic samples, sensitivity assay, specificity assay, reproducibility assay and detection of clinical field strains. WN and YQC analyzed the data and wrote the manuscript. KM and YPC verified the validity and checked the results. All authors read and approved the final version of this manuscript.

Consent for publication
Not Applicable

Competing interests
The authors declare that they have no competing interests.

Author details
[1]Laboratory of Diagnositics Development, China Animal Health and Epidemiology Center, 369 Nanjing Road, Qingdao, Shandong 266032, China. [2]College of Veterinary Medicine, Yangzhou University, 12 East Wenhui Road, Yangzhou, Jiangsu 225009, China. [3]China Institute of Veterinary Drug Control, 8 Zhongguanchun South Street, Beijing 100081, China. [4]Xi'an Jiaotong-Liverpool University, 111 Ren'ai Road, Suzhou, Jiangsu Province 215123, China.

References
1. Atluri VL, Xavier MN, de Jong MF, den Hartigh AB, Tsolis RM. Interactions of the human pathogenic *Brucella* species with their hosts. Annu Rev Microbiol. 2011;65:523–41.
2. Yu D, Hui Y, Zai X, Xu J, Liang L, Wang B, et al. Comparative genomic analysis of *Brucella abortus* vaccine strain 104M reveals a set of candidate genes associated with its virulence attenuation[J]. Virulence. 2015;6:745–54.
3. Perkins SD, Smither SJ, Atkins HS. Towards a *Brucella* vaccine for humans. FEMS Microbiol Rev. 2010;34:379–94.
4. Pappas G, Papadimitriou P, Akritidis N, Christou L, Tsianos EV. The new global map of human brucellosis. Lancet Infect Dis. 2006;6:91–9.
5. Corbel MJ. Brucellosis: an overview. Emerg Infect Dis. 1997;3:213–21.
6. Joint FAO/WHO expert committee on brucellosis. World Health Organ Tech Rep Ser 1986; 740:1–132; PMID: 3097967.
7. Deqiu S, Donglou X, Jiming Y. Epidemiology and control of brucellosis in China. Vet Microbiol. 2002;90:165–82.
8. Huang QY, Wu R, Dong GX. Study of bacteriology. In: Lu CP, editor. veterinary microbiology. 3rd ed. Beijing: China agriculture press; 2001. p. 199–382. Chinese.
9. Kutyavin IV, Lukhtanov EA, Gamper HB, Meyer RB. Oligonucleotides with conjugated dihydropyrroloindole tripeptides: base composition and backbone effects on hybridization. Nucleic Acids Res. 1997;25:3718–23.
10. Jing Z, Yan J, Fan W. Research progress of brucellosis vaccine. Chin J Zoonoses. 2016;32:188–99. (in Chinese)
11. Mi J, Han Y, Lin H, Li X, Ta N, Wei R, et al. Effect of the professional population intervention with the brucellosis bacteria vaccine for 5 years in Arong banner. Inner Mongolia Chin J Zoonoses. 2013;29:633–5. (in Chinese)
12. Gopaul KK, Sells J, Bricker BJ, Crasta OR, Whatmore AM. Rapid and reliable single nucleotide polymorphism-based differentiation of *Brucella* live vaccine strains from field strains. J Clin Microbiol. 2010;48:1461–4.
13. Nan W, Zhang Y, Tan P, Xu Z, Chen Y, Mao K, et al. A rapid cycleave PCR method for distinguishing the vaccine strain *Brucella abortus* A19 in China. J Vet Diagn Investig. 2016;28:214–8.

17

Characterization of recombinant OspA in two different *Borrelia* vaccines with respect to immunological response and its relationship to functional parameters

Deborah A Grosenbaugh[1*], Karelle De Luca[2], Pierre-Yves Durand[2], Bradley Feilmeier[1], Kristopher DeWitt[1], Cecile Sigoillot-Claude[2], Marie-Line Sajous[2], Michael J Day[3] and Frederic David[1]

Abstract

Background: Prevention of Lyme disease in dogs in North America depends on effective vaccination against infection by the tick vector-born spirochete *Borrelia burgdorferi*. Most vaccines effectively prevent spirochete transmission to dogs during tick feeding based on immunization with the outer-surface lipoprotein A (OspA) of *B. burgdorferi*. More recently, vaccines containing additional OspC protein moieties have been introduced. These are designed to enhance protection by forming a second line of defense within the vertebrate host, where OspC expression replaces OspA as the dominant surface antigen. However, supportive data for demonstration of OspC mediated protection is still lacking. Since OspA immunogenicity is of paramount importance to protection against spirochete transmission; this study was designed to compare the immunogenicity of two commercially available vaccines against the *Borrelia burgdorferi* OspA. We further characterized OspA antigen fractions of these vaccines with respect to their biochemical and biophysical properties.

Results: Two groups of beagle dogs ($n = 9$) were administered either: (1) a nonadjuvanted/monovalent, recombinant OspA vaccine (Recombitek® Lyme) or (2) an adjuvanted, recombinant OspA /OspC chimeric fusion vaccine (Vanguard® crLyme). The onset of the anti-OspA antibody response elicited by the nonadjuvanted/monovalent OspA vaccine was significantly earlier than that for the bivalent OspA /OspC vaccine and serum borreliacidal activity was significantly greater at all post-vaccination time points. As expected, only dogs inoculated with the bivalent OspA/OspC vaccine mounted a humoral anti-OspC response. However, only three out of nine dogs in that group had a positive response. Comparison of the OspA vaccine structures revealed that the OspA in the nonadjuvanted/monovalent vaccine was primarily in the lipidated form, eluting (SEC-HPLC) at a high molecular weight, suggestive of micelle formation. Conversely, the OspA moiety of the OspA/OspC vaccine was found to be nonlipidated and eluted as the monomeric protein.

Conclusions: We hypothesize that these structural differences may account for the superior immunogenicity of the nonadjuvanted monovalent recombinant OspA vaccine in dogs over the adjuvanted OspA fraction of the OspA/OspC vaccine.

Keywords: OspA, Lyme vaccine, Borrelia

* Correspondence: Deborah.Grosenbaugh@boehringer-ingelheim.com
[1]Merial Inc., Boehringer Ingelheim, Athens, GA, USA
Full list of author information is available at the end of the article

Background

Canine Lyme disease is caused by the spirochete *Borrelia burgdorferi*, which is transmitted by *Ixodes spp.* ticks. Prevention of disease in dogs is based on tick control and effective vaccination. There are several vaccines on the market. Most of them effectively prevent spirochete transmission to dogs during tick feeding based on immunization with the outer-surface lipoprotein A (OspA) of *B. burgdorferi* [1, 2]. OspA has been shown to mediate humoral-mediated immunity in dogs [3] and cell-mediated immunity in humans and mice [4]. OspA is a major surface antigen of the *B. burgdorferi* spirochete, expressed during midgut colonization of its arthropod vector, and is downregulated when the bacterium enters the vertebrate host [5]. Therefore, the mammalian host antibody response can function as the first line of immunological defense against transmission of disease by neutralizing the organism within the tick vector after attachment and intake of host blood; thereby interfering with transmission.

More recently, vaccines containing OspC protein moieties have been investigated [6–8]. These are designed to enhance protection by forming a second line of defense within the vertebrate host, where OspC expression replaces OspA as the dominant surface antigen and results in a shift to anti OspC antibody production. OspC cell-mediate immunity has been demonstrated in acutely infected humans [9] and may also play and role in canines.

However, supportive data for demonstration of OspC mediated protection is still lacking. Immunization with OspC alone failed to protect mice from challenge by either *B. burgdorferi* isolates or infected wild-tick challenge [10]. Interestingly, canine vaccine efficacy studies only consider protection from challenge in the context of OspC and OspA antigen co-administration [6, 7]. Moreover, the variability among OspC genotypes within the *Borrelia burgdorferi* sensu stricto provides a challenge for the production of a broadly protective OspC-based vaccine [11]. Thus it is critical that the OspA component of either a monovalent OspA or a multivalent OspA/OspC vaccine elicits an immunological response that affords robust protection from spirochete transmission during tick feeding.

Since OspA immunogenicity is of paramount importance to protection against spirochete transmission, we compared immunological response to OspA of two commercially available vaccines: a nonadjuvanted/monovalent, recombinant OspA vaccine (Recombitek® Lyme, Merial, Inc.) and an alum-adjuvanted, recombinant OspA, chimeric OspC vaccine (VANGUARD® crLyme, Zoetis). We followed serological responses to-OspA, OspC as well as borreliacidal activity. Surprisingly, it appeared that the nonadjuvanted OspA elicited a more robust immunological response than the adjuvanted vaccine. In an attempt to understand these results, we further characterized OspA antigen fractions of these vaccines with respect to their biochemical and biophysical properties. It is concluded that the nature of the OspA antigen may dramatically impact its immunogenicity which must be considered in vaccine development.

Methods

Animals

Twenty-one, purpose-bred, male ($n = 11$) and female ($n = 10$) beagle dogs (Marshall BioResources, North Rose, NY 14516) were used in the study. The experimental unit was the single animal. All dogs had received routine core vaccination (canine distemper virus, canine adenovirus, canine parainfluenza virus, canine parvovirus, *Bordetella bronchiseptica*), but no previous vaccination for Lyme disease. Dogs were acclimated to the housing facility and handling procedures prior to entering the study. Dogs were 3 to 4 months of age at first vaccination and weighed between 3.5 and 4.5 kg. All were deemed clinically healthy based on physical examination. All animals were observed daily throughout the study to monitor clinical condition. Upon conclusion of the study, animals were returned to Animal Resources for assignment to other studies.

Dogs were housed separately by sex and weight (3 to 4 dogs/run), and commingled with respect to vaccination status in conventional housing. Dogs were fed an appropriate commercially available adult dog food and water was provided ad libitum. Housing, animal care, and study protocol were approved by the institutional ethics committee (Merial Institutional Animal Care and Use Committee.

Blinding and randomization

Animals were randomized into one of two treatment groups and negative controls using littermates as a factor; and were housed in separate runs by gender, commingled and randomly assigned to pens using treatment as a factor. The random allocation sequence listing was generated by a statistician using SAS v9.4 (SAS Institute, Cary, NC). Treatments were administered in accordance with a randomization table.

All personnel performing clinical assessments, sample collection and laboratory analyses were blinded to the animal/treatment group assignments.

Vaccination

Dogs were vaccinated with one of two recombinant vaccines.

- A nonadjuvanted, purified *B. burgdorferi* outer surface protein A (OspA) antigen derived from a bacterial recombinant vector. The OspA antigen corresponds to the active ingredient of Recombitek® Lyme (Merial, Inc.) and was formulated at the commercial release dose ($n = 9$).

- An alum-adjuvanted, recombinant OspA, chimeric outer surface protein (OspC) consisting of seven OspC subtypes. VANGUARD® crLyme (Zoetis) at the commercial dose ($n = 9$).
- Negative control animals remained unvaccinated ($n = 3$).

Both vaccines were administered in a volume of 1 ml, by subcutaneous injection, in the right and left flank, on Days 0 and 21, respectively, followed by a 5-month booster.

Sample collection

Approximately 10 mL of blood were collected prior to the first and second vaccination, and at 14, 21, 28, 56, 64, 112 days following the second vaccination, and again at 14 days following the 5-month booster. Blood was collected into serum-separator tubes from the jugular vein of unsedated dogs using a 21 g ¾″ Surflo® butterfly catheter (Terumo, Tokyo, Japan). Serum was separated by centrifugation, and stored frozen at – 20 °C.

Serological response

All serum samples were assayed using a fluorescent bead-based multiplex assay for the simultaneous detection of *B. burgdorferi* OspA, OspC, and OspF [12]. These tests were performed by Cornell University Veterinary Diagnostic Laboratory, Ithaca NY.

Serum borreliacidal activity

A modified Borreliacidal Assay was developed and performed based on literature references [13–15]. Briefly, *B. burgdorferi* cultures were maintained in BSK-H Media (Sigma, Ref# B8291-500 mL) at 33 °C under static growth conditions. *B. burgdorferi* cultures were quantified using a Petroff-Hausser counting chamber under dark field microscopy and diluted to a target of 1×10^7 cells/mL in fresh media.

The canine serum samples were filter sterilized using a 0.2 µm membrane prior to use, then heat inactivated at 56 °C for 10 min to prevent endogenous complement activity. Each serum sample was diluted two-fold 14 times (1:2 to 1:16,384) by adding 0.2 mL sera to 0.2 mL fresh BSK-H media in 2 mL cryogenic vials (Corning, Ref# 430659). Guinea pig complement (Calbiochem, MilliporeSigma, Ref# 234395-5ML) was filter-sterilized using a 0.2 µm membrane and then added to the diluted *B. burgdorferi* culture at a ratio of 6.67 mL Guinea pig complement to 100 mL *B. burgdorferi* culture.

To perform the assay, 0.2 mL of the culture-complement mixture was mixed with 0.2 mL of the serum dilutions and incubated at 33 °C for 16 h. After 16 h, an additional 0.8 mL of fresh BSK-H media was added to each vial. A culture-only control (without the addition of complement or dog serum) was set up to ensure normal bacterial growth. Additionally, a culture-complement (without the addition of dog serum) was set up to ensure that the complement was not resulting in indiscriminate *B. burgdorferi* mortality and cell lysis. All dilutions of each of the samples were read after 4 days using dark field microscopy at 400× magnification. The viable and motile *B. burgdorferi* cells were quantified visually using a Petroff-Hausser enumeration chamber. The borreliacidal serum antibody titer was determined by taking the reciprocal of the highest serum dilution needed to induce a minimum of 50% cell lysis relative to the culture complement control.

Measurement of total OspA-specific immunoglobulin G and IgG subclasses

The concentration of OspA specific antibodies of the IgG1, IgG2, IgG3 and IgG4 subclasses and the total anti-OspA IgG antibody relative titers were measured using enzyme-linked immunosorbent assays (ELISA). ELISA techniques were based on detection of anti-OspA IgG by polyclonal rabbit anti-dog IgG antibodies or monoclonal mouse anti-dog IgG1, IgG2, IgG3 or IgG4 subclasses. Briefly, OspA antigen (MERIAL, Lyon, France), in PBS without $Ca_2^+Mg_2^+$, was coated onto the wells of a microtitration plate and incubated overnight at 5 °C. After five washes and a blocking step (5% BSA in PBS), serial dilutions of sera were incubated on the coated plate for 90 min at 37 °C. Biotin-conjugated anti-dog IgG (rabbit anti-dog IgG heavy and light chains [H&L]; Nordic Laboratories, Tilburg, The Netherlands) was then added. Binding of total IgG was detected with streptavidin-HRP (Jackson ImmunoResearch, Europe Ltd., United Kingdom). To detect binding of IgG subclasses, mouse anti-dog IgG1, IgG2, IgG3 or IgG4 subclass monoclonal antibodies were added at dilutions of 1/20000e, 1/70000e, and 1/3000e (IgG3 and IgG4) respectively in 0.05% PBS/Tween and 1% BSA. Subsequent binding was revealed using a peroxidase-conjugated goat anti-mouse IgG antibody (Jackson ImmunoResearch, Europe Ltd., United Kingdom) at a dilution of 1/5000e in 0.05% PBS/Tween and 1% BSA. Secondary and tertiary reagents were incubated for 90 min at 37 °C. Finally, substrate (tetramethylbenzidine) was added to each well. After an incubation period of 30 min at ambient temperature, H_2SO_4 4 N solution was added as a blocking agent. The absorbance in each well was quantified by spectrophotometry. The antibody titers were calculated by regression and expressed as $Log_{10}OD_{50}$.

SPR (surface plasma resonance) assays

SPR assays were performed on a BIAcore T200 (GE Healthcare Bio-Sciences AB, Sweden) using kits and buffers provided by the supplier according to the manufacturer's instructions. A CM5 chip was immobilized with OspA or irrelevant proteins. MAbs or sera on test were diluted in running buffer and injected onto the chip. The resonance unit (RU) obtained with each pair of antigen/antibodies was monitored. The dissociation constants and avidity are calculated from half-lives using the BIAcore software, and expressed in seconds.

OspA lipidation

Samples were analyzed on a Beckman System Gold HPLC (model 126, Beckman Coulter Life Sciences, Brea, CA, USA) with a TDA detector (Model 302, Viscotek, Malvern Instruments Ltd., Worcestershire, UK), using a Zorbax 300SB-C3 column (4.6 × 150 mm; 5 µm) and a Zorbax 300SB-C3 Guard 5 µm pre-column (Agilent, Santa Clara, CA, USA). Mobile phase used for gradient elution: A = 0.1% (*v*/v) TFA in water and B = 0.1% (v/v) TFA in ACN. The elution program comprised a flow rate of 1.5 mL/min with linear gradient from 5% B to 59% B over a period of 2 min, a flow rate of 1.5 mL/min at 59% B for 3 min, a flow rate of 1.5 mL/min with linear gradient from 59% B to 100% B over a period of 2 min and a flow rate of 1.5 mL/min at 100% B for 5 min. The column temperature was controlled at 40 °C. Detection was performed at UV 219 nm. Sample volume injected was 10 µl. OspA desorption from aluminum gel was performed by adding 150 mg of tri-sodium citrate per 1 ml of vaccine and incubation overnight at 5 °C under agitation. Aluminum gel was removed by centrifugation 10 min at 2190 g and supernatant was concentrated using ultrafiltration spinners 10 k MWCO according supplier recommendations (ThermoFischer, Rockford, IL, USA).

Statistical analysis

Statistical analyses were performed using SAS v9.4 (SAS Institute, Cary, NC). The Log_{10} serum antibody responses to OspA and borreliacidal activity were compared between the groups on each day using a linear model with group, day and group by day as fixed effects. All animals had negative or equivocal serology on Day-7, so the baseline serology was not used as covariate. Data from the same animal were recognized by the model using an AR(1) correlation structure. The least squares means (LSM) of Log_{10} serum antibody responses were compared among groups by day. The *p*-values were adjusted for multiple comparisons using Tukey's method. The central values with respect to the ELISA and SPR assays were compared among the two vaccinated groups by day using Student's t-test when applicable, Wilcoxon non parametric test otherwise. Dispersions were compared by mean of F-tests.

Results

Humoral antibody response

In order to evaluate the intensity of the anti-OspA response, serum samples from dogs from both vaccination cohorts ($n = 9$) were assayed for serum antibody to Osp A using a multiplex assay (Fig. 1a). The non adjuvanted/monovalent OspA vaccine produced an early onset response by 18 days following a single vaccination, that was significantly greater than that induced by the adjuvanted OspA/chimeric OspC vaccine ($p = 0.0008$). At all other time points, the mean anti-OspA serum antibody titers in response to vaccination with the nonadjuvanted OspA vaccine was higher than that of the adjuvanted OspA/OspC vaccine but these differences were not statistically significant.

Since IgG subclasses display different functions, we investigated the quality of the anti-OspA response by measuring total IgG titers, as well as IgG1, IgG2, IgG3 and IgG4. In our hands the available commercial ELISAs were not strictly specific to each of the individual IgG subclasses. Consequently, IgG subclass-specific ELISAs were developed internally from previously established methods [16] and illustrated in Fig. 2a & b. The central values of the total IgG titers were significantly higher in the dogs vaccinated with the monovalent vaccine for each time point (D18: $p < 0.001$; D42: $p = 0.004$; D105: $p = 0.006$; D175: $p < 0.001$). There was also a trend of higher dispersion of the response between dogs in the adjuvanted OspA/chimeric OspC vaccine compared to the monovalent OspA vaccine at days 18, 42 and 105, which reached significance at D175 ($p = 0.012$) (Fig. 2a). These results corroborate the multiplex serological results confirming a greater and more consistent anti-OspA humoral response between dogs with the monovalent OspA than with the bivalent vaccine, even after boosting at 5 months ($p < 0.001$) (Fig. 2b). The subclasses displayed the same chronological profiles as the total IgG, with the IgG1 response predominating over IgG2, -3 and -4 for both vaccines, as illustrated, at D175 (Fig. 2b). With the exception of IgG3, which exhibits a highly heterogeneous response, all other subclasses resulted in significantly higher titers in response to inoculation with the monovalent vaccine than with the bivalent vaccine (IgG1: $p < 0.001$; IgG2: $p = 0.002$; IgG4: $p < 0.001$), with the IgG1 response being more homogeneous between the dogs vaccinated with the monovalent vaccine ($p = 0.012$).

Antibody avidity measurements using surface plasmon resonance (SPR) (Fig. 2c) showed that vaccination with the non adjuvanted monovalent OspA resulted in the production of large amounts of specific, high-avidity antibodies, which increased after each vaccination, with all dogs consistently reaching a maximum value after the last vaccination at 5 months. In contrast, the dogs vaccinated

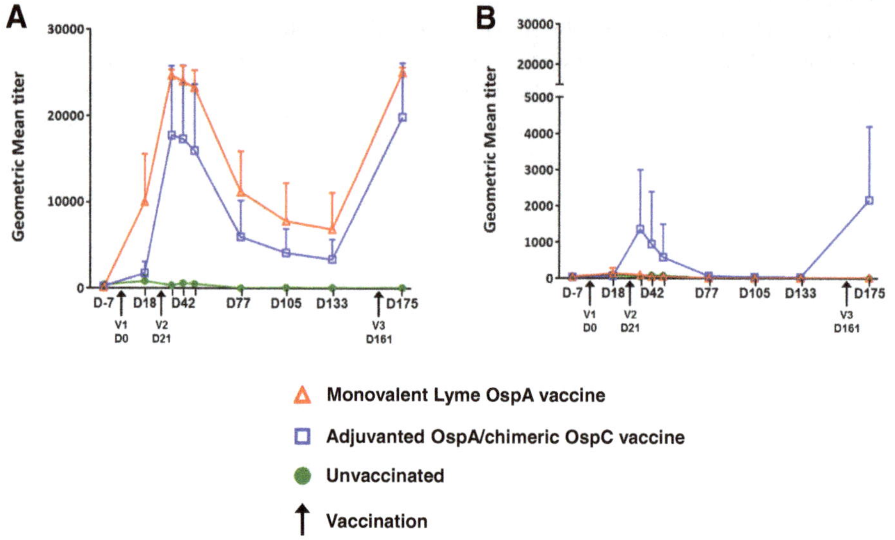

Fig. 1 Humoral Antibody Response. Geometric mean of the borreliacidal serum antibody titers following vaccination with a recombinant, monovalent OspA vaccine and an adjuvanted, recombinant OspA, chimeric OspC vaccine as compared to unvaccinated controls. Serum samples from all dogs were assayed for serum antibody to Osp A (**a**) and Osp C (**b**)

with OspA/chimeric OspC vaccine mounted a production of specific antibodies, but with much lower avidity, which was not improved by the third vaccination at 5 months. At D18, D105 and D175, the avidity response generated in the monovalent group was significantly superior to the OspA/OspC chimeric group (D18: $p = 0.003$; D105: $p = 0.005$; D175: $p < 0.001$). The response by the unvaccinated dogs confirmed the absence of specific anti-OspA antibodies (Fig. 2c). Taken together these results demonstrate a higher avidity response

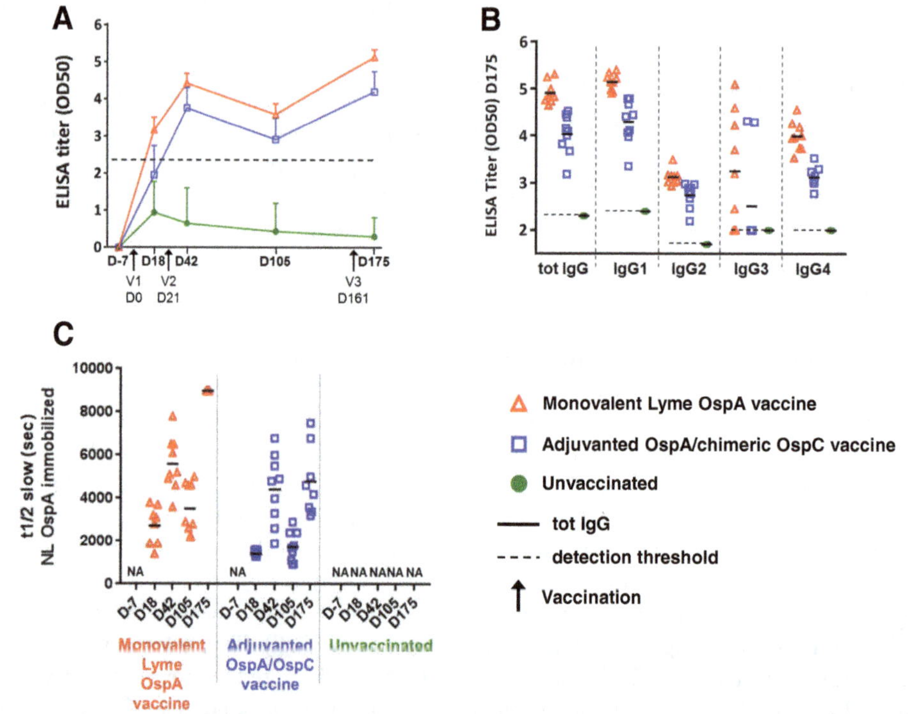

Fig. 2 IgG-Specific Humoral Antibody Response. The total anti-OspA IgG antibody titers along the complete kinetics (**a**), Anti-OspA total IgGs and the four IgG isotypes at D175 (**b**) and antibody avidity by SPR (**c**) following vaccination with a recombinant, monovalent OspA vaccine and an adjuvanted, recombinant OspA, chimeric OspC vaccine on Day 0, Day 21, and Day 161 as compared to unvaccinated controls

elicited by the monovalent OspA compared to that of the bivalent OspA/OspC vaccine.

Since the bivalent vaccine OspA antigen relies on support by a chimeric OspC antigen as its mechanism of action, serum samples from all dogs were also assayed for serum antibody to OspC (Fig. 1b). As expected, the OspC response to the monovalent OspA vaccine was comparable to that of the unvaccinated controls. Response to vaccination to the OspA/chimeric OspC vaccine followed a temporal pattern similar to that of the OspA response, but was highly variable between individual dogs with respect to magnitude. Only three out of nine dogs exceeded the threshold for positivity 2 weeks following the second inoculation.

Serum borreliacidal activity

The functionality of the antibody response was further explored by measuring borreliacidal activity in serum samples from all dogs at selected time points (Fig. 3). Post-vaccination borreliacidal activity of the sera from dogs receiving nonadjuvanted/monovalent OspA were consistently and significantly higher 18 days following the first vaccination ($p = 0.0053$), 14 days following the second vaccination ($p = 0.0011$) and 14 days after the 5 months booster vaccination ($p = 0.0021$) than those from dogs that received the OspA/chimeric OspC vaccine.

OspA biochemical properties and their impact on antigen conformation

To investigate possible causes for the observed difference in the serological response between the two vaccines, the lipidation state of their respective OspA active ingredients were determined by reverse-phase high performance liquid chromatography (RP-HPLC) and compared to a nonlipidated OspA mutant. The latter was created by deleting the N-terminal cystein (OspA nonlipidated control). The OspA active ingredient from the nonadjuvanted/monovalent vaccine eluted as a mix of bi- and tri-lipidated forms. It contained no measurable nonlipidated proteins, whereas the OspA active ingredient from the adjuvanted OspA/chimeric OspC vaccine matched the profile of the non lipidated control (Fig. 4). Size exclusion HPLC (SEC-HPLC) coupled to a tetra-detector array (TDA) composed of a UV-IR-LS-Viscometer indicated a molecular mass of the lipidated OspA from the nonadjuvanted/monovalent vaccine to be 418 kDa, corresponding to a diameter of 18 nm. Molecular mass of the non-lipidated OspA control was measured at 34 kDa for a diameter of 6.4 nm, which is in accordance with the predicted monomeric state.

To further investigate the nature of the size increase of the lipidated OspA active ingredient from the nonadjuvanted/

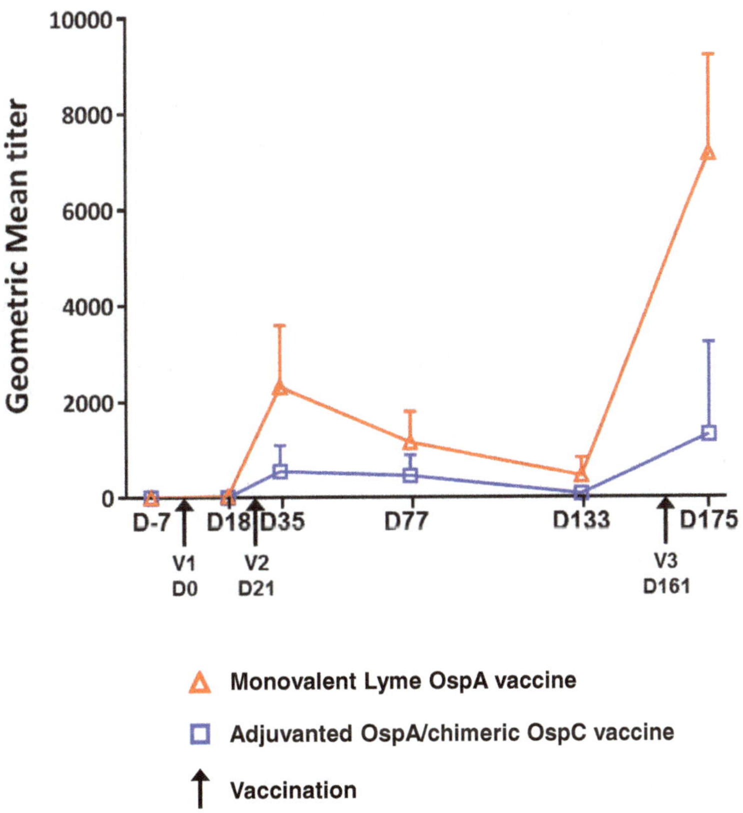

Fig. 3 Serum Borreliacidal Activity. Geometric mean titers of borreliacidal activity following vaccination with a recombinant, monovalent OspA vaccine and an adjuvanted, recombinant OspA, chimeric OspC vaccine

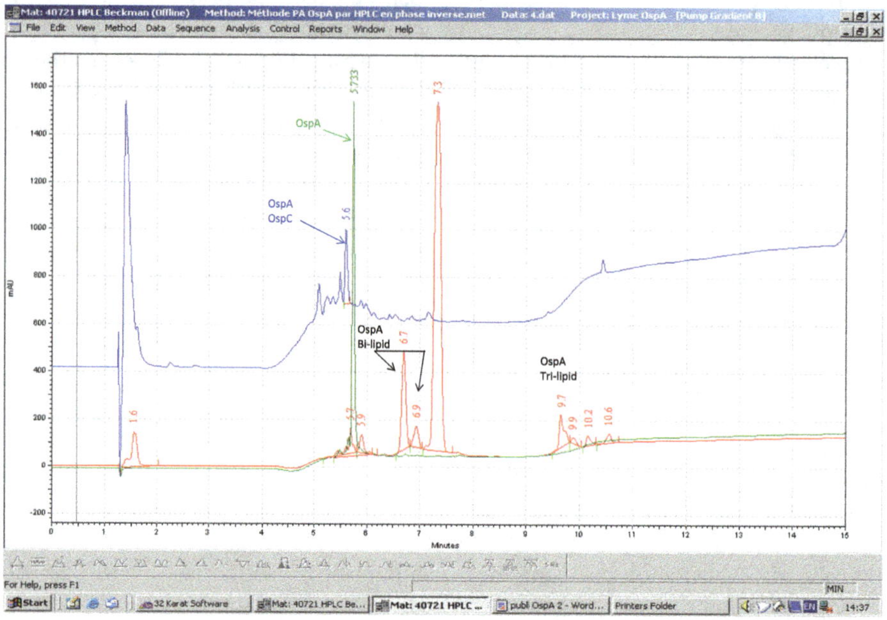

\\eu.boehringer.com\users\lyn\users1\mlsajous\Desktop\lyme\graphe HPLC pour Lyme.xlsx

Fig. 4 OspA biochemical properties and their impact on antigen conformation. HPLC separation (retention time) of the lipidation states of Recombitek ® Lyme and Vanguard ® crLyme compared to a nonlipidated OspA standard

monovalent vaccine, both lipidated recombinant OspA and the nonlipidated OspA control were analysed by Fourier transform infrared spectroscopy (FTIR) to assess secondary structure. Both spectra showed similar percentages of secondary structural elements of both proteins. Moreover, no intermolecular beta-sheets were detected for lipidated OspA. Thus, the lipidated proteins did not appear to form aggregation patterns, suggesting that the multimeric profile of nonadjuvanted/monovalent OspA proteins is due exclusively to the presence of the lipid moities.

Discussion

In this study, we compared the immunogenicity of two different OspA antigens from commercially available canine vaccines: a nonadjuvanted/monovalent, recombinant OspA vaccine (Recombitek® Lyme) and an adjuvanted, recombinant OspA /OspC chimeric fusion vaccine (Vanguard® crLyme).

Our results show that the OspA monovalent, nonadjuvanted vaccine elicited an earlier onset of immunity with a significantly higher antibody response than the adjuvanted vaccine after the first vaccination. Following the second and third vaccinations the average antibody titers were consistently higher at all time points in the dogs receiving the nonadjuvanted vaccine as compared to the dogs receiving the alum-adjuvanted vaccine, although these differences were not significant. Alum is characterized as primarily potentiating a strong Th2 response [17]. It is possible that a different adjuvant, potentiating Th1 responses, may have influenced the results obtained with the recombinant OspA /OspC chimeric fusion antigen.

The humoral response was explored qualitatively by measuring IgG subclasses distribution and functionally by quantifying complement-mediated borreliacidal activity. It is shown that the IgG1 response predominates in both vaccines; but the nonadjuvanted vaccine mounted a more homogenous IgG response with antibodies of greater avidity than that elicited by the adjuvanted vaccine. In addition, the complement-mediated borreliacidal activity induced by the non adjuvanted OspA vaccine was significantly higher than that of the adjuvanted OspA/OspC vaccine at all time points.

The IgG1 subclass described for humans resembles that of the canine IgG-B counterpart [18]. In dogs, it has been identified to be involved in antibody-dependent cell-mediated cytotoxicity (ADCC), cell-mediated cytotoxicity (CDC) and in C1q complement binding. The IgG1 isotype response is pronounced in human patients recovering from subacute *Borrelia* infection and may contribute to clearing of the infection [19].

This may have implications regarding the functionality of the humoral immune response as a whole. Taken together, our results suggest that the greater levels of anti-OspA IgG antibody elicited by the non adjuvanted OspA vaccine and the higher avidity of these antibodies may enhance the ability of this vaccine to trigger complement fixation and, in turn, borreliacidal activity.

HPLC analysis indicates that most of the OspA in the monovalent vaccine was in the form of bi- and tri-lipidated protein, while OspA derived from the adjuvanted OspA/OspC vaccine eluted as a single, nonlipidated peak. The lipidated OspA eluted as a much larger particle (18 nm) than the nonlipidated OspA (6.4 nm). This suggests that the lipidated proteins are organized as particular elements, possibly micelles, based on the tendency of lipoproteins to organize into aggregates that internalize hydrophobic moieties. It has been shown that lipidation of OspA protein is a critical determinant of immunogenicity [20] which may, in part, account for the superior immunogenic profile of the monovalent OspA. Self-assembled micellar nanoparticles appear to increase the efficiency of antigen uptake by dendritic cells [21]. Nanoparticles can also migrate to lymph nodes, and activate nodal dendritic cells, increasing the germinal B cell response [22]. We therefore hypothesize that the lipidation of the OspA antigen present in the monovalent nonadjuvanted vaccine accounts for its superior immunogenic profile over the adjuvanted, nonlipidated OspA from the bivalent vaccine.

With regards to OspC immunogenicity, as expected, the monovalent non-adjuvanted OspA vaccine did not elicit a detectable anti-OspC antibody response. In the OspA/OspC adjuvanted vaccine group, only three out of nine dogs were confirmed positive 2 weeks after the second vaccination.

Since OspC antigens are highly variable [23], this result may be a reflection of a mismatch between the OspC antigens used in the vaccine and the antibody assay [12]. Alternatively, the low rate of seroconversion against OspC elicited by the OspA/OspC vaccine could be related to the inherent variability of OspC antibody responses in dogs [24] or the inability of the OspC chimeric antigen used in the vaccine to elicit an effective antibody response against the native OspC antigen. Whether this low seroconversion to OspC is a reflection of antigenic or immunogenic variability, it illustrates the technical challenge of inducing a broadly protective and consistent immune response against OspC in dogs. Finally, with regards to the OspC immune response, it is also possible that some of the dogs that were negative in the antibody assay performed here would have been positive if tested using assays designed to measure cell mediated immune responses.

The importance of the antibody response to OspA in mediating borreliacidal activity within the tick and consequently blocking transmission to the host has been thoroughly documented [5, 25, 26]. Considering that the protective efficacy of OspC alone remains to be demonstrated [10], the earlier onset of immunity against OspA (after the first dose of vaccine) and the greater ability to generate a borreliacidal activity conferred by the lipidated monovalent OspA vaccine are expected to be an advantageous regarding efficacy. It is acknowledged that humoral mediated immune response may not fully predict vaccine efficacy; but likewise, demonstration of superior clinical efficacy using current *Borrelia* challenge models in a limited number of genetically homogenous dogs is also not likely to reflect vaccine efficacy in the field. However, obtaining this enhanced immunogenicity by expressing a lipidated OspA active ingredient without using an adjuvant is an inherent safety advantage.

Conclusions

Our results show that the OspA monovalent, nonadjuvanted vaccine elicited an earlier onset of immunity with a significantly higher antibody response than the adjuvanted vaccine. The functionality of the antibody response was supported by a greater concurrent increase in serum borreliacidal activity from dogs that receive the nonadjuvanted/monovalent OspA vaccine over those from dogs that received the OspA/chimeric OspC vaccine. The extent of lipidation resulting in structural differences between OspA fractions of the vaccines appear to confer an immunological advantage that obviates the need for the addition of an adjuvant .

Abbreviations

ACN: Acetonitrile; ADCC: Antibody-dependent cell-mediated cytotoxicity; AR: Autoregression; BSA: Bovine serum albumin; CDC: Cell-mediated cytotoxicity; D: Day; ELISA: Enzyme-linked immunosorbent assay; FTIR: Fourier transform infrared spectroscopy; LSM: Least squares mean; MAbs: Monoclonal antibodies; MWCO: Molecular weight cutoff; OD_{50}: Optical density 50%; OspA: Outer-surface lipoprotein A; OspC : Outer-surface lipoprotein C; PBS: Phosphate-buffered saline; RP-HPLC: Reverse phase high performance liquid chromatography; RU: Resonance unit; SEC-HPLC: Size exclusion high performance liquid chromatography; SPR: Surface plasmon resonance; TDA: Tetra-detector array; TFA: Trifluroacetic acid

Acknowledgments

The authors wish to acknowledge the technical assistance of Marsha Royston (management of the in life phase and sample collection), Shabnam Abedi, Anita Norman and Dana Parker (borreliacidal assay); Natalia Bomchil (non-lipidated OspA production and manuscript revision); and Valérie Monget (SPR assays). We would also like to thank Hongyu Ru and Daniel Pialot for the statistical analyses of the data, and Yu-Wei Chiang for valuable discussions regarding the borreliacidal assay.

Funding

This work was financially supported by Merial, which is now a part of Boehringer Ingelheim.

Authors' contributions

DAG and FD conceived the study design. DAG wrote the in-life study protocol and conducted that phase of the study. BF and KDW developed and ran the borreliacidal assay. KDL and P-YD developed and conducted the immunological assays. CS-C and MLS designed and executed studies relative to protein structure and biochemistry. MJD advised on the assays involving the canine IgG subclasses. All authors participated in drafting, revising, and reviewing the manuscript. DAG prepared the final version for submission. All authors read and approved the final manuscript.

Consent for publication
Not applicable.

Competing interests
Merial employees were responsible for study design, data collection, analysis, interpretation of the data, and preparation of the manuscript.

Author details
[1]Merial Inc., Boehringer Ingelheim, Athens, GA, USA. [2]MERIAL S.A.S., Boehringer Ingelheim, Lyon, France. [3]Bristol Veterinary School, University of Bristol, Langford, UK.

References

1. Conlon JAR, Mather TN, Tanner P, Gallo G, Jacobson RH. Efficacy of a nonadjuvanted, outer surface protein a, recombinant vaccine in dogs after challenge by ticks naturally infected with *Borrelia burgdorferi*. Vet Ther. 2000; 1:96–107.
2. Wikle RE, Fretwell B, Jarecki M, Jarecki-Black JC. Canine Lyme disease: one-year duration of immunity elicited with a canine OspA monovalent Lyme vaccine. Intern J Appl Res Vet Med. 2006;4:23–8.
3. Töpfer KT, Straubinger RK. Characterization of the humoral immune response in dogs after vaccination against the Lyme borreliosis agent. A study with five commercial vaccines using two different vaccination schedules. Vaccine. 2007; 25:314–26. https://doi.org/10.1016/j.vaccine.2006.07.031.
4. Alexopoulou L, Thomas V, Schnare M, Lobet Y, Anguita J, Schoen RT, Medzhitov R, Fikrig E, Flavell RA. Hyporesponsiveness to vaccination with *Borrelia burgdorferi* OspA in humans and in TLR1- and TLR2-deficient mice. Nat Med. 2002;8:878–84. https://doi.org/10.1038/nm732.
5. Belperron AA, Bockenstedt LK. Natural antibody affects survival of the spirochete *Borrelia burgdorferi* within feeding ticks. Infect Immun. 2001;69: 6456–62. https://doi.org/10.1128/IAI.69.10.6456-6462.2001.
6. Earnhart CG, Marconi RT. An octavalent lyme disease vaccine induces antibodies that recognize all incorporated OspC type-specific sequences. Hum Vaccin. 2007;3:281–9.
7. LaFleur RL, Dant JC, Wasmoen TL, Callister SM, Jove DA, Lovrich SD, Warner TF, Abdelmagid O, Schell RF. Bacterin that induces anti-OspA and anti-OspC borreliacidal antibodies provides a high level of protection against canine Lyme disease. Clin Vaccine Immunol. 2009;16:253–9. https://doi.org/10.1128/CVI.00373-08.
8. Probert WS, Crawford M, Cadiz RB, LeFebvre RB. Immunization with outer surface protein (Osp) a, but not OspC, provides cross-protection of mice challenged with north American isolates of *Borrelia burgdorferi*. J Infect Dis. 1997;175:400–5 https://academic.oup.com/jid/article-abstract/175/2/400/816707.
9. Vaz A, Glickstein L, Field JA, McHugh G, Sikand VK, Damle N, Steere AC. Cellular and humoral immune responses to Borrelia burgdorferi antigens in patients with culture-positive early Lyme disease. Infect Immun. 2001;69: 7437–44. https://doi.org/10.1128/IAI.69.12.7437-7444.2001.
10. Gilmore RD, Bacon RM, Carpio AM, Piesman J, Dolan MC, Mbow ML. Inability of outer-surface protein C (OspC)-primed mice to elicit a protective anamnestic immune response to a tick-transmitted challenge of *Borrelia burgdorferi*. J Med Microbiol. 2003;52:551–6. https://doi.org/10.1099/jmm.0.05068-0.
11. Earnhart CG, Marconi RT. Construction and analysis of variants of a polyvalent Lyme disease vaccine: approaches for improving the immune response to chimeric vaccinogens. Vaccine. 2007;25:3419–27. https://doi.org/10.1016/j.vaccine.2006.12.051.
12. Wagner B, Freer H, Rollins A, Erb HN. A fluorescent bead-based multiplex assay for the simultaneous detection of antibodies to *B. burgdorferi* outer surface proteins in canine serum. Vet Immunol Immunpathol. 2011;140:190–8. https://doi.org/10.1016/j.vetimm.2010.12.003.
13. Callister SM, Jobe DA, Schell RF, Pavia CS, Lovrich SD. Sensitivity and specificity of the borreliacidal-antibody test during early Lyme disease: a "gold standard"? Clin Diagn Lab Immunol. 1996;3:399–402.
14. Callister SM, Jobe DA, Schell RF, Lovrich S, Onheiber KL, Korshus JB. Detection of borreliacidal antibodies in dogs after challenge with *Borrelia burgdorferi*-infected *Ixodes scapularis* ticks. J Clin Microbiol. 2000;38:3670–4.
15. Rousselle JC, Callister SM, Schell RF, Lovrich SD, Jove DA, Marks JA, Wieneke CA. Borreliacidal antibody production against outer surface protein C of *Borrelia burgdorferi*. J Infect Dis. 1998;178:733–41 https://doi.org/10.1086/515382.
16. Day MJ. Immunoglobulin G subclass distribution in canine leishmaniosis: a review and analysis of pitfalls in interpretation. Vet Parasitol. 2007;147:2–8.
17. Ghimire TR. The mechanisms of action of vaccines containing aluminum adjuvants: an in vitro vs in vivo paradigm. Springerplus. 2015;4:181–99. https://doi.org/10.1186/s40064-015-0972-0.
18. Bergeron LM, McCandless EE, Dunham S, Dunkle B, Zhu Y, Shelly J, Lightle S, Gonzales A, Bainbridge G. Comparative functional characterization of canine IgG subclasses. Vet Immunol Immunopathol. 2013;157:31–41. https://doi.org/10.1016/j.vetimm.2013.10.018.
19. Widhe M, Ekerfelt C, Forsberg P, Bergström S, Ernerudh J. IgG subclasses in Lyme borreliosis: a study of specific IgG subclass distribution in an interferon-gamma-predominated disease. Scand J Immunol. 1998;47:575–81.
20. Erdile LF, Brandt MA, Warakomski DJ, Westrack GJ, Sadziene A, Barbour AG, Mays JP. Role of attached lipid in immunogenicity of *Borrelia burgdorferi* OspA. Infect Immun. 1993;61:81–90.
21. Trimaille T, Verrier B. Micelle-based adjuvants for subunit vaccine delivery. Vaccine. 2015;3(4):803–13. https://doi.org/10.3390/vaccines3040803.
22. Luo Z, Shi S, Jin L, Xu L, Yu J, Chen H, Li X. Cationic micelle based vaccine induced potent humoral immune response through enhancing antigen uptake and formation of germinal center. Colloids Surf B. 2015;135:556–64. https://doi.org/10.1016/j.colsurfb.2015.07.079.
23. Rhodes DVL, Earnhart CG, Mather TN, Meeus PFM, Marconi RT. Identification of *Borrelia burgdorferi* ospC genotypes in canine tissue following tick infestation: implications for Lyme disease vaccine and diagnostic assay design. Vet J. 2013;198:412–8. https://doi.org/10.1016/j.tvjl.2013.07.019.
24. Baum E, Grosenbaugh DA, Barbour AG. Diversity of antibody responses to *Borrelia burgdorferi* in experimentally infected beagle dogs. Clin Vaccine Immunol. 2014;21:838–46. https://doi.org/10.1128/CVI00018-14.
25. Fikrig E, Telford SR, Barthold SW, Kantor FS, Spielman A, Flavell RA. Elimination of Borrelia burgdorferi from vector ticks feeding on OspA-immunized mice. Proc Natl Acad Sci U S A. 1992;89:5418–21.
26. de Silva AM, Telford SR, Brunet LR, Barthold SW, Fikrig E. *Borrelia burgdorferi* OspA is an arthropod-specific transmission-blocking Lyme disease vaccine. J Exp Med. 1996;183:271–5.

18

Evolution of H9N2 avian influenza virus in embryonated chicken eggs with or without homologous vaccine antibodies

Haiyun Jin[1,2†], Wan Wang[1,2†], Xueqin Yang[1,2], Hailong Su[1,2], Jiawen Fan[1,2], Rui Zhu[1,2], Shifeng Wang[3], Huoying Shi[1,2*] and Xiufan Liu[1,2]

Abstract

Background: Vaccines constitute a unique selective pressure, different from natural selection, drives the evolution of influenza virus. In this study, A/Chicken/Shanghai/F/1998 (H9N2) was continually passaged in specific pathogen-free embryonated chicken eggs with or without selective pressures from antibodies induced by homologous maternal antibodies. Genetic mutations, antigenic drift, replication, and pathogenicity of the passaged virus were evaluated.

Results: Antigenic drift of the passaged viruses occurred in the 47th generation (vF47) under selective pressure on antibodies and in the 52nd generation (nF52) without selective pressure from antibodies. Seven mutations were observed in the vF47 virus, with three in PB2 and four in HA, whereas 12 mutations occurred in the nF52 virus, with three in PB2, two in PB1, four in HA, one in NP, one in NA, and one in NS. Remarkably, the sequences of the HA segment from vF47 were 100% homologous with those of the nF52 virus. Both the vF47 and nF52 viruses showed enhanced replication compared to the parental virus F/98, but higher levels of replication and pathogenicity were displayed by nF52 than by vF47. An inactive vaccine derived from the parental virus F/98 did not confer protection against challenges by either the vF47 or nF52 virus, but inactive vaccines derived from the vF47 or nF52 virus were able to provide protection against a challenge using F/98.

Conclusion: Taken together, the passage of H9N2 viruses with or without selective pressure of the antibodies induced by homologous maternal antibodies showed genetic variation, enhanced replication, and variant antigenicity. Selective pressure of the antibody does not seem to play a key role in antigenic drift in the egg model but may impact the genetic variation and replication ability of H9N2 viruses. These results improve understanding of the evolution of the H9N2 influenza virus and may aid in selecting appropriate vaccine seeds.

Keywords: H9N2 influenza virus, Selective pressure of antibody, Mutation, Antigenic drift, Replication

Background

The H9N2 influenza virus has spread rapidly in chickens throughout Asia since the 1990s [1, 2]. This virus, which was initially isolated from chickens in 1994, has caused severe economic losses for the poultry industry in China [2–6]. To control the spread of H9N2 avian influenza, a vaccination program for the H9N2 influenza virus has been widely implemented throughout mainland China over the past two decades [7, 8]. While this immunization program effectively reduced the economic loss caused by H9N2 influenza virus in chickens, it did not prevent the spread of H9N2 avian influenza through much of China [8]. In many Chinese provinces, H9N2 avian influenza now not only circulates in chickens but has also spread to pigs [9, 10] and wild and domestic birds [6, 11].

There are two scenarios under which the transmission of H9N2 avian influenza virus occurs. The first is a sporadic outbreak of H9N2 avian influenza virus in chicken farms occurring despite chicken vaccination, and can

* Correspondence: hyshi@yzu.edu.cn
†Equal contributors
[1]College of Veterinary Medicine, Yangzhou University, Yangzhou, Jiangsu 225009, People's Republic of China
[2]Jiangsu Co-innovation Center for the Prevention and Control of Important Animal Infectious Diseases and Zoonoses, Yangzhou 225009, China
Full list of author information is available at the end of the article

even occur in animals with a high antibody titer against H9N2 influenza [7, 8]. This scenario implies that the existing vaccine may not provide complete protection against infection by the prevalent H9N2 virus. Thus, vaccination against H9N2 influenza virus will not prevent the shedding of a common strain of H9N2 and may play a role in driving the evolution and spread of H9N2 influenza virus. The second scenario under which H9N2 avian influenza virus is transmitted relies on the ability of the H9N2 virus to reassort with other influenza virus subtypes to generate new influenza viruses. In this manner, an H9N2 virus supplied internal genes to an H5N1 virus in 1997 [2, 12, 13] and to H7N9 [14, 15] and H10N8 avian influenza viruses in 2013 [16]. Pu et al. [17] reported genotype 57 of the H9N2 chicken virus as the fittest virus to emerge over the 10 years of co-circulation of multiple H9N2 genotypes, that it had changed antigenicity and improved adaptability in chickens, and finally provided all of their internal genes to the novel H7N9 viruses [17]. The new virus genotype 57 displayed a strong advantage in its ability to escape the selective pressure of hosts.

The immune selective pressure of host drives influenza virus evolution [18]. During this process, antigenic drift can allow an influenza virus to escape recognition by virus-neutralizing antibodies [18, 19]. To date, all reported antigenic variations of H9N2 influenza virus were characterized based on their reactivity with monoclonal antibodies in a cell model [20, 21]. However, the effect of vaccine-induced polyclonal antibodies on the evolution of H9N2 influenza virus has not been quantitatively explored in either embryonated chicken eggs or a chicken model. Overall, chickens are suitable hosts for influenza virus, possess a whole functioning immune system, and can be a good model for studying the influence of vaccine-induced antibody on the evolution of H9N2 avian influenza virus. Moreover, specific pathogen-free (SPF) embryonated chicken eggs have an immature immune system compared with mature chickens. Even though eggs are not natural hosts of avian influenza, they can be a useful artificial model to evaluate the effects of selective pressures from antibodies (SPA) induced by homologous maternal antibodies on the evolution of H9N2 influenza viruses. Given that the H9N2 virus is still widely spreading and vaccination is the only current effective means with which to control H9N2 influenza, it would be useful to evaluate the influence of vaccine-induced antibodies on the evolution of the H9N2 avian influenza virus.

Sun et al. reported that, in China, the prevalent H9N2 avian influenza virus prior to 2000 was the BJ/94-lineage, and after 2004 the F/98-lineage became dominant. Currently, the F/98-lineage is still the prevalent genotype in China [22, 23]. In this study, A/Chicken/Shanghai/F/98 (H9N2, F/98) avian influenza virus, which is used in most regions of China as an early vaccine seed for H9N2 avian influenza [8, 21], was serially passaged in SPF embryonated chicken eggs with or without SPA induced by homologous maternal antibodies. The resulting passaged viruses were analyzed to investigate the effects of selective pressure of the antibody on the antigenic drift, genetic evolution, replication, pathogenicity, and immunogenicity of these viruses.

Methods

Animals

Ten-day-old of incubation SPF embryonated chicken eggs, SPF hens and cocks were purchased from the Shandong Poultry and Breeding Farms, China, and housed under SPF conditions. All animal experiments were approved by the Jiangsu Administrative Committee for Laboratory Animals (permission number SYXK-SU-2007-0005) and complied with the Jiangsu Laboratory Animal Welfare and Ethics guidelines of the Jiangsu Administrative Committee of Laboratory Animals [24].

H9N2 virus, MDCK cells and vaccine preparation

A/Chicken/Shanghai/F/98 (H9N2, F/98) influenza virus was isolated in Shanghai in 1998, purified and stocked by the Animal Infectious Disease Laboratory, School of Veterinary Medicine, and Yangzhou University [25]. The H9N2 avian influenza virus F/98 was propagated in the allantoic cavity of 10-day-old SPF embryonated eggs. The virus preparation was stored at − 70 °C until use. All experiments involving live viruses and animals were carried out in biosafety level (BSL) 2+ containment, as approved by Yangzhou University.

Madin-Darby canine kidney (MDCK) cells were grown in DMEM media (Invitrogen) containing 10% fetal bovine serum (FBS) (Invitrogen), and cultured in an incubator with 5% CO_2, 37 °C.

The F/98 strain was inactive by adding 0.2% formalin (*v*/v) for 24 h at 37 °C. Inactivation was confirmed by the absence of detectable infectivity after two blind passages of formalin-treated allantoic fluid in embryonated eggs. The inactive allantoic fluid was emulsified in two parts of paraffin oil (v/v), which is currently used commercially as an adjuvant for veterinary vaccine production [26].

Hemagglutination (HA) and hemagglutination inhibition (HI) assays, the antisera preparation of F/98 virus, routine HA and HI tests were used as outlined in the OIE *Manual of Diagnostic Tests and Vaccines for Terrestrial Animals* (http://www.oie.int/manual-of-diagnostic-tests-and-vaccines-for-terrestrial-animals/).

Three, four-week-old SPF chickens were immunized by intramuscular injection of 0.3 ml oil-emulsion of inactive whole virus vaccine of the indicated viruses.

Sera were taken in chickens at 3 weeks after immunization and treated with receptor-destroying enzyme (RDE, Cholera filtrate, Sigma, USA) to remove non-specific haemagglutination inhibitors, as above described an HI test was performed. Samples were regarded positive for inhibition of haemagglutination at a dilution ≥1:16.

HI test for yolk antibody

Three ten-day-old of incubation SPF embryonated chicken eggs either directly from SPF hen, or from the vaccinated SPF hens inseminated with SPF cocks. For yolk immunoglobulin extraction using a simplified chloroform polyethylene-glycol procedure, 2 ml of egg yolk was mixed with an equal volume of phosphate-buffered saline, and then added to 4 ml of chloroform. After mixing well, the yolk was centrifuged at 3500 rpm for 10 min. The supernatant was collected and used for antibody tests. The HI test was performed according to the standard procedures recommended by the OIE *Manual of Diagnostic Tests and Vaccines for Terrestrial Animals*. Briefly, the yolk samples were treated with a receptor-destroying enzyme (RDE) (Denka Seiken Co. Ltd., Tokyo, Japan) at 37 °C for 20 h to eliminate non-specific inhibitors of hemagglutination. HI titers obtained from a purified yolk and RDE mixture (25 ml egg yolk + 75 ml RDE provided a starting dilution of 1:1) were defined as the reciprocal of the highest dilution of yolk, which completely inhibited hemagglutination of 4 hemagglutination units of the virus with a 1% solution of chicken red blood cells. Samples with HI titers under 16 were considered negative.

F/98 (H9N2) serial passaged in the SPF embryonated chicken eggs with or without SPA

Three SPF hens were vaccinated three times with oil emulsion vaccine of F/98 strain. When HI titer in the serum diagram for the experiment design of the vaccinated hens was up to 512 [27], the vaccinated SPF hens were artificially inseminated with SPF cocks, resulting in the eggs with 16 or 32 HI titers of the yolk antibody against the parental virus F/98. These eggs were used as the SPA model. Meanwhile, the SPF embryonated chicken eggs directly bought from the same chicken farm served as a control without SPA. Three eggs from either SPA or the SPF embryonated chicken eggs were inoculated with 10^6 the 50% egg infectious dose (EID_{50}) of the F/98 virus. The allantoic fluid of each generation pooled from 3 eggs with or without SPA was collected after 72 h incubation. Part of allantoic fluid was saved at the − 70 °C, part of allantoic fluid were combined and used for the next passage in another three eggs with or the SPF embryonated chicken eggs, respectively, until 80 passages (Fig. 1). The embryo means death time (MDT)

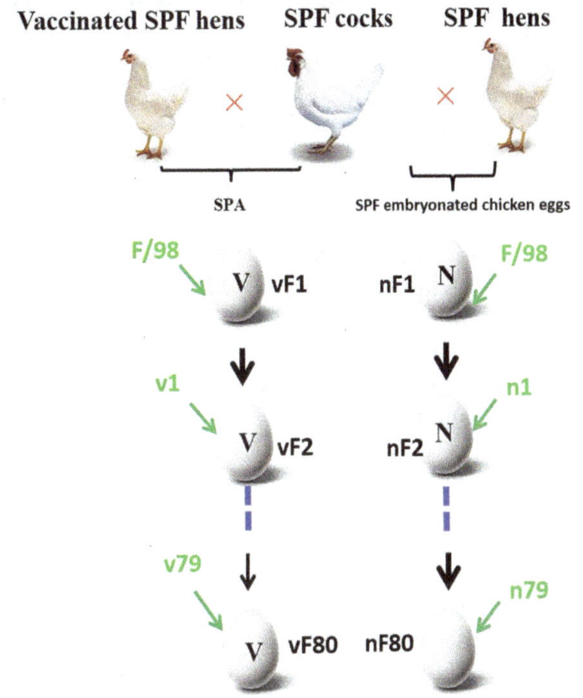

Fig. 1 Virus passage process. These images in Fig. 1 were made by authors and permitted to use

of the indicated passaged virus were calculated as described by Eugster AK. Et al [28], and EID_{50} titers of the indicated passaged virus were determined by serial titration of viruses in SPF embryonated chicken eggs using the Reed and Muench method [29].

Assay of viral antigenic drift

Haemagglutination antibody levels of each passaged virus against F/98 virus were determined by a haemagglutination inhibition (HI) assay. When HI titers of the passaged virus were up to 8-fold difference from that of the parental virus F/98, antigenicity of this passaged virus was believed to be drift [20]. These passaged virus presented in the allantoic fluid were divided two parts. The genes of one part virus were directly deep sequencing, another part virus was plaque purified twice in MDCK cells. Ten clones of each indicated virus were picked up, and passaged once in the allantoic cavities of 10-day-old chicken eggs for 72 h at 37 °C, and did Sanger sequencing for whole genome sequences [30].

Deep sequencing

Viral RNA was extracted from allantoic fluid of the indicated passaged viruses using the High Pure RNA isolation kit (Roche). RNA was subjected to reverse transcription-PCR (RT-PCR) using 18 primer sets that cover the entire viral genome. These primer sets were designed according to the genome sequences of the F/98 virus and by using Primer Premier 5.0 software. The fragments, approximately 600 to 800 nucleotides in length, were sequenced using the Illumina HiSeq2000 sequencing platform in the Chinese National Human Genome Center, Shanghai. Briefly, a library was constructed with TruSeq DNA sample prep kit set A. The DNA library was diluted and hybridized to the paired-end sequencing flow cells. DNA clusters were generated on a cBot cluster generation system with the TruSeq PE cluster generation kit v2, followed by sequencing on a HiSeq 2000 system with the TruSeq SBS kit v2. The threshold for the detection of single-nucleotide polymorphisms (SNP) was set manually at 10% of the population.

Sanger sequencing

Genome RNAs of viral clones were extracted from culture supernatants using the QIAamp viral RNA kit (Qiagen). Genes were reverse transcribed and amplified using a OneStep RT-PCR kit (Qiagen). Primers were the same as those used in the deep sequencing assay. The amplified cDNA products were excised from agarose gels and purified using a QIAquick gel extraction kit (Qiagen). Full-genome DNAs were Sanger sequenced by TAKARA BIOTECHNOLOGY (DALIAN) CO., LTD., and the sequence data were analyzed using GenScan software.

The positions of amino acid substitutions on the HA molecule were analyzed on the 3-dimensional structure obtained from the Protein Databank (PDB accession number, 1JSD) with the RasMol 2.7.3 program.

Replication and transmission in chickens

For studying the viral replication and pathogenicity in chicken, groups of six 4-week-old SPF chickens were oral, intranasally, or intratracheally inoculated with 0.2 ml of 10^6 EID_{50} of the parental virus F/98, the passaged viruses or phosphate buffer solution (PBS) control. Tissue samples (trachea and lung) from the inoculated chickens were collected at 3 days and 5 days post-inoculation (dpi) (28, 40). Briefly, three SPF chickens were euthanatized using CO_2 asphyxiation at designated times and half of the tissues were harvested, washed and ground into 20% (*w*/*v*) suspension in 1 ml PBS. Virus titers in the trachea and lung were determined in 10-day-old SPF embryonated chicken eggs accordingly (43). Another half part of the tissues were fixed with 10% neutral buffered formalin, embedded in paraffin, sectioned at 5 mm and routinely processed for staining with hematoxylin and eosin for histopathological examination (47). These experiments were repeated three times.

For studying the viral transmission, twelve 4-week-old SPF chickens for each virus were divided into: (i) inoculated group (three chickens), (ii) direct contact group (three chickens), (iii) airborne contact group (three chickens), (iv) PBS control group (three chickens) (28, 40). The infected group was inoculated oral, intranasally and intratracheally with 10^6 EID_{50} of indicated virus. The airborne contact group was placed in a cage directly adjacent to the infected group with a distance of 50 cm between cages. At day 3, 5, 7 and 9 post-inoculation, tracheal and cloacal swabs from chickens were collected in 1 ml of PBS containing antibiotics, following freeze/thaws once, and were centrifuged at 3000 rpm for 10 min. Of the resulting supernatant, 0.2 ml were taken and the EID_{50} titers of tracheal and cloacal swabs collected from the indicated passaged virus were determined by serial titration of viruses in SPF embryonated chicken eggs using the Reed and Muench method [29]. Sera collected from each experiment bird at 10 and 20 dpi were tested by HI assay to check the antibody in the serum of chickens against the indicated viruses [31]. The experiment was repeated three times.

Antigenic variant of the passaged viruses in chickens

To study the cross - immunogenicity of the passaged virus, 135 4 - week - old SPF chickens were divided into 5 groups, A, B, C, D and E (Table 3). In group A, each subgroup of 9 chickens were immunized with PBS and challenged with PBS and the indicated 0.3 ml inactivated oil-emulsion virus [32], respectively; in group B, each subgroup of 9 chickens were immunized with the vaccine of F/98 virus, and challenged with the indicated virus, respectively; In group C, or D, or E, each subgroup of 9 chickens were immunized with the indicated passaged virus, and challenged with the indicated virus, respectively (Table 3). On days 3 and 5 post-challenge, the viruses from challenged chickens were isolated from trachea and cloaca. The experiment was repeated three times.

Statistics

Data were presented as the geometric means and standard deviations for all assays. The Mann-Whitney U test (GraphPad Software, Inc., San Diego, CA) was used to evaluate the replication ability of strains and the tissue lesion in chickens challenged with different viruses. A *P* value of 0.05 was considered statistically significant.

Results

Adaption of H9N2 avian influenza virus F/98 passaged in SPF eggs with or without SPA

To explore the role of SPA on the evolution of H9N2 avian influenza virus, the F/98 virus was serially passaged in SPF embryonated eggs in the presence or absence of SPA, and the allantoic fluid of each generation was collected and stocked (Fig. 1). HI titers of the passaged virus in these fluids were determined.

Compared to the parental virus F/98, the HI titers of the passaged viruses were significantly decreased to 32-fold starting with vF47 (vF47: and nF52. In contrast, the HI titer of nF47 was only two-fold lower than that of F/98, indicating that antigenic drift had occurred in the passaged viruses vF47 and nF52 (Table 1). This result indicates that the antigenicity of F/98 H9N2 avian virus changed after being continually passaged either with or without SPA.

The passaged viruses vF47, nF47 and nF52 in the allantoic fluid were further deeply sequenced. We did not determine any viral quasispecies. Simultaneously, the passaged viruses vF47, vF60, vF70, vF80, nF47, nF52, nF60, nF70, and nF80 in the allantoic fluid were twice purified by plaque purification in MDCK cells (10 plaques of each indicated virus were picked up and sequenced to determine the purity of the passage viruses). Those viruses were then passaged once in the allantoic cavities of 10-day-old chicken eggs. A sequence analysis of these viruses confirmed that serial passage in allantoic cavities of the egg model did not lead to the formation of viral quasispecies.

The F/98, nF47, vF47, and nF52 viruses passaged in the allantoic fluid of eggs were selected for further research. We found that the embryo means death time (EMDT) of nF47, vF47, and nF52 in SPF embryonated chicken eggs was reduced by 7 h, 11 h, and 17.5 h, respectively, compared to the 86 h EMDT of the parental F/98 virus. The 50% egg infectious dose (EID_{50}) of nF47, vF47, and nF52 was significantly higher than that of their parental virus F/98 by 9.3-fold, 12.5-fold, and 117.5-fold, respectively (Table 1, $p < 0.01$). Notably, vF47 and nF47 shared similar EID_{50} titers. However, after five more passages, the EID_{50} of the nF52 virus was significantly increased compared to nF47 and vF47 (Table 1, $p < 0.01$).

SPA affects the genetic mutations of H9N2 avian virus

According to HI titers of the passaged viruses, vF47 and nF52 viruses were the first generations that displayed antigenic change compared to the parental virus F/98. To identify the effect of SPA on the genetic mutations of the H9N2 avian virus, the genomes of vF47, vF60, vF70, vF80, nF47, nF52, nF60, nF70, and nF80 virus passaged in the allantoic fluid of eggs were sequenced by Sanger sequencing. Compared to the parent virus F/98, nF47 has four amino acid substitutions, three in the PB2 gene (S155 N, C228Y, K375R) and one in the HA gene (K131R). Conversely, vF47 has seven amino acid mutations, three in the PB2 gene (I185K, C228Y, K375R) and four in the HA gene (K131R, S145 N, G181E, A198V). Additionally, nF52 has 12 amino acid mutations, three in the PB2 gene (S155 N, C228Y, K375R), two in the PB1 gene (T156A, R189K), four in the HA gene (K131R, S145 N, G181E, A198V), one in the NP gene (R99K), one in the NA gene (A459T), and one in the NS1 gene

Table 1 Adaptation of H9N2 avian influenza virus in SPF embryonated chicken eggs with or without SPA

Characters	F/98	nF47	nF52	vF47
HI titer	512	256	16	16
Change in HI titer compare to F/98		2-fold	32-fold	32-fold
EMDT (h)[a]	86	79	68.5	75
Change in EMDT(h)compare to F/98		7	17.5	11
EID_{50} (log10 EID_{50}/0.2 ml)	6.67	7.64	8.74	7.77
Changed in EID_{50} compare to F/98 (log10 decrease)		9.3-fold**	117.5-fold**##	12.5 fold**
Mutations[b] compare to F/98 (start-end passage of mutant)		PB2: S155 N, C228Y, K375R (nF46-nF80)	PB2:S155 N, C228Y, K375R (nF46-nF80)	PB2: I185K, C228Y, K375R (vF43-vF80)
		PB1: none	PB1:T156A, R189K (nF49-nF80)	PB1: none
		PA: none	PA: none	PA: none
		HA: K131R (nF30)	HA: K131R(nF30-nF80), S145 N, G181E, A198V (nF52-nF80)	HA: K131R, S145 N, G181E, A198V (vF47-vF80)
		NP: none	NP: R99K (nF50-nF80)	NP: none
		NA: none	NA: A459T (nF52-nF80)	NA: none
		M: none	M: none	M: none
		NS1: none	NS1: A143T (nF50-nF80)	NS1: none

[a]EMDT: Embryo mean death time
[b]each gene represent results from 10 clones
**$P < 0.01$ for the 50% egg infectious dose of nF47, vF47, and nF52 was significantly higher than that of their parental virus F/98
##$P < 0.01$ for the 50% egg infectious dose of nF52 was significantly higher than that of nF47 and vF47

(A143T) (Table 1). The genome sequences of vF60, vF70, and vF80 were each the same as that of vF47. The nF60, nF70, and nF80 genome sequences were each the same as that of nF52. The sequencing results show that vF47 has three more mutations in the HA gene (S145 N, G181E, A198V) and one different mutation in the PB2 gene (S155 N) compared with nF47. However, after five more passages, additional mutations distributed in the NA, PB1, NP, and NS1 genes of the nF52 virus were observed. Interestingly, vF47 and nF52 shared the same mutations in the HA gene, even though vF47 and nF52 resulted from the different eggs with and without SPA (Table 1).

To determine whether the amino acid changes observed in vF47 or nF52 occur in H9N2 wild-type isolates, sequences from the National Institute of Allergy and Infectious Diseases database (http://www.fludb.org) between 1994 and 2015 (from 1 January 1994 to 20 December 2015) were analyzed. Most H9N2 wild-type isolates shared common mutations with vF47 or nF52. Over the past 20 years, the mutations C228Y and K375R of the PB2 gene that we observed in the passaged viruses displayed high mutation frequencies of 92–100% in wild-type viruses. Additionally, the mutation frequencies of K131R, S145 N, G181E, and A198V in the HA gene that we observed in the vF47 and nF52 viruses were 96.3–99.4%, 3.7–18.1%, 0–72%, and 30.2–42.4% in wild-type viruses, respectively. In comparison, the A143T mutation in the NS1 gene that we observed in the nF52 virus had a mutation frequency of 18.8–43.2% in wild-type viruses. Notably, the mutations S145 N and G181E in HA were significantly increased in wild-type isolates, with 18.1% and 54% over recent years.

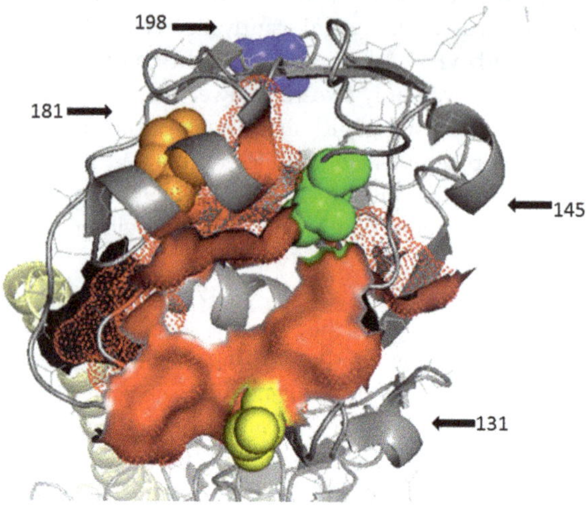

Fig. 2 Mutants mapping of HA. Schematic representation of monomer structures of the H9 haemagglutinin molecule showing the locations of amino acid substitutions on HA1. Amino acid changes of escape mutants selected with or without homologous vaccine antibody against Ck/SH/F/98 (H9N2). The positions of the mutations sites are shown as yellow for 131 site, green for 145 site, apricot yellow for 181 site, and blue for 198 site. Red for receptor binding pocket of HA1 in H9 virus. Amino acid positions correspond to H9 numbering. Images were created with RasMol 2.7.3

Mutants mapping of the H9 HA molecule

As described above, vF47 and nF52 shared the same mutations carrying K131R (yellow), S145 N (green), G181E (apricot yellow), and A198V (blue) in the HA gene. The locations of the amino acid substitution in the HA of H9 are illustrated on the three-dimensional map of F/98 HA (Fig. 2). The results show that all mutants distributed close to the hemagglutinin receptor-binding site (red). Interestingly, substitution of S145 N provided one more potential glycosylation site in both the vF47 and nF52 viruses.

H9N2 viruses passaged with or without SPA display different replication and pathogenicity in chickens

We further examined the replication and pathogenicity of the viruses passaged with or without SPA by comparing the virus titers and pathology parameters in chickens. The results show that the viral load of the passaged viruses in the trachea were 100–10,000-fold higher than that of their parental virus F/98 (Fig. 3a, $p < 0.01$) at 3 and 5 days post-infection (dpi). The titers of vF47 in the trachea were significantly lower than those of nF47 at 3 and 5 dpi (Fig. 3a, $p < 0.01$), and they were also lower than that of nF52 at 5 dpi (Fig. 3a, $p < 0.01$). Additionally, the titers of nF47 and nF52 at 5 dpi were not only higher than their corresponding titers at 3 dpi (Fig. 3b, $p < 0.01$), but they were also higher than those of their parental virus F/98 and of vF47 (Fig. 3b, $p < 0.01$). The titer of vF47 decreased in the lung (Fig. 3b, $p < 0.01$) to a level similar to that of the parental virus F/98.

The histopathological lesions of the trachea and lung in chickens infected with one of the passaged viruses, or with the wildtype virus F/98, had similar levels of severity at 3 dpi (Fig. 3c - k). At 5 dpi, the passaged virus vF47 displayed an increased level of pathogenicity only in the trachea (Fig. 3c, Fig. 3i, $p < 0.01$), whereas the passaged viruses nF47 and nF52 showed enhanced pathogenicity levels in both the trachea and lung (Fig. 3c - d, $p < 0.01$; Fig. 3g - h, k- l) compared with those of the parental virus F/98. Additionally, nF47 and nF52 each showed a higher pathological score than that of vF47 at 5 dpi (Fig. 3d, $p < 0.01$).

SPA improves the airborne transmission characteristics of H9N2 influenza virus

We set up transmission experiments with the passaged viruses nF47, vF47, nF52 and their parental virus F/98 to further explore the effect of SPA on the transmission route of the H9N2 influenza virus [31]. The results show that all tested viruses could spread by direct contact. In

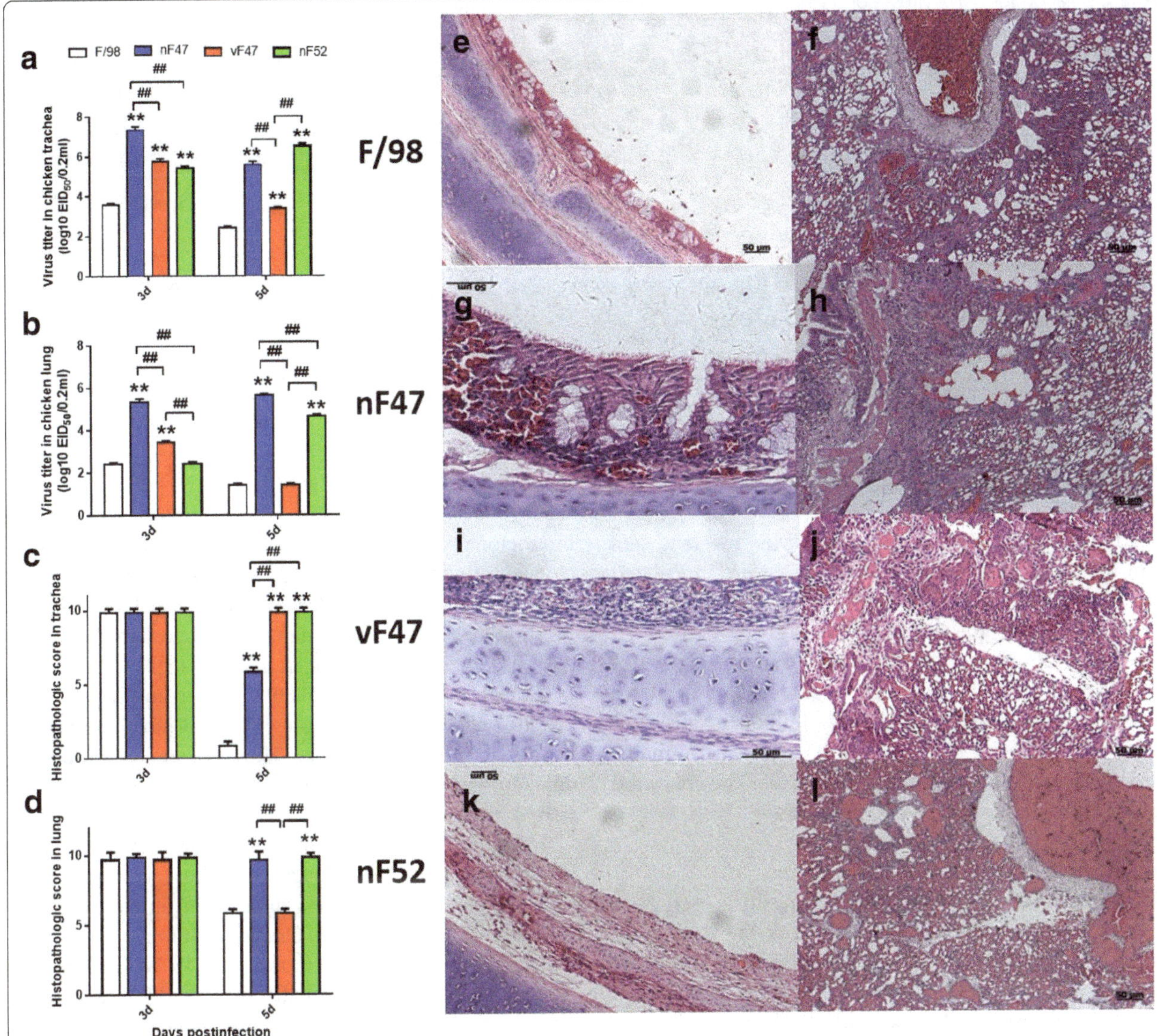

Fig. 3 Replication and pathological changes of the viruses in chickens. Groups of three chickens were inoculated orally, intranasally, and intratracheally with 10^6 EID_{50} of F/98 or the passaged viruses. **a-b** Replication ability of the viruses in trachea and lung of chickens were evaluated at 3 and 5 dpi. For virus titration in SPF eggs. The average of each group is shown, with error bars representing the SD. **, $P < 0.01$ compared with the value for the parental virus F/98 group; ##, $P < 0.01$ for the passaged viruses group compared each other. Data are representative of three independent experiments. **c-d** Histology scores of viruses in the trachea (**c**) and lung (**d**) chickens at 3 and 5 days after inoculated with H9N2 virus. Horizontal lines show the mean, error bars represent the SD, and data are representative of three independent experiments. **e-l** Representative H&E histology sections of the viruses at 5 d after inoculated with different virus. **e-f** F/98 virus-infected trachea and lung; **g-h** nF47 virus-infected trachea and lung; **i-j** vF47 virus-infected trachea and lung; **k-l** nF52 virus-infected trachea and lung. The histopathological changes were scored as follows. For trachea, 0: normal; 1: congestion; 2: cilia loss; 3: a few inflammatory cell infiltration; 7: a lot of inflammatory cell infiltration; for lung, 0: normal; 1: congestion; 2: hemorrhage; 3: inflammatory cell infiltration in bronchial submucosa; 7: a lot of inflammatory cell infiltration in bronchial submucosa and alveolus

the directly inoculated group, the shedding of vF47 was detected at 3 and 5 dpi in the trachea of chickens and was measured at 5, 7 and 9 dpi in the cloaca of chickens. This is the same shedding pattern observed for the parental virus F/98. In contrast, the nF47 virus could be isolated at 3, 5, 7, and 9 dpi, and the nF52 virus was isolated at 3, 5, and 7 dpi in the trachea of chickens, thus indicating that nF47 and nF52 each displayed a longer shedding period than vF47 and F/98 did in the trachea of chickens. In the airborne contact group, the F/98, nF47, and vF47 viruses could spread by airborne transmission, whereas nF52 lacked the ability to undergo airborne transmission (Table 2). These features were further confirmed by the result of the serologic analysis of HI assays, in which serum collected from the airborne contact chickens that were inoculated with nF52 showed

Table 2 Isolation for H9N2 viruses of tracheal and cloacal swabs in chickens in transmission experiment

Virus	Ways of infection	Tracheal swabs (virus titers[b])				Cloacal swabs (virus titers[b])				Mean HI titers of chickens (2^n)	
		3 d	5 d	7 d	9 d	3 d	5 d	7 d	9 d	10 d	20 d
F/98	Directly inoculation[a]	9/9(3.3 ± 0.2)	6/9(1.85 ± 0.2)	0/9	0/9	0/9	2/9(1.65 ± 0.1)	6/9(1.8 ± 0.4)	3/9(<1[c])	5 ± 0.7	9 ± 0.5
	Airborne contact[a]	2/9(1.7 ± 0.1)	4/9(<1[c])	2/9(<1[c])	0/9	0/9	4/9(1.1 ± 0.1)	2/9(<1[c])	0/9	3 ± 1.9	9 ± 0.3
nF47	Directly inoculation[a]	9/9(5.3 ± 0.4)	9/9(3.45 ± 0.3)	9/9 (1.65 ± 0.2)	6/9(<1[c])	0/9	4/9(2.4 ± 0.3)	7/9(1.3 ± 0.1)	3/9(<1[c])	6 ± 0.4	10 ± 0.2
	Airborne contact[a]	5/9(3.5 ± 0.1)	7/9(2.5 ± 0.3)	2/9(<1[c])	2/9(<1[c])	0/9	3/9(1.6 ± 0.2)	0/9	0/9	7 ± 1.5	9 ± 2.9
VF47	Directly inoculation[a]	9/9(4.2 ± 0.3)	9/9(2.5 ± 0.3)	0/9	0/9	0/9	2/3(2.45 ± 0.3)	7/9(1.5 ± 0.1)	2/9(1.15 ± 0. 2)	7 ± 0.2	10 ± 0.6
	Airborne contact[a]	5/9(2.2 ± 0.4)	7/9(1.2 ± 0.1)	6/9(<1[c])	0/9	0/9	3/9(1.9 ± 0.1)	7/9(1.1 ± 0.5)	3/9(<1[c])	7 ± 2.6	10 ± 1.1
nF52	Directly inoculation[a]	9/9(3.8 ± 0.2)	9/9(4.1 ± 0.2)	6/9 (2.6 ± 0.1)	0/9	0/9	4/9(2.9 ± 0.3)	6/9(2.2 ± 0.3)	3/9(<1[c])	7 ± 0.8	10 ± 1.7
	Airborne contact[a]	0/9	0/9	0/9	0/9	0/9	0/9	0/9	0/9	0	0

[a]number of positive tracheal or cloacal/total number of chickens
[b]Virus titers in tracheal or cloacal swabs are expressed as mean log10 EID_{50}/ml ± SD
[c]Lower than the detection limit of 10 EID_{50}

negative reactivity against the nF52 virus, whereas sera from the airborne contact chickens that were inoculated with F/98, nF47, or vF47 viruses displayed positive reactivity against the indicated viruses at 10 and 20 dpi (Table 2). This finding implies that the presence of SPA during serial passaging might be beneficial for preserving the ability of H9N2 influenza virus to spread via airborne transmission as well as for maintaining the same shedding pattern as the parental virus F/98.

Immunogenic drift of the passaged viruses

The immunization and challenge procedure used here is described in Table 3. These results show that all chickens immunized with PBS shed the indicated virus at 3 or 5 dpi (Table 3). In chickens immunized with F/98, those challenged with F/98 or nF47 were observed to shed less from the trachea and cloaca, respectively (Table 3). Conversely, chickens challenged with vF47 or with nF52 were found to shed more (Table 3). However, in groups immunized with one of the passaged viruses (nF47, vF47, nF52), less shedding was detected in the trachea and cloaca of chickens challenged with F/98 or their respective homolog viruses (Table 3).

Discussion

Previous work studying the evolution of influenza focused on performing sequence analyses of field isolates [1, 6, 8, 11, 12, 16, 17, 22, 23, 25, 32]. However, given the extensive use of vaccines in both humans and animals, it is also important to investigate the role of vaccine-induced antibody activity on influenza virus evolution. To date, there have been few reports about influenza virus escape mutants; the reported mutants were selected by host SPA in MDCK cells, by monoclonal antibodies in mice [20, 21, 33], or by polyclonal antibodies in pigs [18, 34]. While those reports show that SPA plays an important role in the evolution of influenza virus [22], neither embryonated chicken eggs nor chickens have been used to explore the effect of SPA on the evolution of H9N2 avian influenza virus, despite chickens being one of the most important hosts of influenza virus. Herein, we developed a chicken egg model to characterize the evolution of H9N2 avian influenza virus F/98, the vaccine seed in China and to serially passage this virus in SPF embryonated chicken eggs with or without SPA. Three groups of mutations distributed in the passaged viruses nF47, vF47 and nF52 were found.

Group one, containing mutants S145 N, G181E, and A198V in HA, was found in both the vF47 and nF52 virus. The antigenicity of the vF47 and nF52 viruses were changed with 32-fold HI titers lower than the parental virus F/98. Those changes resulted in low levels of protection against the passaged viruses vF47 and nF52 in chickens that were immunized with the vaccine based on the parental virus F/98 (Tables 1 and 3). In comparison, the results of the HI titer of nF47 was only 2-fold lower than the parental virus F/98 and resulted in good protection against the nF50 in chickens immunized with parental virus F/98. This indicates that mutants S145 N, G181E, A198V in HA may contribute to the antigenic drift of the v47 and n52 virus. These mutants are close to the hemagglutinin receptor-binding site and are consistent with the fact that substitutions near the hemagglutinin receptor-binding site determine the antigenic evolution of influenza A H3N2 viruses [35]. Since the vF47 and nF52 were adaptive virus with or without SPA, selective pressure of the antibody seems not to play the main role on antigenic drift in the egg model.

Table 3 Isolation of H9N2 viruses in vaccinated chickens after challenged with the passaged viruses

Group	Challenge virus	HI mean titer(2^n) (Homologous antigen 2^n)	3dpi Tracheal swab[a] (Virus titers [b])	3dpi Cloacal swab[a] (Virus titers[b])	5dpi Tracheal swab[a] (Virus titers [b])	5dpi Cloacal swab[a] (Virus titers [b])
A (None-immune)	BSG	0	0/6	0/6	0/6	0/6
	F/98	0	6/6 (3.2 ± 0.3)	1/6 (1.6 ± 0.1)	3/6 (1.8 ± 0.2)	0/6
	nF47	0	6/6 (5.2 ± 0.1)	6/6 (3.1 ± 0.3)	2/6 (3.2 ± 0.1)	2/6 (1.1 ± 0.1)
	vF47	0	6/6(4.1 ± 0.2)	3/6 (2.1 ± 0.1)	6/6 (1.5 ± 0.3)	2/6 (<1[c])
	nF52	0	6/6 (3.6 ± 0.1)	2/6 (3.8 ± 0.2)	6/6 (4.1 ± 0.2)	2/6 (1.6 ± 0.3)
B (Immune F/98)	F/98	7	1/6 (1.2 ± 0.1)	0/6	0/6	0/6
	nF47	7	1/6(3.1 ± 0.1)	0/6	2/6 (1.3 ± 0.3)	0/6
	vF47	7.3	6/6 (4.3 ± 0.1)	4/6 (2.2 ± 0.2)	6/6 (2.7 ± 0.2)	5/6 (1.0 ± 0.2)
	nF52	7	6/6 (3.9 ± 0.3)	2/6 (1.6 ± 0.1)	6/6 (2.1 ± 0.1)	3/6 (<1[c])
C (immune nF47)	F	7	0/6	0/6	0/6	0/6
	nF47	7	0/6	0/6	0/6	0/6
D (immune vF47)	F	6.7	0/6	0/6	0/6	0/6
	vF47	6.7	0/6	0/6	0/6	0/6
E (immune nF52)	F	7	1/6(1.9 ± 0.3)	0/6	0/6	0/6
	nF52	7	0/6	0/6	0/6	0/6

[a]number of positive tracheal or cloacal swabs /total number of chickens

[b]Virus titers in tracheal or cloacal swabs are expressed as mean log10 EID_{50}/ml ± SD

[c]Lower than the detection limit of 10 EID_{50}

Group two included K131R in HA, C228Y and K375R in PB2, which appeared in three viruses: nF47, nF52, and vF47. The EID_{50} of each of the passaged viruses (nF47, vF47, and nF52) was significantly higher than that of the parental virus F/98 (Table 1). The replication abilities of the passaged viruses nF47, vF47, and nF52 in the trachea of chickens were significantly higher compared to the parental strain F/98 (Fig. 3a). This implies that the mutants K131R in HA, C228Y and K375R in PB2 may contribute to the enhanced replication of the passaged viruses. This result is consistent with previous reports of viruses passaged in mice and swine [18, 30, 36–38].

Interestingly, group three, consisting of A459T in NA, T156A and R189K in PB1, R99K in NP, and A143T in NS1, only appeared in the nF52 virus. Compared to the vF47 virus, the nF52 has a 9.3-fold higher incidence of EID_{50} (Table 1), significantly higher replication ability in the trachea and lung of chickens (Fig. 3a-d), and specifically lost the characteristic of airborne transmission. These differences between the vF47 and nF52 may result from the mutants of group three, which were not present in the vF47 virus generated in SPA. In other words, SPA induced by homologous maternal antibodies limited the vF47 virus to possess the mutants of group three (A459T in NA, T156A and R189K in PB1, R99K in NP and A143T in NS1), implying that SPA may regulate the genetic variation and replication ability of H9N2 viruses in the egg model.

Conclusions

In summary, our findings suggest that the antigenic drift of H9N2 influenza virus occurs during serial passaging with SPA or SPF embryonated chicken eggs. The virus produced by passaging in the presence of SPA has fewer amino acid substitutions and displays earlier antigenic drift than the virus produced by passaging in SPF embryonated chicken eggs. In contrast, the virus passaged in SPF embryonated chicken eggs developed more genetic changes. These mutations lead to the virus having enhanced replication and pathogenicity in SPF chickens and changed the feature of airborne spread compared to the SPA-passaged virus. The vaccine prepared from the parental virus did not provide protection against the passaged viruses, but the vaccines produced from the passaged viruses conferred complete protection against the parental virus. Our findings broaden the understanding of antigenic drift and the selection of vaccine seeds for H9N2 influenza viruses.

Abbreviations

BSL: Biosafety level; dpi: Days post-inoculation; EID_{50}: The 50% egg infectious dose; EMDT: Embryo means death time; F/98: A/Chicken/Shanghai/F/98 (H9N2); FBS: Fetal bovine serum; h: Hour; HA: Haemagglutinin; HI: Haemagglutination inhibition; MDCK: Madin-Darby canine kidney; nF47: The 47nd generation without selective pressure from antibodies; nF52: The 52nd generation without selective pressure from antibodies; OIE: Office international des epizooties; PBS: Phosphate buffer solution; RDE: Receptor-destroying enzyme; RT-PCR: Reverse transcription- polymerase chain reaction; SNP: Single-nucleotide polymorphisms; SPA: Selective pressures from antibodies; SPF: specific pathogen-free; vF47: The 47th generation under selective pressure on antibodies

Acknowledgements
Not applicable

Funding
This work was supported by the National Natural Science Foundation of China (31672516, 31172300, 30670079), supported by the Grant No. BE2016343 from Jiangsu province, the Jiangsu University and College Natural Science Foundation (12KJA230002), the Doctoral Program of Higher Education of China (20133250110002) and a project funded by the Priority Academic Program Development of Jiangsu Higher Education Institutions (PAPD).

Authors' contributions
Conceived and designed the experiments: HJ, WW, HSH and XL. Performed the experiments: HJ, WW, XY, HS, JF, RZ. Wrote the paper: HJ, WW, XY, HS, JF, RZ, SW, HSH. All authors read and approved the final manuscript.

Consent for publication
Not applicable.

Competing interests
The authors declare that they have no competing interests.

Author details
[1]College of Veterinary Medicine, Yangzhou University, Yangzhou, Jiangsu 225009, People's Republic of China. [2]Jiangsu Co-innovation Center for the Prevention and Control of Important Animal Infectious Diseases and Zoonoses, Yangzhou 225009, China. [3]Department of Infectious Diseases and Pathology, College of Veterinary Medicine, University of Florida, Gainesville, FL 32611-0880, USA.

References

1. Naeem K, Ullah A, Manvell RJ, Alexander DJ. Avian influenza A subtype H9N2 in poultry in Pakistan. Vet Rec. 1999;145(19):560.
2. Guo YJ, Krauss S, Senne DA, Mo IP, Lo KS, Xiong XP, Norwood M, Shortridge KF, Webster RG, Guan Y. Characterization of the pathogenicity of members of the newly established H9N2 influenza virus lineages in Asia. Virology. 2000;267(2):279–88.
3. Alexander DJ. A review of avian influenza in different bird species. Vet Microbiol. 2000;74(1–2):3–13.
4. Li KS, Xu KM, Peiris JS, Poon LL, Yu KZ, Yuen KY, Shortridge KF, Webster RG, Guan Y. Characterization of H9 subtype influenza viruses from the ducks of southern China: a candidate for the next influenza pandemic in humans? J Virol. 2003;77(12):6988–94.
5. Liu H, Liu X, Cheng J, Peng D, Jia L, Huang Y. Phylogenetic analysis of the hemagglutinin genes of twenty-six avian influenza viruses of subtype H9N2 isolated from chickens in China during 1996-2001. Avian Dis. 2003;47(1): 116–27.
6. Xu KM, Li KS, Smith GJ, Li JW, Tai H, Zhang JX, Webster RG, Peiris JS, Chen H, Guan Y. Evolution and molecular epidemiology of H9N2 influenza A viruses from quail in southern China, 2000 to 2005. J Virol. 2007;81(6):2635–45.
7. Li C, Yu K, Tian G, Yu D, Liu L, Jing B, Ping J, Chen H. Evolution of H9N2 influenza viruses from domestic poultry in mainland China. Virology. 2005; 340(1):70–83.
8. Zhang P, Tang Y, Liu X, Peng D, Liu W, Liu H, Lu S, Liu X. Characterization of H9N2 influenza viruses isolated from vaccinated flocks in an integrated broiler chicken operation in eastern China during a 5 year period (1998-2002). J Gen Virol. 2008;89(Pt 12):3102–12.
9. Cong YL, Pu J, Liu QF, Wang S, Zhang GZ, Zhang XL, Fan WX, Brown EG, Liu JH. Antigenic and genetic characterization of H9N2 swine influenza viruses in China. J Gen Virol. 2007;88(Pt 7):2035–41.
10. Cong YL, Wang CF, Yan CM, Peng JS, Jiang ZL, Liu JH. Swine infection with H9N2 influenza viruses in China in 2004. Virus Genes. 2008;36(3):461–9.
11. Wang B, Chen Q, Chen Z. Complete genome sequence of an H9N2 avian influenza virus isolated from egret in Lake Dongting wetland. J Virol. 2012; 86(21):11939.
12. Zhao G, Gu X, Lu X, Pan J, Duan Z, Zhao K, Gu M, Liu Q, He L, Chen J, et al. Novel reassortant highly pathogenic H5N2 avian influenza viruses in poultry in China. PLoS One. 2012;7(9):e46183.
13. Gu M, Chen H, Li Q, Huang J, Zhao M, Gu X, Jiang K, Wang X, Peng D, Liu X. Enzootic genotype S of H9N2 avian influenza viruses donates internal genes to emerging zoonotic influenza viruses in China. Vet Microbiol. 2014;174(3–4):309–15.
14. Cui L, Liu D, Shi W, Pan J, Qi X, Li X, Guo X, Zhou M, Li W, Li J, et al. Dynamic reassortments and genetic heterogeneity of the human-infecting influenza A (H7N9) virus. Nat Commun. 2014;5:3142.
15. Gao R, Cao B, Hu Y, Feng Z, Wang D, Hu W, Chen J, Jie Z, Qiu H, Xu K, et al. Human infection with a novel avian-origin influenza A (H7N9) virus. N Engl J Med. 2013;368(20):1888–97.
16. Ye G, Liang CH, Hua DG, Song LY, Xiang YG, Guang C, Lan CH, Ping HY. Phylogenetic analysis and pathogenicity assessment of two strains of avian influenza virus subtype H9N2 isolated from migratory birds: high homology of internal genes with human H10N8 virus. Front Microbiol. 2016;7:57.
17. Pu J, Wang S, Yin Y, Zhang G, Carter RA, Wang J, Xu G, Sun H, Wang M, Wen C, et al. Evolution of the H9N2 influenza genotype that facilitated the genesis of the novel H7N9 virus. Proc Natl Acad Sci U S A. 2015;112(2):548–53.
18. Murcia PR, Hughes J, Battista P, Lloyd L, Baillie GJ, Ramirez-Gonzalez RH, Ormond D, Oliver K, Elton D, Mumford JA, et al. Evolution of an Eurasian avian-like influenza virus in naive and vaccinated pigs. PLoS Pathog. 2012; 8(5):e1002730.
19. Van de Sandt CE, Kreijtz JH, Rimmelzwaan GF. Evasion of influenza A viruses from innate and adaptive immune responses. Viruses. 2012;4(9):1438–76.
20. Wan Z, Ye J, Xu L, Shao H, Jin W, Qian K, Wan H, Qin A. Antigenic mapping of the hemagglutinin of an H9N2 avian influenza virus reveals novel critical amino acid positions in antigenic sites. J Virol. 2014;88(7):3898–901.
21. Zhu Y, Yang D, Ren Q, Yang Y, Liu X, Xu X, Liu W, Chen S, Peng D, Liu X. Identification and characterization of a novel antigenic epitope in the hemagglutinin of the escape mutants of H9N2 avian influenza viruses. Vet Microbiol. 2015;178(1–2):144–9.
22. Sun Y, Pu J, Jiang Z, Guan T, Xia Y, Xu Q, Liu L, Ma B, Tian F, Brown EG, et al. Genotypic evolution and antigenic drift of H9N2 influenza viruses in China from 1994 to 2008. Vet Microbiol. 2010;146(3–4):215–25.
23. Zhang P, Tang Y, Liu X, Liu W, Zhang X, Liu H, Peng D, Gao S, Wu Y, Zhang L, et al. A novel genotype H9N2 influenza virus possessing human H5N1 internal genomes has been circulating in poultry in eastern China since 1998. J Virol. 2009;83(17):8428–38.
24. Zhong L, Wang X, Li Q, Liu D, Chen H, Zhao M, Gu X, He L, Liu X, Gu M, et al. Molecular mechanism of the airborne transmissibility of H9N2 avian influenza A viruses in chickens. J Virol. 2014;88(17):9568–78.
25. Lu JH, Liu XF, Shao WX, Liu YL, Wei DP, Liu HQ. Phylogenetic analysis of eight genes of H9N2 subtype influenza virus: a mainland China strain possessing early isolates' genes that have been circulating. Virus Genes. 2005;31(2):163–9.
26. Jansen T, Hofmans MP, Theelen MJ, Schijns VE. Structure-activity relations of water-in-oil vaccine formulations and induced antigen-specific antibody responses. Vaccine. 2005;23(8):1053–60.
27. Edwards S. OIE laboratory standards for avian influenza. Dev Biol (Basel). 2006;124:159–62.
28. A.K. E, et al. Prev Vet Med. 1998;34(1):77–8. 1996
29. Reed L, Muench LEH. A simple method of estimating fifty percent endpoints. Am J Hyg. 1938;27:493–7.
30. Li Q, Wang X, Zhong L, Wang X, Sun Z, Gao Z, Cui Z, Zhu J, Gu M, Liu X, et al. Adaptation of a natural reassortant H5N2 avian influenza virus in mice. Vet Microbiol. 2014;172(3–4):568–74.
31. Shi H, Ashraf S, Gao S, Lu J, Liu X. Evaluation of transmission route and replication efficiency of H9N2 avian influenza virus. Avian Dis. 2010; 54(1):22–7.

32. Zhong L, Zhao Q, Zhao K, Wang X, Zhao G, Li Q, Gu M, Peng D, Liu X. The antigenic drift molecular basis of the H5N1 influenza viruses in a novel branch of clade 2.3.4. Vet Microbiol. 2014;171(1–2):23–30.
33. O'Donnell CD, Vogel L, Wright A, Das SR, Wrammert J, Li GM, McCausland M, Zheng NY, Yewdell JW, Ahmed R, et al. Antibody pressure by a human monoclonal antibody targeting the 2009 pandemic H1N1 virus hemagglutinin drives the emergence of a virus with increased virulence in mice. MBio. 2012;3(3):e00120–12.
34. Degen WG, Smith J, Simmelink B, Glass EJ, Burt DW, Schijns VE. Molecular immunophenotyping of lungs and spleens in naive and vaccinated chickens early after pulmonary avian influenza A (H9N2) virus infection. Vaccine. 2006;24(35–36):6096–109.
35. Lewis NSAT, Kitikoon P, Skepner E, Burke DF, Vincent AL. Substitutions near the hemagglutinin receptor-binding site determine the antigenic evolution of influenza A H3N2 viruses in U.S. swine. J Virol. 2014;88(9):4752–63.
36. Li Q, Wang X, Sun Z, Hu J, Gao Z, Hao X, Li J, Liu H, Wang X, Gu M, et al. Adaptive mutations in PB2 gene contribute to the high virulence of a natural reassortant H5N2 avian influenza virus in mice. Virus Res. 2015;210: 255–63.
37. Liu Q, Chen H, Huang J, Chen Y, Gu M, Wang X, Hu S, Liu X, Liu X. A nonpathogenic duck-origin H9N2 influenza A virus adapts to high pathogenicity in mice. Arch Virol. 2014;159(9):2243–52.
38. Liu Q, Liu K, Xue C, Zhou J, Li X, Luo D, Zheng J, Xu S, Liu GD, Cao Y. Recombinant influenza H1, H5 and H9 hemagglutinins containing replaced H3 hemagglutinin transmembrane domain showed enhanced heterosubtypic protection in mice. Vaccine. 2014;32(25):3041–9.

19

Avian influenza A (H5N1) outbreaks in different poultry farm types in Egypt: the effect of vaccination, closing status and farm size

Jean Artois[1*], Carla Ippoliti[2], Annamaria Conte[2], Madhur S. Dhingra[1,3], Pastor Alfonso[4], Abdelgawad El Tahawy[5], Ahmed Elbestawy[5], Hany F. Ellakany[5] and Marius Gilbert[1,6]

Abstract

Background: The Avian Influenza A (H5N1) virus is endemic in poultry in Egypt. The winter of 2014/2015 was particularly worrying as new clusters of HPAI A (H5N1) virus emerged, leading to an important number of AI A (H5N1) outbreaks in poultry farms and sporadic human cases. To date, few studies have investigated the distribution of HPAI A (H5N1) outbreaks in Egypt in relation to protective / risk factors at the farm level, a gap we intend to fill. The aim of the study was to analyse passive surveillance data that were based on observation of sudden and high mortality of poultry or drop in duck or chicken egg production, as a basis to better understand and discuss the risk of HPAI A (H5N1) presence at the farm level in large parts of the Nile Delta.

Results: The probability of HPAI A (H5N1) presence was associated with several characteristics of the farms. Vaccination status, absence of windows/openings in the farm and the number of birds per cycle of production were found to be protective factors, whereas the presence of a duck farm with significant mortality or drop in egg production in the village was found to be a risk factor.

Conclusions: Results demonstrate the key role of several prevention and biosecurity measures to reduce HPAI A (H5N1) virus circulation, which could promote better poultry farm biosecurity in Egypt.

Keywords: Avian influenza A (H5N1), Egypt, Poultry farms, Risk or protective factors, Biosecurity

Background

The highly pathogenic avian influenza (HPAI) A (H5N1) virus has been enzootic in Egyptian poultry for about ten years [1, 2]. Despite years of efforts to control and prevent HPAI A (H5N1) outbreaks, including surveillance, vaccination and culling, the virus continues to spread in the poultry production and trade systems. All along the value chain, from the producers to the end consumers, the risk of exposure of Egyptian farmers to infected poultry is persistent, resulting in sporadic human cases [3–5], some of which lead to severe illness-complications and death (34% case-fatality rate for the severe human cases in Egypt from 2006 to 2015 [5]). The winter of 2014/2015 was particularly significant as the number of human cases in Egypt reached levels never observed before, with 165 new human cases leading to 51 fatalities [4]. This period also marked the emergence of a new cluster of HPAI A (H5N1) virus within the clade 2.2.1.2 [6]. In 2016, the situation more or less returned to the previous levels, with only 10 human cases reported [7].

After nearly 10 years of continued evolution of the HPAI A (H5N1) virus, several distinct antigenic clusters have emerged in Egypt within the clade 2.2, notably the clades 2.2.1, 2.2.1.1 and 2.2.1.2 [1]. The diversity of viral HA gene found in Egypt [1, 5, 8, 9] may be partially explained by the wide range of poultry production systems coexisting in the Nile river delta, ranging from backyard

* Correspondence: jeanarto@gmail.com
[1]Spatial Epidemiology Lab. (SpELL), Université Libre de Bruxelles, Brussels, Belgium

and household ownership to large commercial and industrial farms. Each system is associated with specific mixes of domestic species, different levels of biosecurity, differences in vaccine coverage, different production cycles and value chains [10] resulting in a wide diversity of selection pressures for the HPAI A (H5N1) virus. Although gallinaceous species dominate the commercial and industrial meat and egg production, ducks, geese, turkeys, pigeons and quails are also intensively reared and are very essential and palatable sources of meat in Egypt. The survival, transmission rate and susceptibility for HPAI A (H5N1) infection varies considerably between poultry species, with notably ducks showing less mortality and clinical signs of infection than chickens, turkeys and geese for the clade 2.2.1.2 circulating in 2014/2015 [11]. In such a context, avian influenza (AI) outbreaks in Egyptian poultry industry are difficult to control and economically disruptive on account of direct losses to poultry stock and indirect costs due to the introduction of biosecurity measures in farms. More importantly, they impact the food security of the country.

A comprehensive review of risk factors of HPAI A (H5N1) at different levels (farm, pixel, administrative unit) in countries other than Egypt [12] found duck population density, indicators of human population density or activity, and indicators of water presence or abundance as being the factors most consistently found across studies and scale. At the farm level, the risk or protective factors of HPAI A (H5N1) infection have rarely been assessed with statistical models in Egypt. The high under reporting rate of HPAI A (H5N1) outbreaks due to the lack of compensation measures for poultry lost [13, 14] and/or indirect effects of vaccination campaigns [15], made it difficult to get reliable data. In household and backyard poultry production, the improper disposal of dead poultry and poultry faeces [16] creates lapses in biosecurity. In addition the limited understanding and poor biosecurity procedures during vaccination of household poultry by vaccine injectors [13] are also known to be risk factors of HPAI A (H5N1) infections. A risk assessment of HPAI A (H5N1) virus in Egypt [10] concluded that for commercial farms, the risk associated with movement of people is high and probably the most important mode of transmission of AI between farms. External injectors, part-time day farm workers, visiting veterinary practitioners, feed delivery, egg-collecting and litter collecting drivers - there are many transmission pathways for AI virus introduction and spread in the commercial farms. These results were confirmed by the study of spatial patterns of genetic relatedness of HPAI A (H5N1) in Egyptian poultry from 2006 to 2013 [17]. Genetic information suggests that wild birds play an important role in viral diffusion between backyard farms, while commercial farms experience human-mediated diffusion via the road network. However, the contacts between external visitors and poultry cannot alone explain the spread of HPAI A (H5N1) between farms. The role of biosecurity practices should also be taken into account as these are able to mediate the virus circulation in poultry production systems. Many authors have investigated risk factors at the farm level and reported significant factors linked to the biosecurity categorized into isolation, sanitation and traffic control [18] in the review of the literature presented in Table 1. This review shows that a set of biosecurity risks and biosecurity practices should be considered to estimate the overall level of biosecurity of poultry farms.

The aims of this study were to analyse the risk of HPAI A (H5N1) presence at the farm level in a large part of the Nile Delta, with a particular emphasis on simple factors such as the type of poultry production system, vaccination status, closed vs. open status of the farm, farm size and the presence or absence of duck

Table 1 Literature review of biosecurity risks and biosecurity practises against HPAI A (H5N1) virus assessed at farm level

Biosecurity practices Positive impacts
Isolation
• Chicken and ducks in different shelters at night [31]
Traffic control
• Designated vehicle for sending eggs to a vendor or market [32]
• Not allowing traders to enter the farm [33]
Sanitation
• Owners used a disinfectant to clean poultry areas [34]
• Farm staff washing their hands before handling birds [33]
Biosecurity risks
Isolation
• Farm accessible to feral and wild animals [32]
• Footbath at entry to farm/shed [32]
• Dead crow seen at or near farm [35]
• Improperly dispose farm waste [36]
• Having contact with pigeons [31]
Traffic control
• Family and friends visiting [24]
• Exchanging eggtrays with market vendors [35]
• Receiving visitors on farm premises [37]
• Purchased live poultry/products [37]
• Farm workers live outside the premises [37]
• Owners bought live chickens from another backyard farm [34]
• Having a neighbouring poultry farm [33]
• High frequency of veterinary visits [38]
• Had visitors in their farm within the past month [36]

farms reporting abnormal mortality or drop in egg production in the village in which the farms were located.

Methods

Case definition

The study was based on passive surveillance data recorded from 2014 to 2015 in commercial poultry farms in the Western-side of Nile delta in Egypt. Suspected premises were visited following reporting of sudden and high mortality in broiler or duck flocks, or of a drop of egg production in layers or breeders. During investigation of the suspected cases, 3–5 pooled samples from sick or freshly dead birds were tested for HPAI A (H5N1) virus by laboratory tests and confirmed by reverse transcription polymerase chain reaction (RT-PCR). The samples which consisted of a set tracheal and cloacal swabs and organs from trachea, lung and kidneys were processed for virus isolation according to the OIE manual [19]. Each farm was categorized as 'infected' if the presence of the HPAI A (H5N1) was confirmed, and as 'non-infected' otherwise. All surveyed farms had therefore reported abnormal mortality or a drop in egg production.

Study area and disease data collection

The study area is located on the Western-side of Nile delta, on the Mediterranean coast of Egypt, ranging from 29°25′ to 31°20′ East, 30°12′ to 31°36' North. The samples were collected from 2014 to 2015 in five governorates (regions), namely Alexandria, Behera, Kafr El-Shikh, Gharbia, Menoufia (Fig. 1). Both chicken ($n = 746$) and duck ($n = 364$) farms were visited and the following information were collected at the time of the visit: species (chicken or duck), farm type (broiler chickens, layer chickens, laying ducks, meat ducks), location (name of the village), date of report, number of animals in the farm, average age and weight of the birds, number of dead birds at the time of the visit, preventive measures implemented in the farm (open vs. closed farm, vaccinated vs. not vaccinated). In an open farm system, windows for the purpose of ventilation are present in the farm structure. Such open farm systems are generally lacking in rodent and peri-domestic bird control. In the closed farm system, ventilation is provided by electric fans or pad cooling systems. The advantage of such a system is improved biosecurity in farms.

With regard to vaccination, presently inactivated vaccines are being used for the control of H5N1, H5N2 or H5N3. In vaccinated flocks, all birds were vaccinated and the recommendations for time of vaccination were provided to the poultry farmers based on the advice of the vaccine manufacturer and Egyptian veterinarian services (Damanhour University, Egypt): i) broiler chickens: day 5–10 (first round); ii) layer chickens: day 10, 40 and 110; iii) meat ducks: day 5, 10; and iv) layer ducks: day 10, 50 and 100. The number of booster doses and the vaccine strain were not available for our dataset. For the geographical coordinates of the farms included in this study, we used the village centroids for protection of privacy.

Statistical analyses

In order to test the effect of a list of independent variables on the probability of presence of HPAI A (H5N1) virus at farm level ($n = 1110$ farms), a binomial generalized linear model (GLM) was formulated. Initially investigated variables were the type of poultry production (egg or meat) and species (chicken or duck) information, which were combined into a single variable describing the production type ("Ptype": broiler chicken farms, layer chicken farms, meat duck farms, laying duck farms). The other independent variables included the presence or absence of vaccination for influenza A (H5Nx) virus ("Vaccination"), the closed vs. open farm status ("Closure"), the number of birds per production cycle in the farm ("Nb_Birds"), the presence (1) or absence (0) of at least one visited duck farm in the village (hence reporting abnormal mortality or drop in egg production) in which the farm was located ("HasDuck"). A multivariate GLM binomial model was developed using all individual risk factors. In addition, the bivariate interactions between production type and vaccination, production type and closure status, and production type and the number of birds were tested. The average age and weight of birds of the flocks were not tested because the largest part of the variability in age and weight was confounded by the poultry type variable. We quantified the effects of all simple and interaction terms from a full model (including all the variables interactions) using an analysis of deviance upon removal and a chi-squared test with type II sum of squares procedure. Insignificant variables and interactions were then taken out according to the Akaike's information criteria (AIC) to derive the final most parsimonious model with a stepwise selection procedure. The final model was also used to visualise the role of each explanatory variable on the prediction, having adjusted for other variables presented in model [20]. The predictive accuracy of the final model was assessed using the Receiver Operating Characteristic curve (ROC). The area under the ROC curve (AUC), sensitivity and specificity indices were computed using a cross-validation (CV) method using 70% of the data to fit the model and the remaining 30% of the data for external validation. A stratified random sampling of the dataset into training and testing sets was used to preserve the virus prevalence inside each subsample during the CV procedure. Finally, the AUC was bootstrapped with 50 different data splits. The presence of spatial autocorrelation in the

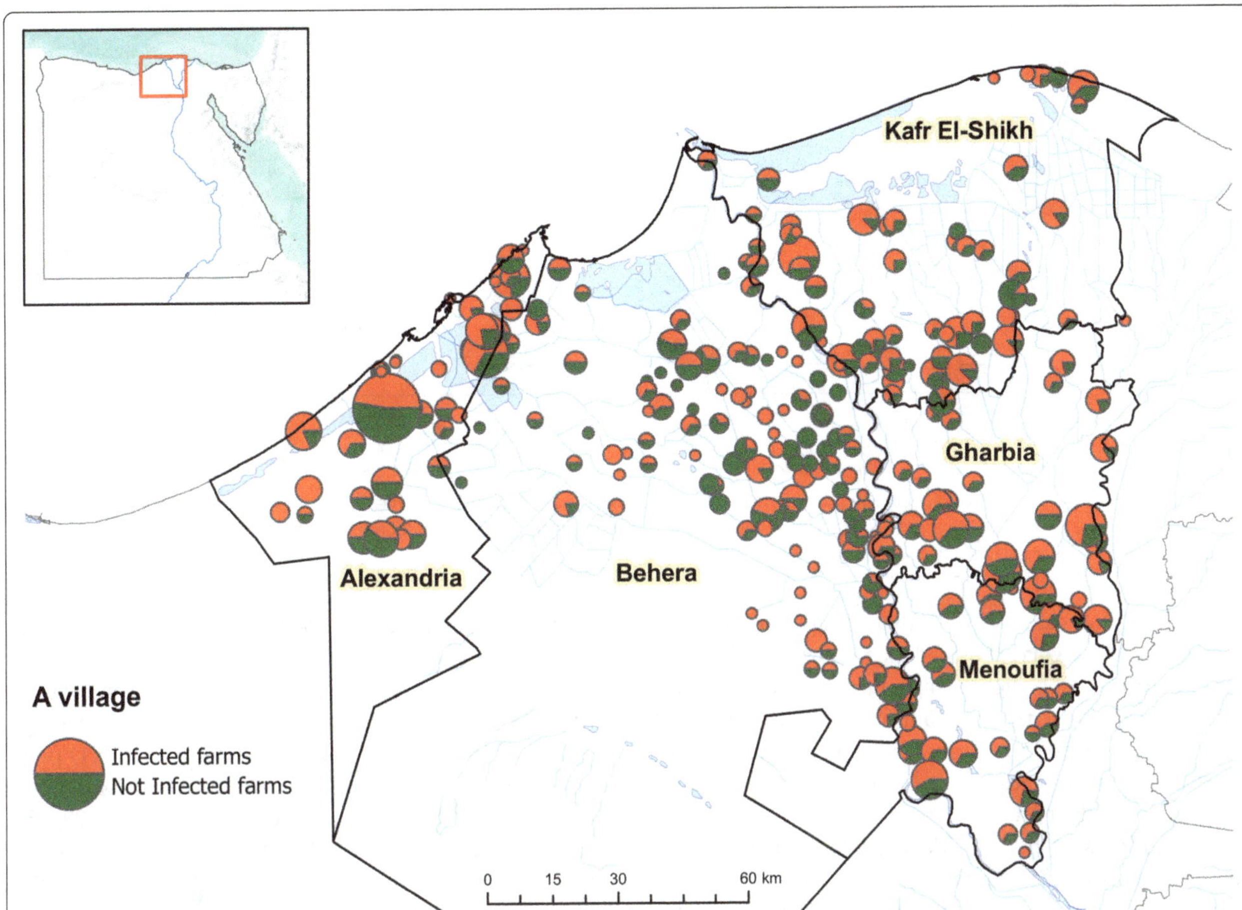

Fig. 1 Map of study area (Nile river delta, Egypt), location of farms (the coordinates refers to villages) and village prevalence to HPAI A (H5N1) virus. The size of the circle depends on the number of farms in the village and the colour represents the proportion of positive (red) and negative (green) farms for Avian Influenza in the years 2014–2015

model residuals was evaluated visually using maps, and quantitatively using spline correlograms [21] and Moran's I statistics [22].

Results

A total number of 1110 farms were visited, based on passive reporting of suspected HPAI A (H5N1) in the years 2014–2015 in 5 Egyptian provinces in the delta of Nile River (Fig. 1): 746 chicken farms (501 broiler farms and 245 layer farms) and 364 duck farms (192 meat farms and 172 laying farms). The proportion of HPAI A (H5N1) positive farms was 62.16% (690/1110). This figure was nearly similar for chicken (62.33%, 465/746) and duck (61.81%, 225/364) farms. However, there were notable differences in the proportion of HPAI A (H5N1) positive farms between the poultry types, with 64.87% broiler chicken farms, 57.14% layer chicken farms, 58.33% meat duck farms, and 65.70% laying duck farms being diagnosed as positive. A map of the number of farms per village with the village-level proportion of positive farms can be seen in Fig. 1, highlighting the widespread distribution of HPAI A (H5N1) positive farms in the Nile Delta and the strong spatial heterogeneity of the proportion of positive farms at the village level.

The proportion of farms vaccinated against HPAI A (H5Nx) virus was about 42.43% (471/1110): 43.91% (220/501) for the broiler chicken farms, 48.57% (119/245) for the layer chicken farms, 40.63% (78/192) for the meat duck farms and 31.40% (54/172) for the laying duck farms. The proportion of closed farms was 44.05%: 50.10% (251/501) for broiler chicken farms, 38.37% (94/245) for layer chicken farms, 43.75% (84/192) for meat duck farms and 34.88% (60/172) for laying duck farms.

The mean number of birds per farm ranged from 101 to 1.3×10^5 in broiler chicken farms, from 2349 to 8.7×10^4 in layer chicken, from 2401 to 9.9×10^4 in meat duck farms and from 2588 to 7.7×10^4 in laying duck farms. Figure 2 shows the distribution of bird numbers per farm type according to their vaccination status. The median number of birds per farm was higher in layer chicken farms compared to other type of poultry

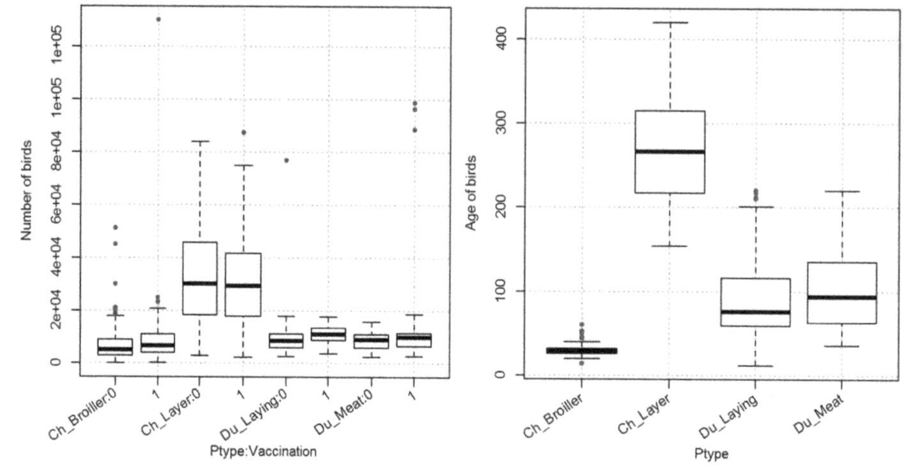

Fig. 2 Distribution at farm level of number of birds per cycle (left) and the mean ages of birds (right). The number of birds is split into 8 categories according to the presence (1) or the absence (0) of vaccination in the farms and the four types of the poultry production. The mean age of birds is divided into the four categories of the poultry production

production. One can also note that except for the layer chicken farm category, the median number of birds per farm appeared to be slightly higher in vaccinated farms. Figure 2 also shows the distribution of the mean age of birds per farm type at the time of the visit. Large differences in the mean ages of birds can be noted between the poultry production types.

The goodness of fit of GLM model was high with a mean AUC value of 0.93 and the model residuals showed no evidence of spatial autocorrelation (see Additional files 1 & 2). The analysis of deviance of GLM model run with all the variables and interactions is presented in Table 2, while the estimates of the final model coefficients with the odds ratios (OR) is presented in Table 3. The GLM model found significant differences between the probability of presence of HPAI A (H5N1) virus according to the vaccination status and this probability increases in farms without vaccination. The strongest change in deviance was found for the vaccination status variable (Table 2). This factor was followed by the closure status, the number of birds (the farm size), and

Table 2 Analysis of deviance from the logistic regression and chi-squared tests

	Deviance	Df	*P*-values
Vaccination	453,326	1	< 0,001
Closure	61,767	1	< 0,001
Nb_Birds	36,159	1	< 0,001
Ptype	28,788	3	< 0,001
HasDuck	11,971	1	0,001
Vaccination:Ptype	29,608	3	< 0,001
Nb_Birds:Ptype	3410	3	0,33
Closure:Ptype	1638	3	0,65

the presence/absence of duck farms reporting abnormal mortality or egg losses in the village. The only significant interaction term was the interaction between poultry farm type and vaccination status, indicating that vaccination may affect the probability of HPAI A (H5N1) presence differently in the different farm types. The single term revealed that vaccination status (OR: 0.08, CI: 0.05–0.13), farm closure (OR: 0.22, CI: 0.14–0.32) and bird numbers (OR: 0.17, CI: 0.09–0.30) were protective factors, whereas the presence of duck farms reporting abnormal mortality or egg losses in the village was a risk factor (OR: 2.31, CI: 1.49–3.64). Figure 3 illustrates these relationships, together with the effect of the poultry farm type on the predicted probability of HPAI A (H5N1) presence. The probability of presence of HPAI A (H5N1) virus was significantly higher in chicken layer farms (OR: 15.62, CI: 4.75–71.69) compared to other farm types. Interestingly, this pattern changed in vaccinated farms and the interactions between the types of production variable against the vaccination variable were important in explaining the response variable (Fig. 3). In vaccinated farms, the probability of farm infection is higher in chicken (broiler and layer) farms compared to the duck farms (meat and laying).

Discussion

The results show that the type of poultry production, HPAI vaccination status and the biosecurity level of farms have a strong influence on the presence or absence of HPAI A (H5N1) virus at poultry farm level. In this study, the biosecurity level of farms was estimated through a list of biosecurity practices and biosecurity risks: the absence of windows/openings in farm, the number of birds per cycle of production (practices) and the presence of duck farms in the village (risk). Every

Table 3 Estimation of model coefficients and odds ratios from the logistic regression with 95% credible intervals

	Estimate	Std. Error	Odds ratio	2.5%	97.5%
(Intercept)	9,22	1,24	–	–	–
Vaccine	−2,57	0,26	0,08	0,05	0,13
Closure	-1,53	0,2	0,22	0,14	0,32
Nb_Birds	-1,8	0,32	0,17	0,09	0,3
HasDuck	0,84	0,23	2,31	1,49	3,64
Ptype - Ch_Layer	2,75	0,67	15,62	4,75	71,69
Ptype - Du_Laying	0,04	0,42	1,04	0,46	2,47
Ptype - Du_Meat	0,19	0,45	1,21	0,52	3,08
[Vaccine:Ptype] - 1:Ch_Layer	−2,95	0,71	0,05	0,01	0,18
[Vaccine:Ptype] - 1:Du_Laying	−2,01	0,65	0,13	0,03	0,45
[Vaccine:Ptype] - 1:Du_Meat	-2,14	0,63	0,12	0,03	0,38

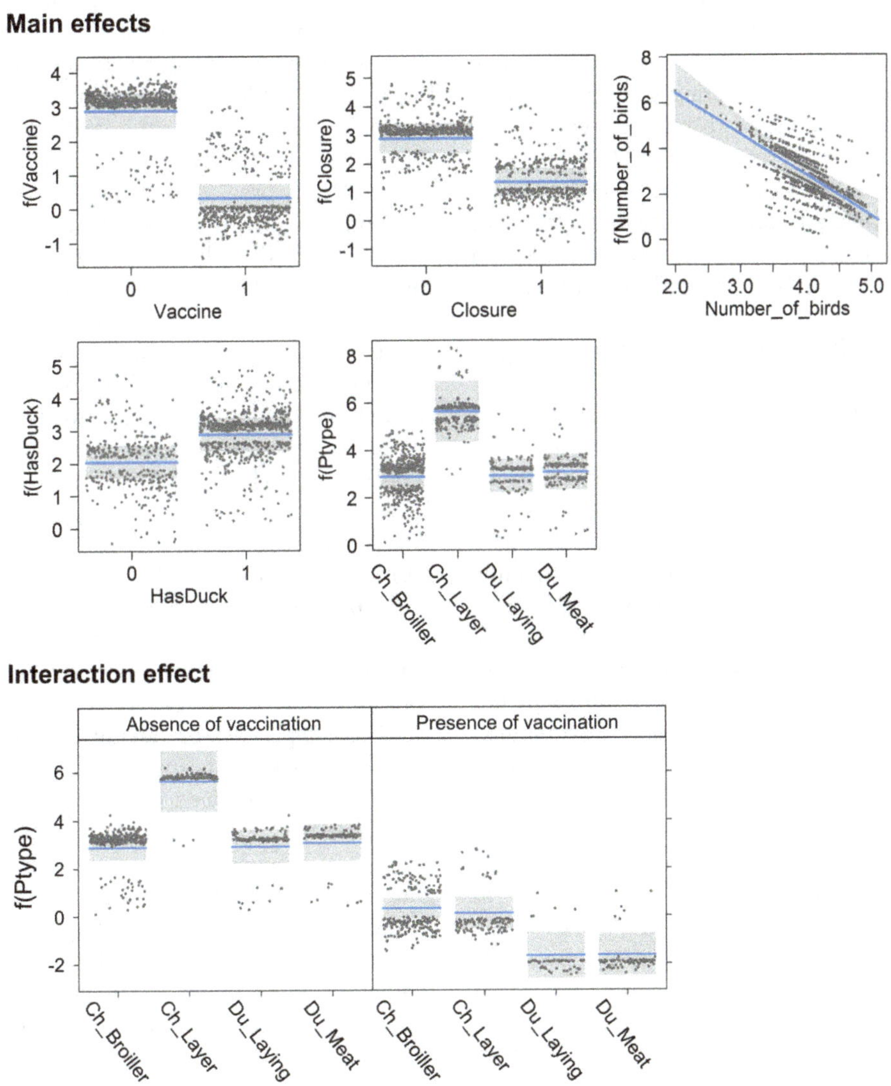

Fig. 3 Conditional plots between the probability of presence of AI A (H5N1) virus and the independent variables of GLM (top) or the type of poultry production according to the presence or the absence of vaccination (bottom). Shading represents 95% confidence intervals and points are partial residuals

variable tested in the GLM model were found significant to explain the probability of HPAI A (H5N1) presence and the discriminatory capacity of model was good with AUC about 0.93. It should be recalled that the model is based only on five independent variables. Figure 1 shows no clear spatial pattern in the distribution of the HPAI A (H5N1) virus among farms and the virus was detected in nearly every village.

Vaccination for HPAI was associated with a decrease in the probability of presence of HPAI A (H5N1) virus and can explain the high goodness of fit of the GLM model. Indeed, the virus was detected in 22.08% (104/471) of vaccinated farm while 91.71% (586/639) of unvaccinated farms were infected showing the good discriminatory capacity of this factor. However, in a few cases (104/471) vaccination failed to prevent the virus from being introduced into the farm. The absence of information about the number of booster doses and the vaccine strain used creates difficulties in interpreting this result. Vaccination in poultry using a non-matching virus vaccine strain to the circulating strain and lack of booster doses have been shown to possibly reduce clinical disease signs, without reducing the effect on virus transmission [23, 24]. Although the cost-benefits of vaccination seem positive at individual farm level, the virus is still persisting in Egypt. The residual circulation of virus in vaccinated farm is an obstacle to prevent the HPAI A (H5N1) virus spreading in Nile river delta.

Then, the risk of HPAI A (H5N1) infection was higher in farms with windows/openings than farms without such types of ventilation in GLM models. This result may suggest that a strict isolation of poultry from wildlife is needed to prevent the farms from infection by the HPAI A (H5N1) virus. Indeed, bridging host species may exist in the peri-domestic populations (terrestrial birds, crows, doves, pigeon, egrets and rodents) frequently found around the poultry farms and some are susceptible to HPAI A (H5N1) [25]. In Egypt, crows, cattle egret and pigeons are naturally infected by H5 viruses [26]. Bridge hosts provide a link through which pathogens can be transmitted from maintenance host populations (from farms and/or wildlife) to receptive populations (the commercial farms) [27]. A FAO report has already pointed the importance [10] of regularly checking and repairing broken windows and the wire screening on the sides of the poultry house to prevent wild bird access to the farms. Moreover, farms without an efficient or modern ventilation system may be an indicator of lack of other investments in the farm infrastructure resulting in overall lower levels of biosecurity.

In the study area 97.57% of studied farms had less than 20,000 birds per cycle with the exception of layer chicken farms, (Fig. 2). Rather, the layer chicken farm production is more intensive and 69.80% of layer chicken farms have more than 20,000 birds per cycle. The results of model showed that the risk of HPAI A (H5N1) infection decreases significantly with the number of birds per cycle of production. The number of birds per cycle provides a figure for estimating the farm size and is a good surrogate of various aspects of the biosecurity level of farms. For example, management practices of farmers can change according to the size and the level of intensification of the poultry production of farms [28]. In this study of 267 broiler chicken farms in the Gharbia Governorate, the farms with more than 20,000 birds per cycle use notably more automatic feeders/waters and assess more systematically the health status of birds before selling, than the farms of more moderate size. Moreover, it was reported in the study by Eltholth et al. (2016) that the farmers of such large farms do not visit other farms whereas they are more inclined to do so in farms of a more moderate size.

The probability of presence of the HPAI A (H5N1) virus in poultry is dependant of the type of poultry production. The GLM predicted that the probability of virus presence was higher for the layer chicken farms while the observed prevalence for this category was lowest (57.14%) compared to other poultry type. The observed virus prevalence is the result of a sum of multiple factors and cannot be directly interpreted. A multiple regression model was needed to separate the effects affecting the probability of farm infection. For example, layer chicken farms have a higher number of poultry per production cycle in average, and the effects associated with this factor can be predominant compared to some other effects linked to the type of poultry production. The higher probability of HPAI A (H5N1) virus in layer chicken farms may be linked to the higher mean age of birds (Fig. 2) in this production system (the age is not taken into account in the model).

The presence of a duck farm reporting abnormal mortality or a drop in egg production in the village where the farm is located was associated with a higher probability of presence of the HPAI A (H5N1) virus in the GLM. In Egypt, duck production is mainly in small commercial or backyard farms with relatively low biosecurity levels. Ducks have long been considered an important risk factor for HPAI A (H5N1) virus presence, and show various levels of clinical signs at the individual level, ranging from high mortality to the absence of clinical signs accompanied with virus shedding [29]. Recent experimental infection of poultry with a HPAI A (H5N1) contemporary virus strain circulating in 2014/2015 [11] shows that unvaccinated ducks showed no symptoms of infection and survived the duration of the experiment. However, this is only theorised here as the authors of this study didn't test the effect of infection on egg production. This recent virus strain may cause much fewer clinical signs of infection in ducks, allowing virus persistence and spread to other poultry farms, a risk that has already been previously identified [30]. In the specific context of this study, silent circulation in duck farms in the absence of clinical signs could not be formally assessed, because farms reporting no clinical signs were simply not surveyed and identified in the villages. However, given the variability in clinical signs, and the overall high prevalence of HPAI H5N1 in the area, one could reasonably assume that a number of farms with silent circulation could have represented an equivalent, if not greater, risk of transmission to their neighbourhood as those reporting abnormal mortalities or drops in egg production.

The study analysed data from passive surveillance and all surveyed farms had therefore reported abnormal mortality or drop in egg production. So, the results this study should be considered in that specific context, which entails a number of limitations. First, the virus was detected in 62.16% of the tested farms and this figure can therefore not be compared to prevalence figures obtained through cross-sectional surveys that consider all farms. Two types of farms may not have reported abnormal mortality or drops in egg production, for entirely different reasons. On the one hand, some farms with very high biosecurity and thorough implementation of vaccination may never report clinical signs. On the other hand, farms with domestic ducks or specific chicken breeds that have lower susceptibility may also not present clinical signs in birds, and would not be included. So, depending on the relative abundance of those two situations, our apparent farm-level prevalence of 62.16% may be an overestimation or an underestimation of the true prevalence. For the same reason, our measure of the benefits of vaccination at the farm level could be underestimated if many vaccinated farms never report any clinical signs to be included in the survey, or/and were not infected at all, or, conversely, overestimated, if inefficiently vaccinated farms had silent circulation of the virus. Other factors may be at play in influencing the vaccination coverage. For example, in parts of the Nile Delta other than the survey area that experienced fewer recent HPAI A (H5N1) outbreaks, farmers may have a lower perception of the usefulness of vaccination, which could result in lower vaccination coverage.

Conclusions

The analysis focuses on only a relevant but limited subset of protective or risk factors at the farm level for different type of poultry production systems. However, many other potentially important factors could be considered, such as, for example, the presence of other pathogens, the number of visits to the farms, the turnover of poultry production, the extent of inward (inputs) and outward (outputs) movements, or the position of the farm in the poultry value-chain network. Future investigations could consider such information to provide a more comprehensive assessment of the local risk of AI transmission in poultry.

Additional files

Additional file 1: Receiver operating characteristic from the logistic regression computed with the training data (black line) and computed with a cross-validation (CV) method (blurred lines). A stratified random sampling of the dataset into training and test sets was used for the CV and the AUC was bootstrapped with 50 different data splitting. (PNG 84 kb)

Additional file 2: The results used in assessing spatial autocorrelation. A) Map of residual deviances of GLM (top): the dot sizes are proportional to the deviance value of each farm. The red dots represent negative residual deviances while the blue dots are the positive residual deviances. B) Correlogram of model residuals (bottom-left). C) Moran's test for spatial autocorrelation using a spatial weights matrix based on the neighbourhood relations showed in the figure (bottom-right). Two farms were linked together if the distance between these two farms was less than 0.08°. (PNG 202 kb)

Abbreviations

AI: Avian influenza; AIC: Akaike's information criteria; AUC: Area under the receiver operating characteristic curve; Closure: Predictor variable related to the closed vs. opened status of the farm; CV: Cross-validation; GLM: Generalized linear model; HasDuck: Predictor variable related to the presence or absence of at least one duck farm reporting abnormal mortality or drop in egg production in the village in which the farm was located; HPAI: Highly pathogenic avian influenza; Nb_Birds: Predictor variable related to the number of birds per production cycle in the farm; OR: Odds ratio; Ptype: Predictor variable related to the type of poultry production; ROC: Receiver operating characteristic curve; RT-PCR: Reverse transcription polymerase chain reaction; Vaccination: Predictor variable related to the presence or absence of vaccination for influenza A (H5Nx) virus

Funding

This study was supported by grants from the US National Institutes of Health (1R01AI101028-02A1). MG is supported by the Fonds National de la Recherche Scientifique (FNRS, Brussels, Belgium). The manuscript contents (the design of the study, data collection, analysis, and interpretation of data) and the opinions expressed in this publication are solely the responsibility of the author(s) and do not necessarily represent the official views of the NIH/FNRS.

Authors' contributions

JA, CI, AC and MG analyzed the data and wrote the manuscript. AET, AE, HFE designed the study and collected the survey data. All authors contributed to the final discussion and revisions of the manuscript. All authors read and approved the final manuscript.

Ethics approval and consent to participate

No experimentation on animals was carried and no data on human was used during this study. All farmers participated voluntarily to the study as part of the routine surveillance of poultry disease in Egypt that is made at the farmers request when they experience abnormal mortality. Inclusion criteria included evidence of the AIV H5N1 and the informed oral consent of the farm manager to provide the required data. All tests and procedures complied with general guidelines of poultry disease surveillance and were approved by the Local Ethic Commission of the Animal health and welfare of Damanhour University with respect to care of animals under study and all efforts were made to minimize suffering.

Consent for publication

Not applicable.

Competing interests
The authors declare that (1) MG is a member of the editorial board of BMC Veterinary Research; (2) they have no other competing interests.

Author details
[1]Spatial Epidemiology Lab. (SpELL), Université Libre de Bruxelles, Brussels, Belgium. [2]Istituto Zooprofilattico Sperimentale dell'Abruzzo e del Molise 'G. Caporale', Teramo, Italy. [3]Food and Agriculture Organization of the United Nations, Rome, Italy. [4]National Center for Animal and Plant Health (CENSA), OIE Collaborating Center for Reduction of the Risk of Disasters in Animal Health, 32700 San José de las Lajas, Mayabeque, Cuba. [5]Faculty of Veterinary Medicine, Damanhour University, Damanhour, Egypt. [6]Fonds National de la Recherche Scientifique, Brussels, Belgium.

References

1. Abdelwhab EM, Hassan MK, Abdel-Moneim AS, Naguib MM, Mostafa A, Hussein ITM, et al. Introduction and enzootic of a/H5N1 in Egypt: virus evolution, pathogenicity and vaccine efficacy ten years on. Infect Genet Evol. 2016;40:80–90. Available from: http://linkinghub.elsevier.com/retrieve/pii/S1567134816300545 [cited 7 Nov 2017]
2. Arafa A, El-Masry I, Khoulosy S, Hassan MK, Soliman M, Fasanmi OG, et al. Predominance and geo-mapping of avian influenza H5N1 in poultry sectors in Egypt. Geospat Health. 2016;11 Available from: http://geospatialhealth.net/index.php/gh/article/view/492 [cited 27 Nov 2017]
3. Kandeel A, Manoncourt S, el Kareem EA, Ahmed A-NM, El-Refaie S, Essmat H, et al. Zoonotic transmission of avian influenza virus (H5N1), Egypt, 2006–2009. Emerg Infect Dis. 2010;16:1101–7. Available from: http://wwwnc.cdc.gov/eid/article/16/7/09-1695_article.htm [cited 7 Nov 2017]
4. Refaey S, Azziz-Baumgartner E, Amin MM, Fahim M, Roguski K, Elaziz HAEA, et al. Increased number of human cases of influenza virus a(H5N1) infection, Egypt, 2014–15. Emerg Infect Dis. 2015;21:2171–3. Available from: http://wwwnc.cdc.gov/eid/article/21/12/15-0885_article.htm [cited 7 Nov 2017]
5. Kayali G, Kandeil A, El-Shesheny R, Kayed AS, Maatouq AM, Cai Z, et al. Avian influenza a(H5N1) virus in Egypt. Emerg Infect Dis. 2016;22:379–88. Available from: http://wwwnc.cdc.gov/eid/article/22/3/15-0593_article.htm [cited 7 Nov 2017]
6. Arafa AS, Naguib MM, Luttermann C, Selim AA, Kilany WH, Hagag N, et al. Emergence of a novel cluster of influenza a (H5N1) virus clade 2.2. 1.2 with putative human health impact in Egypt, 2014/15. Eur Secur. 2015;20:21085. Available from: https://www.eurosurveillance.org/content/10.2807/1560-7917.ES2015.20.13.21085.
7. WHO/GIP. Cumulative number of confirmed human cases for avian influenza A(H5N1) reported to WHO, 2003–2017. 2017. Available from: http://www.who.int/influenza/human_animal_interface/2017_12_07_tableH5N1.pdf
8. Balish AL, Davis CT, Saad MD, El-Sayed N, Esmat H, Tjaden JA, et al. Antigenic and genetic diversity of highly pathogenic avian influenza a (H5N1) viruses isolated in Egypt. Avian Dis. 2010;54:329–34. Available from: http://www.jstor.org/stable/40601080 [cited 29 Oct 2015]
9. Arafa A, Suarez D, Kholosy SG, Hassan MK, Nasef S, Selim A, et al. Evolution of highly pathogenic avian influenza H5N1 viruses in Egypt indicating progressive adaptation. Arch Virol. 2012;157:1931–47. Available from: http://link.springer.com/article/10.1007/s00705-012-1385-9 [cited 24 Sep 2015]
10. Ali AM, Ankers P, DeHaan N, Saad A, Hussein S, Lubroth J, et al. Mapping influenza A (H5N1) virus transmission pathways and critical control points in Egypt. Rome: Food and Agriculture Organization of the United Nations; 2013. Available from: http://www.fao.org/docrep/017/i3272e/i3272e00.htm.
11. Kandeil A, Mostafa A, El-Shesheny R, El-Taweel AN, Gomaa M, Galal H, et al. Avian influenza H5N1 vaccination efficacy in Egyptian backyard poultry. Vaccine. 2017;35:6195–201. Available from: http://linkinghub.elsevier.com/retrieve/pii/S0264410X17312690 [cited 7 Nov 2017]
12. Gilbert M, Pfeiffer DU. Risk factor modelling of the spatio-temporal patterns of highly pathogenic avian influenza (HPAIV) H5N1: a review. Spat Spatiotemporal Epidemiol. 2012;3:173–83. Available from: http://linkinghub.elsevier.com/retrieve/pii/S1877584512000032 [cited 30 Sep 2016]
13. Peyre M, Samaha H, Makonnen YJ, Saad A, Abd-Elnabi A, Galal S, et al. Avian influenza vaccination in Egypt: limitations of the current strategy. J Mol Genet Med. 2009;3:198–204. Available from: http://www.ncbi.nlm.nih.gov/pmc/articles/PMC2805840/
14. Abdelwhab EM, Hafez HM. An overview of the epidemic of highly pathogenic H5N1 avian influenza virus in Egypt: epidemiology and control challenges. Epidemiol Infect. 2011;139:647–57. Available from: http://www.journals.cambridge.org/abstract_S0950268810003122 [cited 3 Dec 2017]
15. Vergne T, Grosbois V, Jobre Y, Saad A, El Nabi AA, Galal S, et al. Avian influenza vaccination of poultry and passive case reporting, Egypt. Emerg Infect Dis. 2012;18:2076. Available from: https://wwwnc.cdc.gov/eid/article/18/12/12-0616_article.
16. Sheta BM, Fuller TL, Larison B, Njabo KY, Ahmed AS, Harrigan R, et al. Putative human and avian risk factors for avian influenza virus infections in backyard poultry in Egypt. Vet Microbiol. 2014;168:208–13. Available from: http://linkinghub.elsevier.com/retrieve/pii/S0378113513005099 [cited 29 Nov 2017]
17. Young SG, Carrel M, Kitchen A, Malanson GP, Tamerius J, Ali M, et al. How's the flu getting through? Landscape genetics suggests both humans and birds spread H5N1 in Egypt. Infect Genet Evol. 2017;49:293–9. Available from: http://linkinghub.elsevier.com/retrieve/pii/S1567134817300473 [cited 27 Nov 2017]
18. Cardona CJ, Kuney DR. Biosecurity on chicken farms. Commercial chicken meat and egg production. 5th ed; 2002. p. 543–56. Available from: https://link.springer.com/chapter/10.1007/978-1-4615-0811-3_28.
19. OIE. Manual of diagnostic tests and vaccines for terrestrial animals, avian influenza: World organisation for animal health; 2014. Available from: http://www.oie.int/fileadmin/Home/fr/Health_standards/tahm/2.03.04_AI.pdf
20. Breheny P, Burchett W. Visualization of regression models using visreg. R Package; 2013. p. 1–15. Available from: http://myweb.uiowa.edu/pbreheny/publications/visreg.pdf.
21. ON BØ, Falck W. Nonparametric spatial covariance functions: estimation and testing. Environ Ecol Stat. 2001;8:53–70. Available from: https://link.springer.com/article/10.1023/A:1009601932481 [cited 30 May 2017]
22. Cliff A, Ord JK. Spatial processes models and applications. London: Pion; 1981. ISBN 0850860814.
23. van der Goot JA, van Boven M, de Jong MCM, Koch G. Effect of vaccination on transmission of hpai h5n1: the effect of a single vaccination dose on transmission of highly pathogenic avian influenza h5n1 in Peking Ducks. Avian Dis. 2007;51:323–4. Available from: http://www.bioone.org/doi/abs/10.1637/7658-060206R.1 [cited 1 Dec 2017]
24. Henning KA, Henning J, Morton J, Long NT, Ha NT, Meers J. Farm- and flock-level risk factors associated with highly pathogenic avian influenza outbreaks on small holder duck and chicken farms in the Mekong Delta of Viet Nam. Prev Vet Med. 2009;91:179–88. Available from: http://linkinghub.elsevier.com/retrieve/pii/S0167587709001688 [cited 1 Dec 2017]
25. Kaplan BS, Webby RJ. The avian and mammalian host range of highly pathogenic avian H5N1 influenza. Virus Res. 2013;178:3–11. Available from: http://linkinghub.elsevier.com/retrieve/pii/S0168170213002967 [cited 3 Dec 2017]
26. Fadel HM, Afifi R. Investigation of avian influenza infection in wild birds in Ismailia and Damietta cities, Egypt. Vet World. 2017;10:695–701. Available from: http://www.veterinaryworld.org/Vol.10/June-2017/20.html [cited 27 Nov 2017]
27. Caron A, Cappelle J, Cumming GS, de Garine-Wichatitsky M, Gaidet N. Bridge hosts, a missing link for disease ecology in multi-host systems. Vet Res. 2015;46 Available from: http://www.veterinaryresearch.org/content/46/1/83 [cited 28 Nov 2017]
28. Eltholth M, Mohamed R, Elgohary F, Elfadl E. Assessment of biosecurity practices in broiler chicken farms in Gharbia Governorate, Egypt. Alexandria J Vet Sci. 2016;49:68. Available from: http://www.scopemed.org/fulltextpdf.php?mno=220886 [cited 7 Nov 2017]
29. Pantin-Jackwood M, Swayne DE, Smith D, Shepherd E. Effect of species, breed and route of virus inoculation on the pathogenicity of H5N1 highly pathogenic influenza (HPAI) viruses in domestic ducks. Vet Res. 2013;44:62. Available from: https://www.ncbi.nlm.nih.gov/pmc/articles/PMC3733953/ [cited 7 Nov 2017]
30. Kim J-K, Negovetich NJ, Forrest HL, Webster RG. Ducks: the "Trojan Horses" of H5N1 influenza. Influenza Other Respir Viruses. 2009;3:121–8. Available from: http://doi.wiley.com/10.1111/j.1750-2659.2009.00084.x [cited 12 Jan 2018]
31. Biswas PK, Christensen JP, Ahmed SSU, Das A, Rahman MH, Barua H, et al. Risk for infection with highly pathogenic avian influenza virus (H5N1) in backyard chickens, Bangladesh. Emerg Infect Dis. 2009;15:1931–6. Available from: http://wwwnc.cdc.gov/eid/article/15/12/09-0643_article.htm [cited 4 Dec 2017]
32. Biswas PK, Christensen JP, Ahmed SSU, Barua H, Das A, Rahman MH, et al. Risk factors for infection with highly pathogenic influenza A virus (H5N1) in commercial chickens in Bangladesh. Vet Rec. 2009;164:743–6. Available
31\. Shi H, Ashraf S, Gao S, Lu J, Liu X. Evaluation of transmission route and replication efficiency of H9N2 avian influenza virus. Avian Dis. 2010; 54(1):22–7.

of potential risk factors associated with highly pathogenic avian influenza subtype H5N1 outbreak occurrence in Lagos and Kano States, Nigeria, during the 2006–2007 epidemics: avian influenza in Nigeria. Transbound Emerg Dis. 2013;60:87–96. Available from: http://doi.wiley.com/10.1111/j.1865-1682.2012.01322.x [cited 4 Dec 2017]

34. Paul M, Wongnarkpet S, Gasqui P, Poolkhet C, Thongratsakul S, Ducrot C, et al. Risk factors for highly pathogenic avian influenza (HPAI) H5N1 infection in backyard chicken farms, Thailand. Acta Trop. 2011;118:209–16. Available from: http://linkinghub.elsevier.com/retrieve/pii/S0001706X11000672 [cited 4 Dec 2017]
35. Biswas PK, Rahman MH, Das A, SSU A, Giasuddin M, Christensen JP. Risk for highly pathogenic avian influenza H5N1 virus infection in chickens in small-scale commercial farms, in a high-risk area, Bangladesh, 2008: risk for HPAI in chickens in small-scale commercial farms, Bangladesh. Transbound Emerg Dis. 2011;58:519–25. Available from: http://doi.wiley.com/10.1111/j.1865-1682.2011.01235.x [cited 4 Dec 2017]
36. Liu H, Zhou X, Zhao Y, Zheng D, Wang J, Wang X, et al. Factors Associated with the Emergence of Highly Pathogenic Avian Influenza A (H5N1) Poultry Outbreaks in China: Evidence from an Epidemiological Investigation in Ningxia, 2012. Transbound Emerg Dis. 2017;64:746–53. Available from: http://doi.wiley.com/10.1111/tbed.12433 [cited 4 Dec 2017]
37. Fasina FO, Rivas AL, Bisschop SPR, Stegeman AJ, Hernandez JA. Identification of risk factors associated with highly pathogenic avian influenza H5N1 virus infection in poultry farms, in Nigeria during the epidemic of 2006–2007. Prev Vet Med. 2011;98:204–8. Available from: http://linkinghub.elsevier.com/retrieve/pii/S0167587710003302 [cited 4 Dec 2017]
38. Osmani MG, Thornton RN, Dhand NK, Hoque MA, Milon SMA, Kalam MA, et al. Risk Factors for Highly Pathogenic Avian Influenza in Commercial Layer Chicken Farms in Bangladesh During 2011. Transbound Emerg Dis. 2014;61:e44–51. Available from: http://doi.wiley.com/10.1111/tbed.12071 [cited 4 Dec 2017]

20

Characteristics of owned dogs in rabies endemic KwaZulu-Natal province, South Africa

Melinda Hergert[1*], Kevin Le Roux[2] and Louis H. Nel[3,4]

Abstract

Background: Canine rabies has been enzootic in the dog population of the KwaZulu-Natal province of South Africa since the mid-1970s and has been associated with high rates of human exposures and frequent transmissions to other domestic animal species. Several decades of control efforts, consisting primarily of mass vaccination programs, have previously failed to sufficiently curb rabies in the province. Despite this history of canine rabies, the target canine population has never been extensively studied or quantified. For efficient and effective vaccination campaign planning, the target population must be evaluated and understood. This study reports evaluated observations from survey records captured through a cross sectional observational study regarding canine populations and dog owners in rabies enzootic KwaZulu-Natal province, South Africa. The objective of this study was to aid government veterinary services in their current and ongoing efforts to eliminate canine rabies in the province by gaining information about the size and distribution of the owned dog population.

Results: Thirty-eight percent of the households owned one or more dogs, with rural areas surveyed containing a significantly higher number of owned dogs than urban areas. The mean dog/person ratio for this study was 1:7.7 (range 1:5.4–1:31). The provincial sex ratio was 1.5:1 male to female, with the percentages for male dogs across the communities ranging from 53 to 61.5%. The age structure of this dog population indicates a high turnover rate. Dogs were kept mostly for guarding homes or livestock. Eighty-four percent of dogs had received a rabies vaccine at some point in their lifetime, almost all during a rabies campaign.

Conclusions: The study indicates the majority of owned dogs can be handled by at least one member of the household, thus can be made readily accessible for rabies vaccination during a campaign. Characteristics of owned dogs in the province were similar to those studied in other African countries; however, there were remarkable differences in age, sex and husbandry practices compared to dogs in eastern or northern Africa. These geographical differences lend credence to the theory that canine populations are heterogeneous; therefore, target populations should be evaluated prior to intervention planning.

Keywords: Canine, Rabies, South Africa, Population study

Background

In developing countries the domestic dog (*Canis familiaris*) is both the principal reservoir and the primary vector for rabies in humans and other domestic animal species [1] and exposure to infectious dogs result in over 99% of human rabies cases worldwide [2–4]. In a recent study, this number was conservatively estimated at 59,000 cases per year [5], but the burden is likely to be higher, considering that half of the global human population lives in canine rabies endemic areas of the poverty stricken developing world. Canine (dog) rabies is endemic throughout Africa [6] and the continent carries an estimated 36.4% of the global burden of human rabies [5].

It is well established that the key to the prevention of human rabies, lies in the control of the disease in the canine reservoir [7, 8]. This objective is readily achievable through mass vaccination [3, 9]. However, to be truly effective, thorough knowledge of the characteristics of

* Correspondence: melindahergert@yahoo.com
[1]Department of Paraclinical Sciences, Faculty of Veterinary Science, University of Pretoria, Onderstepoort 0110, South Africa
Full list of author information is available at the end of the article

the canine population (including the true size of the population) is necessary for efficient planning and allocation of campaign resources [10, 11].

The World Health Organization (WHO) suggests that canine ecology surveys should be composed of two parts: one questionnaire for gathering information on the household, and another for collecting information on each dog owned by the household [12]. Household associated queries provide information about the member composition of the household, socioeconomics, religion, culture, number of owned dogs, dog bite histories, knowledge of rabies and other human related points of interest. The individual dog questionnaire gains descriptive statistics on each of the dogs owned by the household, as well as purpose, management and husbandry style. Non-dog owning community members can contribute with respect to the household questionnaire, thus gaining general information about the entire community. Area culture and infrastructure may affect the methodology employed in marketing and scheduling tactics of vaccination campaigns for rabies control. Central point vaccinations may be conducive to a township configuration, whereas rural areas may require house-to-house delivery of vaccine. Optimal frequency of vaccination campaigns which target at risk dog sub-populations, while considering economics and measurable outcomes are critical to the planning and sustainability of dog rabies control programs in developing countries [8, 13].

Two rabies virus variants are recognized in South Africa, respectively recognized in herpestids (mongooses, genets) and canines [14–17]. Historically, the largest percentage of human rabies cases in South Africa has occurred in KwaZulu-Natal (KZN) where canine variant is circulated and maintained within the large provincial population of domestic dogs [18–21]. Despite the long history of endemic canine rabies in KZN, extensive canine ecology studies have not been performed as part of the provincial disease control program and there is an inadequate understanding of the dog population – particularly in reference to population figures and ownership practices. Door-to-door mass rabies vaccination campaigns are conducted annually by KZN government veterinary services (GVS) with the cooperation of staff from the Departments of Health and Environmental Health using bright yellow trucks and loud hailer systems announcing their arrival. The objective of this study was to aid GVS in their current and ongoing efforts to eliminate canine rabies in the province by gaining information about the size and distribution of the owned dog population.

Methods

Study area and sampling procedure

From September 2009 through January 2011, household surveys were conducted in six different communities across KZN province, covering three land use types (Fig. 1). Distribution of the 1992 households completing the surveys was 52% rural, 33% urban and 15% peri-urban. Rabies was enzootic in all areas, with the exception of the peri-urban community of Wembezi. Affluent urban and suburban areas where people keep dogs in confined spaces were excluded, as these dogs most likely have lower rabies risk due to fewer effective contacts between animals and access to private veterinary services [8]. Study areas were selected with the assistance of KZN DAERD GVS division, and consisted of high density townships and rural areas as described in Hergert et al. [22].

Simple random sampling and systematic surveys are difficult in developing countries due to logistical reasons; therefore, a cluster or 'area' design was used because rural area homesteads are not numbered, and informal housing settlements within townships are frequently haphazardly arranged [23, 24]. Clusters for this survey were identified using Google Earth maps at 4.6 km eye altitude with a grid in order to maintain consistent sampling methodology which allows for the random systematic selection of similar sampling units between differing geographical areas [10]. Clusters were numbered from left to right and selected by sampling with replacement using an online random number generator [22, 25]. There is potential for extrapolating survey results into the entire study area permitting generalizations providing that the geographical, socioeconomic and culture settings are the same or very close, which was true for each area type [10]. The desired minimum sample size for each area was 323 households.

Questionnaire interviews

Utilizing WHO [26] canine rabies control guidelines, the questionnaires were composed of two parts; a household survey for collecting respondent demographics, and an individual dog survey for descriptive statistics of the owned dog population. The surveys were translated into isiZulu and then back translated to English. The surveys and interviewing methods were piloted in a township with comparable human demographics and a history of canine rabies. KZN DAERD Animal Health Technicians and students, Department of Health workers, Environmental Health workers and SPCA employees were trained to perform the surveys and acquire informed verbal consent from respondents. Only respondents who verbally agreed to the survey were interviewed. Any children between the ages of 14 and 18 years of age who answered the survey on behalf of the family had an adult family member present during the interview to provide verbal consent. All interviews were conducted on weekdays between the hours of 9 am and 3 pm.

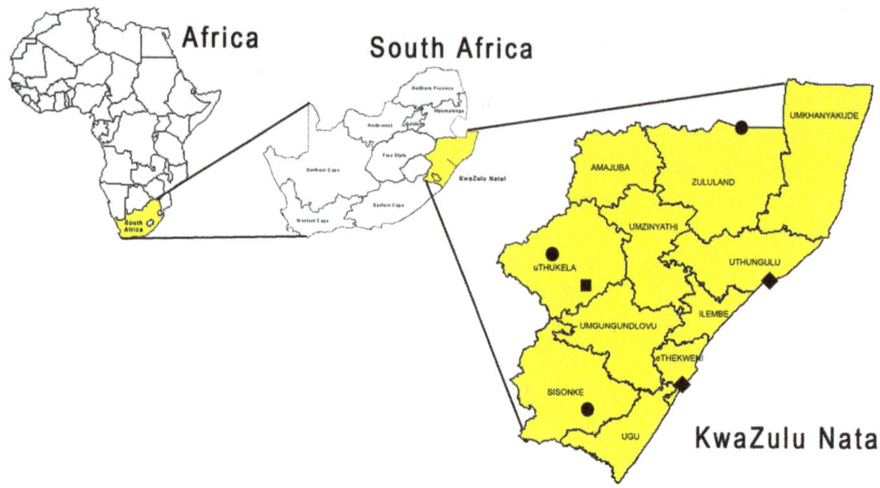

Fig. 1 Geographical location of KwaZulu-Natal with the six study areas indicated. Note: Black square = Wembezi (peri-urban rabies free), black diamonds = Umlazi and Esikhawini (urban rabies enzootic), black circles = Ixopo, Pongola and St. Chads (rural rabies enzootic)

Data analysis

The data from each area was entered into a Microsoft Excel spreadsheet and then imported into SAS version 9.3 (SAS Institute, Inc., Cary, North Carolina, USA). Descriptive statistics were generated, and cross tabulations calculating Pearson's Chi Square (χ^2) were performed in tests of association. Area dog population numbers were calculated by multiplying the owned dog per person ratio by the most recent human census counts for the local municipality.

Results

Questionnaire interviews

A total of 1992 households consisting of 13,756 people (occupant range 1–34, median = 6) completed the surveys within the three targeted community types. Response rates ranged from 92 to 100% in the six areas surveyed. Survey questions were answered by a person defined as head of the household (68%, $n = 1361$), other adult (22%, $n = 435$), child over the age of 14 (9%, $n = 183$), and children under 14 with grandparent present (1%, $n = 11$). Category for respondent was missing in two cases. The sex of the respondent was not recorded.

Ninety-nine percent of the population was of Zulu culture. Eighty-four percent reported to be Christians, with 13% equally divided between Traditional African beliefs and the Shembe religion, a combination of Christianity and Zulu culture. Only two households reported to be of Muslim faith.

Eighty-four percent of houses were built of blocks or brick construction, with the remaining 16% being made of locally sourced materials like mud, manure, sticks or tin. Forty-three percent of households had a flush toilet, 52% had a pit latrine and 4% had no toilet facilities. Twenty-seven percent of houses had solid fences, most of which were found in urban communities. A pit near the house, or community dump was used for refuse removal by 55% of households surveyed. Twelve percent of the population surveyed owned cattle or goats, and 31% kept chickens. Fifty-five percent of households had at least one member working away from the home.

Thirty-eight percent (757/1992) of all of the households owned one or more dogs (range 1–19, median = 2). Individual descriptive statistics was attempted for every owned dog over suckling age; however, some records were missing substantial data points. Data were collected on 1667 individual dogs, of which 99 % were at home during some time of interview. The most common reason given (52%) for why a household did not own dogs was that they did not like them. Sixteen percent of households previously had dogs that died and wanted to replace them. Other reasons cited for not owning dogs were religion, lack of fencing, avoidance of conflict with neighbors and landlords, or that they could not afford them.

Dog demographics

Age structure and sex ratios

Age structure of the owned dogs varied between areas. The rabies negative community of Wembezi reported the largest percentage of dogs three years or younger with a value of 79% (provincial average 66%). The largest age group in Wembezi was 1–2 years of age, which is suggested a high population turnover. The two urban townships showed the greatest disparity in range of elderly dogs. The urban township of Umlazi had the highest percentage of dogs over the age of five years at 29%, while the urban township of Esikhawini had the lowest percentage of dogs older than five years with a value of

13.7%. Of the thirty respondents who did not know the age of the dog, seventeen were not the owner. Where dog owners could recall the lifespan of dogs they no longer had, the average lifespan was reported as 4.9 to 6.5 years across the areas surveyed.

The provincial sex ratio was 1.5:1 male to female, with the percentages for male dogs across the communities ranging from 53 to 61.5%. Lactating females with litters of puppies present were most commonly seen in the rural areas. Geographically, there was no significance between sex of the dog and area surveyed, determined by the Chi Square test for independence (Chi Square = 1.8917, DF = 5, $p = 0.86$, Cramer's V = 0.034).

Reproductive history of female dogs

Of the breeding age females ($n = 293$), 46% had whelped previously. Ninety-three percent (272/293) had given birth within the last 12 months. Data on litter size were missing for 21 cases and disposition from one case. Based upon owner recollection there were 1239 pups born in 251 litters giving an average litter size of 4.9 pups per litter (range 1–14). From these litters 32% of pups died before weaning age, 9% were sold, 26% were given away, and 32% remained in the original household. One litter was reported as stolen and another had been killed by the bitch. No owners reported killing or abandoning the puppies. Of the 25 litters that were sold, 48% were born to bitches that had been bought and 44% from bitches that were received as gifts (Table 1). Only two of the litters born to bitches reported as being kept for breeding were sold, and two of the litters were reported as having died. It is unknown if any puppy deaths were husbandry related, including exposure to elements, insufficient diet, overwhelming parasites, or infectious diseases (ex. Parvo, distemper, canine herpes, or *Brucella canis*). None of the litters from the hunting bitches were reported as sold. The breed of the dogs was not recorded because overwhelmingly, the community's dogs were of the Africanis or 'local' land race [27, 28].

Table 1 Cross-tabulation of disposition of 271 litters of pups with the purpose of the bitch in surveyed communities KZN September 2009 – January 2011

Disposition of Pups	Purpose of Dog						Total
	Breeding	Guard house	Guard livestock	Hunting	Other	Pet	
Died	2	73	5	4	2	1	87
Gave away	1	58	1	4	1	4	69
Bitch killed	0	1	0	0	0	0	1
Sold	2	21	0	0	0	2	25
Still have	5	73	4	5	0	1	88
Stolen	0	1	0	0	0	0	1
Total	10	227	10	13	3	8	271

Desire and value of dog sterilization

Out of the 1794 total dogs observed, only 7 (5 males, 2 females) were reported as having been sterilized. One dog from the urban community of Umlazi had been sourced from the SPCA where adoption policy dictates that animals must be sterilized prior to leaving the shelter. As population turnover is an important characteristic in dog ecology and rabies control, respondents were asked if they would like to have their dogs sterilized to which 60 % (944/1552) responded positively. Odds ratio calculation (1.097) showed no influence or protective factor regarding sex of dog and owner desire for sterilization. Dog owners were further asked what monetary value they would place on sterilization surgery. There were four categorical responses to the question ranging from 0 to > 100 South African Rand (SAR). Less than 7% of respondents placed a value on this service of > 50 SAR (Table 2). The categories of 51–100 SAR and > 100 SAR were collapsed into the category of > 50 SAR for analysis and reporting.

Dog densities and population estimates

Rural areas surveyed contain a significantly higher number of owned dogs than urban areas. Dog owning households varied from 45 to 64% in the three rural communities versus 12–15% in the two urban communities (Table 3). The peri-urban community of Wembezi is interesting in that it parallels human densities seen in urban areas with an average of six persons per household; whereas the dog statistics are more similar to the rural communities with 39% of households owning dogs and a dog/human ratio of 1:6. The mean dog/person ratio for this study was 1:7.7 (range 1:5.4–1:31). Area dog population numbers were calculated based upon the most recent human census counts for the local municipality [29, 30].

Dog management and husbandry

Dog management and husbandry comprises many variables including food source and frequency, handling of the dog, dog purpose, level of restriction, and provision of shelter. Most of the owned dogs were reported as guard dogs (87%), either for the homestead (85%) or livestock (2%). Less than 5% were considered as pets. Three percent of dogs were used for breeding and 5% for hunting. Only 17% of the dogs in the survey were reported as being fully restricted to the household by a chain or tether. Twenty percent of dogs were restricted for at least part of the day. The remaining 63% were never restricted and allowed to roam at will. Twenty-three percent of the dogs wore collars regardless of their level of restriction. Some type of shelter was provided for 59% of the dogs.

Over 94% of dog owners believed that they provided enough food for their dogs. Nine respondents admitted

Table 2 Owner valuation of sterilization services in South African Rand (SAR)

	Percent Owner Valuation of Veterinary Sterilization Service		
	0 SAR	*1–50 SAR*	*> 50 SAR*
Ixopo	42	56	2
Pongola	69	26	5
St. Chad's	59	38.5	2
Umlazi	49	40	11
Esikhawini	57	33	10
Wembezi	62	31	7
Provincial Average	56.33%	37.42%	6.17%

they did not feed their dogs every day. Although 19% of owners reported purchasing commercial dog food for their animals, the majority of owned dogs (73%) were fed left-over human food from the household. The remaining dogs were left to scavenge from rubbish pits or given butcher's waste. Thirty-four percent of respondents said they fed dogs that they did not own on their property. Of those, 65% knew these dogs which were scavenging meals at their house; the remaining 35% were unknown dogs but were not considered strays by the respondents. No dogs were identified by respondents as community owned, neighborhood or stray dogs.

Seventy-two percent of the dogs were reported as owned by the head of the household. The remaining dogs were owned by other adult males or females (18%), the household children (7%), or shared ownership by everyone in the household (3%). Twenty-two percent of dogs could only be handled by their owner, 11 % could be handled by the children, and 65 % could be handled by everyone in the household. Less than 2% of dogs were reported as unmanageable.

Most of the dogs were either bought (44%) or received as gifts (38%). Seventeen percent of dogs appeared to be locally sourced, as they had come either from a neighbor or from the owners own bitch. Less than 2% of dogs had come to the current residence with a family member who had moved from another location, and only one dog was reported as adopted from the SPCA.

Rabies vaccination status of dogs

The individual dog survey allowed for the collection of the rabies vaccination status of each dog over suckling age in the household; however, rabies data points were missing for 47 of the 1667 animals. Eighty-four percent (1361/1620) of dogs with complete records had received a rabies vaccine at some point in their lifetime, and almost all of these dogs had last been vaccinated by an animal health technician during a rabies campaign. Less than 2% of dog owners reported that their dog had been vaccinated by a private veterinarian. Sixty-four percent (1043/1620) of the dogs were reported as having been immunized within the last one year. Owners said they could provide proof of vaccination cards in 82% of cases.

Respondents who had not presented their dogs at the last government vaccination campaign were asked why. Lack of owner awareness and campaign timing contributed the most to this failure ($n = 137$, 61.5%). Extraneous reasons ($n = 85$, 38.5%) commonly given for why dog owners said they had not presented their dogs for vaccination were: dog new to the household, dog thought to be too young for vaccination, or the dog had run away from the technicians. Respondents who said they did not want the vaccine were not queried further as to why.

Table 3 Dog densities calculated from six surveyed communities KZN 2009–2011

	Rural			Urban		Peri-urban
	St. Chad's	Ixopo	Pongola	Umlazi	Esikhawini	Wembezi
[a]HH Interviewed	357	342	346	334	318	300
%[a]DOHH	52%	64%	45%	12%	15%	39%
Persons/HH	7.42	7.4	8.56	6.34	5.54	5.91
Total Dogs	467	473	412	69	77	296
Dogs/HH	1.31	1.39	1.19	0.21	0.24	0.99
Dogs/DOHH	2.54	2.16	2.64	1.68	1.64	2.55
Dogs/Person	1:5.7	1:5.4	1:7.2	1:31	1:23	1:6
Dogs/Km^2	276	9.2	5.2	476	495	324
Estimated Dog Population	2159[c]	1112[c] 14,982[b]	17031[b]	24,194[c]	3086[c]	2916[c]
Male dogs	261	267	217	37	37	125
Female dogs	170	180	155	28	30	78
Sex ratio M:F	1.5	1.5	1.4	1.3	1.2	1.6

[a]*HH* Household, *DOHH* Dog owning household; [b]Dog populations calculated for municipality; [c]Dog populations calculated for local area

Rabies vaccination status in cats

From 2001 to 2011, 539 cat brain samples were submitted to the provincial laboratory, with only thirty positive results by fluorescent antibody test [KZNDAERD personal communications 2012]. Seventeen percent of households surveyed owned a total of 542 cats (range of 1–10, median = 1). The ratio of dogs to cats in KZN surveyed households was 3.3:1. Sixty-three percent (n = 342) of the owned cats were reported as vaccinated against rabies, of which 226 (66%) were from homes where the dogs had been rabies vaccinated during the most recent government campaign. Cat owners were not asked for proof of vaccination.

Discussion

The personal interview method employed for conducting these door-to-door surveys produced a high return rate of 98% for this study. Developing countries frequently do not have infrastructure for landline telephone systems and mail delivery for every eligible household; therefore, home-based interviews are most suitable for data collection [31, 32].

Rural populations surveyed owned considerably more dogs than the urban and peri-urban communities. Dog owning households varied from 45 to 65% in the three rural communities versus 12–15% in the two urban communities. Similar findings were reported from Zambia where 11% of households in urban Mutendere owned dogs and 42% in rural Palabana kept dogs [33]. Reports from urban Tanzania show 13% of households kept dogs [34]. In rural Sri Lanka, 57% of surveyed households owned dogs [35]. In contrast, Oboegbulem and Nwakonobi [36] found that 38.2% of urban households in Lagos, Nigeria owned dogs, compared to 20% of rural households. Fifty-two percent of households that did not own dogs in the surveys said it was because they did not like them. This consideration is unlike results from Kenya where only 7% of respondents said they did not like dogs [13]. Other reasons provided for not owning dogs included avoiding conflict with landlords and neighbors, and not having a fence to contain the dog. Fear of reprisal from neighbors, and not having fences were also common reasons for not owning dogs by Zambian residents [33].

The mean dog/person ratio for this study was 1:7.7 (range 1:5.4–1:31), generally similar to ratios from rural (1:6.7) and urban (1:45) Zambia reported by De Balogh et al. [33]. Dog densities measured in this study varied from 6.3 to 495 dogs per square kilometer, with highest densities seen in the urban townships. The estimated national averages for Zimbabwe were 1:6.5 dogs/person and 3.4 dogs/km^2 [31]. In rural Kenya, dog densities were estimated at 6 to 21/km^2 [13]. Urban Tanzania reported dog densities as 1:14 dogs/person and 334 dogs/km^2 [34]. Densities from 30 dogs/km^2 up to 3000/km^2 have been reported for rural and urban/suburban Sri Lanka respectively with human dog ratios of 1:7 to 1:16 [35, 37]. Beran and Frith [38] concur with large urban dog densities when they reported 681 to 2388 dogs/km^2 from the city of Guayaquil, Ecuador. However, the dog to human ratio for Guayaquil (1:7.2) was more comparable to rural areas rather than urban centers of Africa, which was a similar finding to the unique peri-urban area of Wembezi in this study. The high dog densities of urban areas correspond to high human densities in urban areas, and as dogs are dependent upon humans directly or indirectly for their food resources the dog population will grow with human populations as long as the people remain tolerant of the dogs [39, 40]. Western countries generally report dog/human ratios of 1:6 to 1:10 [37]. Despite some similarities in the African countries studied these variations in dog densities clearly point to the heterogeneity of dog populations across the world. Compared to Latin American and Asian examples, lower dog densities and human:dog ratios prevail in the African countries where such studies were done.

High dog densities in urban areas suggest the probability of high effective contact rates between dogs; however, solid fencing was found in over 40% of urban households visited in KZN. Fencing was seen at less than 16% of households in rural areas. In contrast, only 9% of houses in urban Mutendere, Zambia had solid fences [33] and only one household in the communal lands of Zimbabwe had a dog-restricting fence [40]. In our study, over half of the surveyed households utilize a pit by the house for rubbish removal, which can be an attractant for roaming dogs. In urban areas with municipal services respondents frequently commented that dogs were disturbing rubbish bins; a similar finding by McCrindle et al. [41] from the Johannesburg township of Soweto. The quantity of random dump-sites on roadsides and discarded litter in urban townships provides resources for scavenging dogs. Rural area roadsides and pathways were cleaner despite the utilization of open pits by homes. Though none of the dogs in the study were referred to as neighborhood or community dogs by respondents, many free-ranging dogs were purposely fed on non-owners' property suggesting communal care. In Zimbabwe, 78.6% of households reported foreign dogs scavenging in the open pits containing human-derived food waste on their property [40]. It is possible that many scavenging dogs in this study were owned since 62% of owned dogs were allowed to roam for scavenging and socialization at all times. Over 70% of the owned dogs in the Eastern Cape Province of South Africa and 79% of owned dogs in Antananarivo, Madagascar were reported as being allowed to roam freely [42, 43]. Only 17% of KZN dogs were reported as always restricted to the yard and another 20% were only chained for part of the day. Many owners reported they let their dogs off the chain to roam and scavenge at night, which was also described from Lagos, Nigeria [36]. Over 53% of houses in Zimbabwe do not have toilets, allowing for the scavenging of human waste by roaming dogs [40]. Some respondents in this survey said they were afraid to visit the pit toilet at night for fear of the scavenging dogs.

For safety and logistical reasons, we relied on respondent knowledge to gain age data on the owned dogs. We found that more than 60% of the owned dog population was 3 years of age or younger, indicating a high population turnover. Similar numbers were reported from a local municipality in the Eastern Cape Province where they found 64% of the dogs were 3 years of age or younger [42]. This is close to the mean age of 2.6 years found by in rural Bophuthatswana, South Africa [44], with 2.8 years reported from Kenya [13] and 2.6 years from the Thungsong District of Thailand [45]. Canine ecology studies conducted in Zimbabwe, Zambia and Tanzania have reported a lower median age for the dog population of 1.9 to 2.2 years [31, 33, 34, 40, 46]. Dogs in rural Sri Lanka had a higher mean age of 3.5 years, with the male dogs living slightly longer, 3.7 years, compared to females at 3.1 years [35]. Brooks [31] also reported male dogs in Zimbabwe living six months longer than female dogs. Dog owners in this survey estimated the average lifespan for their dogs to be 5.5 years, a year older than was estimated for dogs in Zimbabwe [31].

Historically sex ratios in recorded dog populations of Africa are skewed towards males [32, 34, 40, 43]. As seen in other canine studies, this study showed that male dogs out number females with a sex ratio of 1.5:1. This is in close agreement with the Eastern Cape Province of South Africa where the ratio was 1.7:1 as well as urban Madagascar 1.5:1 [42, 43]. Tanzania and Zimbabwe have reported ratios of 1.3:1 [31, 34]. The Thungsong District of Thailand revealed a 2:1 M:F ratio in the owned dog population [45]. The Mirigama area of Sri Lanka also had a preponderance of male dogs (73.6%) [35]. In Kenya, Kitala et al. [13] found that male members of the household believed that male dogs make better guard dogs and hunters, thus the tendency to provide better husbandry practices for male dogs. Male dogs are the preferred choice for guard dogs in urban United States [47]. Residents of all socioeconomic classes in Guayaquil, Ecuador preferred male dogs 56 to 68% [38]. Results showing more male dogs than females in all age brackets are consistent with findings from other countries except Nigeria where a sex ratio biased towards females in both rural (0.8:1) and urban (0.9:1) areas was reported [36]. Perhaps the fact that the head of the household, or males in general, more frequently own the dogs, leads to this tendency for male favored sex bias. The select killing of female pups in Tunisia creates a skewed sex ratio that may be more about population control than sex preference [26].

Controlling reproduction in owned dogs is not a wide spread practice, as only seven dogs in the survey were reported as castrated or spayed. Although over 60% of dog owners said they would like to have their dogs sterilized, 57 % said they would not consider paying for the surgery. Respondents either did not value the service or could not comprehend the associated costs. Ninety-three percent of the breeding age females were reported to have whelped within the last 12 months. In Kenya and Zambia, 85% and 83% of reproductive age bitches had whelped in the last year [13, 33]. In contrast, nearly 64% of female dogs in Guayaquil over the age of one year had never whelped and only 50% of owned females in Antananarivo had been pregnant in the last year [38, 43].

In KZN, 1239 pups were born to 251 litters giving an average litter size for the province of 4.9 puppies per litter with a range of 1 to 14 across the six communities. Thirty-two percent of puppies born to bitches in this survey died prior to weaning age, which is similar to 38% seen in Guayaquil [38]. This figure is higher than the 22% reported from Kenya, but less than the 53% pre-weaning mortality of communal Zimbabwe [13, 40]. De Balogh et al. [33] reported from Zambia that over 50% of the puppies born died within a year, while nearly 30% had been given away or sold, leaving less than 20% remaining in households. In this study 35% of puppies were either sold or given away, while 32% remained in the household. One owner reported his litter had been stolen, while another reported that the bitch had killed the pups. No respondents reported killing or abandoning the pups unlike in Tunisia where 61% of unwanted puppies were killed as a form of population control [26].

As less than 10 % of the puppies were sold, the question arises of why some dogs are considered worthy of purchase. Of the 25 litters that were sold, 48% were born of bitches that had been bought and 44% from bitches that were received as gifts. Although in some communities greyhound type dogs were seen, a comment cannot be made about if the dogs reported as breeders were of pure bred origin. It would be expected that dogs of pure bred origin would be more valuable monetarily, thus the puppies from these litters would be kept or sold rather than given away. In this study, most litters from bitches reported as being kept for breeding were not sold. None of the litters were sold from hunting bitches. Of all of the litters reported as sold, 84% came from bitches whose purpose was to guard the house.

Over 80% of dogs in KZN were either purchased or acquired as gifts. Unlike dogs from the Machakos District of Kenya where Kitala et al. [13] found 35% of dogs originated within the household, less than 12% of KZN dogs came from household bitches. Despite increased human mobility via taxis and buses, less than 2% of the dogs came to the present household with a family member who moved. In Guayaquil, dogs appear to migrate more as Beran and Frith [38] report that 100 to 200 dogs (~ 26% of the population) were brought into the city daily being presented as gifts or with people moving. Despite some respondent complaints about dogs in the community, 16% of households that did not own dogs wanted to get dogs. This desire for dogs was commonly recorded by Kitala et al. [13] in Kenya and by Butler and Bingham [40] in Zimbabwean communities.

There appears to be little difference in the general husbandry and management of dogs between the three community types surveyed. The urban area of Umlazi reported the most dogs kept as pets at 18.5%, with the other urban are of Esikhawini and peri-urban Wembezi trailing at 12% and 9% respectively. The majority of owned dogs in KZN are kept to guard homes or livestock (87%). Less than 5% of dogs in rural areas were kept as pets, and dogs used for hunting were uncommon (4%) as was also reported by Butler [48] in Zimbabwean communal lands. Unlike in Nigeria, no dogs were reported as used for a meat source or for scavenging the homestead in this study [36, 49]. In Guayaquil, Ecuador 70% of canines were kept as guard dogs and 17.9% were kept as mascots or pets [38]. The role of guard dog corresponds with findings in other developing countries including Zimbabwe reporting 60% guard dogs [31, 40], Kenya over 99% guard dogs [13], Antananarivo reported 81% [43] and Thailand with 83% guard dogs [45]. Although the majority of dogs in Thailand are meant to guard the house, only 56% were fed food from the resident household, few were provided shelter and most are permitted to roam freely during the day.

Dog owners in KZN report that they feed their dogs adequately. Observations of owned dogs and dogs roaming streets showed them to be in reasonable body condition as was also reported from Antananarivo [43]. Dogs in rural areas were primarily fed left over human food from the household. In urban Umlazi nearly 70% of dogs were fed commercial dog food. Although the other urban and peri-urban communities also reported feeding commercial food, more than 50% of the dog's diet was left over human food. Dogs in communal lands of Zimbabwe were fed maize meal porridge at least once a day and sometimes milk or bones [40]. Dogs in confinement in urban settings of Nigeria were more likely to directly receive food from their owners, whereas dogs in rural areas that were allowed to roam were somewhat self sufficient, being irregularly fed by their owners and scavenging the neighborhood for the remainder of their needs [36]. Dogs in Madagascar were fed with family food 81%, or a commercial diet 12%, and 7.1% were not fed by their owners [43]. Only nine respondents from this study stated that they did not feed their dogs and left them to scavenge. Kitala et al. [32] reported only 5 % of dogs being fed commercial dog food and the remainder fed on household leftovers and waste.

Accessibility of dogs for vaccination should not be an issue for KZN, as 76% of the dogs were reported as being able to be handled either by everyone in the household or at least the children. GVS should be able to vaccinate these dogs during a campaign provided a family member who can handle the dogs is home during the campaign. De Balogh et al. [33] reported good accessibility of dogs for parenteral vaccination in Zambia at central point locations as children could locate and present the dogs for vaccination. Although 98.6% of the owned dogs in this survey were at home during the visit, many owners reported their dogs would run away once the vaccinations begin. Door-to-door campaigns are currently conducted in KZN, which was also the suggested method for larger settlements in Zambia, especially for those households with many dogs [33].

The study indicates that most of the owned dog population of KZN is adequately rabies vaccinated with coverage of 74% using a vaccine that is labeled with three-year duration of immunity. However, there were two areas, rural Pongola (62%) and urban Umlazi (57%), with coverage levels under the recommended 70% [10, 22]. Thirty-five percent of the dogs in Antananarivo were reported as vaccinated against rabies, but only 7.2% had a valid certificate or vaccination card [43]. In Thungsong District of Thailand, 70% of the owned dog population had been vaccinated in the last 6 months [45]. For some of the areas in this survey, vaccination campaigns had not been conducted for over one year.

Conclusion

The response rate from this survey showed that household surveys are an effective tool for gathering information about communities and the dogs they own. Government vaccination campaigns should be continued in KZN, as most of the dogs and cats in the study had been previously vaccinated by GVS. In order to increase rabies vaccination coverage, consideration should be given to holding vaccine campaigns over many days with varied hours and possibly on weekends in the high risk urban area of Umlazi where many dog owners work away from the household. Although most dogs in KZN are allowed to roam at will, they can be handled by most household members and can be made readily accessible for rabies vaccination during a campaign. Evidence that most of the dogs across the province were left to roam freely and appear to have a high population turnover and inadequate vaccination coverage in high risk areas might help explain why canine rabies persists despite current methods employed by veterinary services. Population characteristics of the dogs in this survey are similar to dogs studied in other southern African countries; however, there were notable differences in age, sex and husbandry compared to dogs in eastern or northern Africa. Populations of stray or unowned dogs cannot be properly assessed through the use of household questionnaires, and our study focused solely on owned dogs, which is a limitation of the study. While it appears that stray dogs are few in this province, data was not gathered to substantiate this claim.

Abbreviations

DAERD: Department of Agriculture, Environment, and Rural Development; GVS: Government Veterinary Services; KZN: KwaZulu-Natal; SAR: South African Rand; WHO: World Health Organization

Acknowledgments

The authors would like to acknowledge the Managing Veterinarians of the KwaZulu-Natal Department of Agriculture, Environment and Rural Development Dr. Dumasani Mtshali and Dr. Temba Sikhakhane, the KZNDAERD Epidemiology staff Dr. Keith Perrett, Mrs. Tokkie Tischendorf, Mrs. Debbie Cooke and Ms. Vigie Govendor, and State Veterinarians and Control Animal Health Technicians Ms. Joey Peens, Mr. Amos Mateta, Mr. Carel Burger, Mr. Hadebe, Dr. Mbaga Lukubisa, Dr. Shavetha Dhanilall, Dr. Johan Blignaut, Dr. Alan Rowe and Dr. Rob Paterson for providing equipment and personnel which aided in the completion of this study. We sincerely appreciate the assistance of personnel from the Department of Health, Department of Environmental Health and the SPCA. We would also like to express sincere appreciation to Dr. Frans Kanfer and Mrs. Jaqui Sommerville of the statistics department at the University of Pretoria, Hatfield campus.

Funding

Funding was provided by the University of Pretoria, Onderstepoort, and The Humane Society International.

Authors' contributions

MH Principal Investigator, conception & design, data acquisition, analysis and interpretation, manuscript draft and critical revision. KLR and LHN design, data acquisition, manuscript draft and critical revision. All authors read and approved the final manuscript. All authors agree to be accountable for all aspects of the work.

Consent for publication

Not applicable.

Competing interests

The authors declare that they have no competing interests.

Author details

[1]Department of Paraclinical Sciences, Faculty of Veterinary Science, University of Pretoria, Onderstepoort 0110, South Africa. [2]KwaZulu-Natal Department of Environment, Agriculture and Rural Development, Government Veterinary Services, 458 Townbush Road, Pietermaritzburg 3202, South Africa. [3]Department of Biochemistry, Genetics and Microbiology, Faculty of Natural and Agricultural Sciences University of Pretoria, Pretoria 0002, South Africa. [4]Global Alliance for Rabies Control, 529 Humboldt St., Suite 1, Manhattan, KS 66502, USA.

References

1. Nel LH, Markotter W. Lyssaviruses. Crit Rev Microbiol. 2007;33:301–24.
2. Blancou J. Epizootiology of Rabies: Eurasia and Africa. In: Campbell JB, Charlton KM, editors. Rabies. London: Kluwer Academic Publishers; 1988.
3. Fekadu M. Canine rabies. Onderstepoort J Vet Res. 1993;60:421–7.
4. World Health Organization. WHO Expert Consultation on Rabies. In: Technical Report Series 931. Geneva: World Health Organization; 2005.
5. Hampson K, Coudeville L, Lembo T, Sambo M, Kieffer A, Attlan M, et al. Estimating the global burden of endemic canine rabies. PLoS Negl Trop. 2015;9(4):e0003709. https://doi.org/10.1371/journal.pntd.0003709.
6. Nel LH, Rupprecht CE. Emergence of lyssaviruses in the Old World: the case of Africa. Curr Top Microbiol Immunol. 2007;315:161–93.
7. Bogel K, Meslin FX. Economics of human and canine rabies elimination: Guidelines for programme orientation. In: World Health Organization Bulletin 68. Geneva: World Health Organization; 1990. p. 281–91.
8. Perry BD. Dog ecology in eastern and southern Africa: implications for rabies control. Onderstepoort J Vet Res. 1993;60:429–36.
9. Hampson K, Dushoff J, Bingham J, Bruckner G, Ali YH, Dobson A. Synchronous cycles of domestic dog rabies in sub-Saharan Africa and the impact of control efforts. PNAS. 2007;104:7717–22.
10. World Health Organization. Guidelines for dog rabies control. VPH/83.43 Rev. 1. Geneva: World Health Organization; 1987.
11. Taylor LH, Wallace RM, Balaram D, Lindenmayer JM, Eckery DC, Mutonono-Watkiss B, Parravani E, Nel LH. The role of dog population management in rabies elimination—a review of current approaches and future opportunities. Front Vet Sci. 2017;4:109.
12. World Health Organization. Guidelines for Dog Rabies Control VPH/83.43. Geneva: World Health Organization; 1984.
13. Kitala PM, McDermott JJ, Kyule MN, Gathuma JM, Perry B, Wandeler AI. Dog ecology and demography information to support the planning of rabies control in Machakos District. Kenya Acta Trop. 2001;78:217–30.
14. King AA, Meredith CD, Thomson GR. Canid and viverrid rabies viruses in South Africa. Onderstepoort J Vet Res. 1993;60:295–9.
15. Von Teichman BF, Thomson GR, Meredith CD, Nel LH. Molecular epidemiology of rabies virus in South Africa: evidence for two distinct virus groups. J Gen Virol. 1995;76:73–82.
16. Nel LH, Sabeta CT, Von Teichman B, Jaftha JB, Rupprecht CE, Bingham J. Mongoose rabies in southern Africa: a re-evaluation based on molecular epidemiology. Virus Res. 2005;109:165–73.
17. Van Zyl N, Markotter W, Nel LH. Evolutionary history of African mongoose rabies. Virus Res. 2010;150:93–102.
18. Swanepoel R, Barnard BJH, Meredith CD, Bishop GC, Bruckner GK, Foggin CM, Hubschle OJB. Rabies in southern Africa. Onderstepoort J Vet Res. 1993;60:325–46.
19. Department of Health, Republic of South Africa. Statistical notes: Human rabies in South Africa. Pretoria: Department of Health South Africa; 2006.
20. Nel LH, Le Roux K, Atlas R. Meeting the rabies control challenge in South Africa. Microbe. 2009;4:61–5.
21. Bishop GC, Durrheim DN, Kloeck PE, Godlonton JD, Bingham J, Speare R. The Rabies Advisory Group. Rabies: Guide for the Medical, Veterinary and Allied Professions. 2nd ed. Pretoria: Government Printer; 2010.
22. Hergert M, Le Roux K, Nel LH. Risk factors associated with non-vaccination rabies status of dogs in KwaZulu-Natal, South Africa Vet Med: Res Rep. 2016;7:75–83.
23. Suzuki K, Pereira JAC, Frias LA, Lopez R, Mutinelli LE, Pons ER. Rabies-vaccination coverage and profiles of the owned-dog population in Santa Cruz de la sierra. Bolivia Zoonosis and Public Health. 2008;55:177–83.
24. Garson, GD. Sampling. http://www.statisticalassociates.com/sampling.pdf. (2009) Accessed May 2009.
25. Random.org www.random.org. Accessed Aug 2009 – Feb 2011.

26. World Health Organization. Report of dog ecology studies related to rabies. WHO/Rab.Res/88.25. Geneva: World Health Organization; 1988.
27. Gallant J. The story of the African dog. Pietermaritzburg: University of Natal Press; 2002.
28. Greyling L, Grobler P, Van der Bank H, Kotze A. Genetic characterisation of a domestic dog *Canis familiaris* breed endemic to South African rural areas. Acta Therio. 2004;49(3):369–82.
29. Stats SA Census. 2001 Census in brief. second ed. Pretoria: Statistics South Africa; 2003.
30. Stats SA. Statistics in brief: midyear population estimates. Pretoria: Statistics South Africa; 2007.
31. Brooks R. Survey of the dog population of Zimbabwe and its level of rabies vaccination. Vet Rec. 1990;127:592–6.
32. Kitala PM, McDermott JJ, Kyule MN, Gathuma JM. Features of dog ecology relevant to rabies spread in Machakos District. Kenya Onderstepoort J Vet Res. 1993;60:445–9.
33. de Balogh KKIM, Wandeler AI, Meslin FX. A dog ecology study in an urban and semi-rural area of Zambia. Onderstepoort J Vet Res. 1993;60:437–43.
34. Gsell A, Knobel DL, Cleaveland S, Kazwala RR, Vounatsou P, Zinsstag J. Features of domestic dog demography relevant to rabies control planning in Tanzania. J Vet Behav: Clin App and Res. 2009;4(2):63.
35. Matter HC, Wandeler AI, Neueschwander BE, Harischandra LPA, Meslin FX. Study of the dog population and the rabies control activities in the Mirigama area of Sri Lanka. Acta Trop. 2000;75:95–108.
36. Oboegbulem SI, Nwakonobi LE. Population density and ecology of dogs in Nigeria: a pilot study. Rev Sci Tech Off Int Epiz. 1989;8:733–45.
37. Wandeler AI, Budde A, Capt S, Kappeler A, Matter HC. Dog ecology and dog rabies control. Rev Inf Dis. 1988;0 Suppl 684-S688.
38. Beran GW, Frith M. Domestic animal rabies control: An overview. Rev Inf Dis. 1988;10 Suppl 672-S677.
39. Wandeler AI, Matter HC, Kappeler A, Budde A. The ecology of dogs and canine rabies: a selective review. Rev Sci Tech Off Int Epiz. 1993;12:51–71.
40. Butler JRA, Bingham J. Demography and dog-human relationships of the dog population in Zimbabwean communal lands. Vet Rec. 2000;147:442–6.
41. McCrindle CME, Cornelius ST, Schoeman HS, Gallant J. Changing roles of dogs in urban African society – a South African perspective. In: The International Association of Human-Animal Interaction Organization, editor. Human-animal interactions and zoonoses prevention and control in developing countries. Prague: WHO/IAHAIO; 1998. p. 62.
42. Van Sittert SJ, Raath J, Akol GW, Miyen JM, Mlahlwa B, Sabeta CT. Rabies in the eastern cape province of South Africa- where are we going wrong? J S Afri Vet Assoc. 2009;81:207–15.
43. Ratsitorahina M, Rasambainarivo JH, Raharimanana S, Rakotonandrasana H, Andriamiarisoa MP, Rakalomanana FA, Richard V. Dog ecology and demography in Antananarivo, 2007. BMC Vet Res. 2009;5:21. https://doi.org/10.1186/1746-6148-5-21.
44. Rautenbach GH, Boomker J, DeVilliers IL. A descriptive study of the canine population in a rural town in southern Africa. J S Afri Vet Assoc. 1991;62:158–62.
45. Kongkaew W, Coleman PG, Pfieffer DU, Chongmas A, Anyarat T. Vaccination coverage and epidemiological parameters of the owned-dog population in Thungsong District. Thailand Prev Vet Med. 2004;65:105–15.
46. Gascoyne S. Rabies in the Serengeti region of Tanzania. ODA/NRRD Animal Health Programme Final Report. London: Institute of Zoology, Regent's Park and London School of Hygiene and Tropical Medicine; 1994. p. 51.
47. Daniels TJ, Beckoff M. Population and social biology of free-ranging dogs. Canis familiaris J Mammol. 1989;70:754–62.
48. Butler JRA. Domestic dogs in communal lands: implications for CAMPFIRE schemes. CASS Occasional Paper – Natural Resource Management Series, CPN87; University of Zimbabwe, Center for Applied Social Sciences; 1997.
49. Aiyedun JO, Olugasa BO. Identification and analysis of dog use, management practices and implications for rabies control in Ilorin. Nigeria Sokoto J Vet Sci. 2012;10:1–6.

21

Effects of subclinical inflammation on C-reactive protein and haptoglobin levels as well as specific humoral immunity in dogs vaccinated against canine distemper and parvovirus

Przemysław Romiszewski[2], Krzysztof Kostro[1*] and Urszula Lisiecka[1]

Abstract

Background: The aim of the present study was to assess the effects of subclinical inflammation on specific humoral immunity in dogs vaccinated with Nobivac® DHP based on serum levels of CRP and Hp. Dogs from the group I were administered Nobivac® DHP, the vaccine against distemper, infectious hepatitis and parvovirus whereas group II animals received subcutaneous turpentine oil to induce subclinical inflammation, followed by Nobivac® DHP after 24 h. Animals in group III received only turpentine oil in the way and amount identical to that as in group II.

Results: Nobivac DHP relatively poorly induced the immune inflammatory response showing good immunogenic properties, which was evidenced by only a double increase in mean CRP and Hp levels associated with antigenic stimulation in group I. In group II, serum neutralization (SN) and haemagglutination inhibition (HI) results were quite closely correlated with serum levels of CPR and Hp.

Conclusions: Our findings suggest that the efficacy of vaccinations in dogs can be significantly affected by subclinical inflammations, which is indicated by a correlation between serum CRP and Hp levels versus antibody titres for canine distemper and parvovirus in both experimental groups of dogs (group I and II). The correlation of mean CRP and Hp values in dogs with subclinical inflammation and after vaccination with the kinetics of increasing antibody titres against distemper and parvovirus in group II dogs reflects the severity of inflammatory response and the extent of specific humoral immunity. Routine determinations of serum CRP and Hp levels as the indices of inflammation severity can be the essential biochemical markers for assessment of dogs' health in the period preceding specific immunoprophylaxis and efficacy of the vaccine.

Keywords: Dogs, Vaccine, Specific humoral immunity, Subclinical inflammation, C-reactive protein, Haptoglobin

Background

The extent and nature of post-vaccination immunity are strictly dependent on the vaccine composition and route of administration, possible suppressive effects of vaccine components and health of vaccinated animals [1, 16, 17, 19–21, 23, 24]. The efficacy of vaccinations is markedly affected by autoimmune diseases, acquired and congenital immunodeficiency, impaired hormonal profiles of immunized animals, particularly thyroid dysfunction, neoplastic diseases, infections with immunosuppressive viruses and environmental factors such as inappropriate living conditions, stress, mineral-vitamin deficiencies, food additives and immunosuppressive drugs [4, 5, 12, 15, 18, 22]. The above conditions result in increased susceptibility to infections, especially with opportunistic microorganisms, and low efficacy of properly administered specific immunoprophylaxis.

* Correspondence: krzysztof.kostro@up.lublin.pl
[1]Department of Epizootiology and Clinic of Infectious Diseases, Faculty of Veterinary Medicine, University of Life Sciences in Lublin, 20-612 Lublin, Poland

To date, the data concerning the relation between vaccination outcomes and negative effects of subclinical inflammations have not been numerous. The aim of the present study was to assess the influence of subclinical inflammation on specific humoral responses in dogs vaccinated against canine distemper and parvovirus based on serum levels of C-reactive protein (CRP) and haptoglobin (Hp).

Methods

Animals

The study encompassed 21 mongrels from a private kennel and informed consent was obtained from the owner. Dogs were chosen for the study based on clinical examinations, hematological results and parasitic status clearance. Nine dogs were excluded from the study because they failed to meet inclusion criteria.

The dogs, aged above 12 weeks, of both genders and comparable body weight, were divided into two experimental groups (group I and II) and control group (group III), 7 individuals each. Group I dogs were administered Nobivac® DHP, the vaccine against distemper, infectious hepatitis and parvovirus whereas group II animals received subcutaneous turpentine oil (1 ml/10 kg b.w.) [9] to induce subclinical inflammation, followed by Nobivac® DHP after 24 h. Animals in group III received only turpentine oil in the way and amount identical to that as in group II.

Serum levels of CRP and HP were determined in animals of group I, II and III; in group I and II, increases in specific antibodies against distemper and parvovirus were also analysed. The levels of CRP and Hp were measured on day 0, 1, 2, 3, 7, 14, 21 and 28 whereas the levels of specific antibodies against distemper and parvovirus on day 0, 7, 14, 21 and 28 after induction of inflammation and/or vaccination.

Vaccine

The polyvalent vaccine Nobivac® DHP (Intervet) was used containing attenuated strains of canine distemper virus (CDV) (strain Onderstepoort), canine adenovirus type 2 (CAV2) and canine parvovirus (CPV) (strain Manhattan LPV 3). The vaccine was administered according to the manufacturer's recommendations.

Acute phase proteins (APPs)

Serum levels of CRP were determined using ELISA (Canine CRP, Tridelta Dev.t Ltd., Ireland) and of Hp using non-species specific, colorimetric assay for the determination of haptoglobin (Tridelta Dev.t Ltd.,). The concentration of CRP was expressed in μg/ml and of Hp in mg/ml.

Specific humoral response

The titres of specific antibodies in serum were determined by the β-seroneutralisation (SN) test on Nunc microplates (Denmark) using the increasing twofold dilutions of sera previously thermally inactivated at 56 °C/30 min. Each serum dilution was mixed with a constant dose of parvovirus (100 $CCID_{50}$), stored at 4 °C for 48 h and at 37 °C for 1 h. The mixture was applied to inoculate the continuous line cells CCC clone 81, using 8 plate wells per each serum dilution. The SN titres were determined based on the inverse of the highest serum dilution resulting in cytopathic effect inhibition for 50% of inoculated cell cultures.

The levels of antibodies inhibiting haemagglutination directed against parvovirus were determined with the β haemagglutination inhibition (HI) method using increasing twofold dilutions of sera mixed with 4 units of HA virus. Non-specific haemagglutination inhibitors (NSIs) and natural haemagglutinins were removed by thermal inactivation of sera (56 °C for 30 min.), absorption with 25% kaolin and saturation with pig erythrocytes.

Results were statistically analysed by calculating a mean and standard deviation; significance of intergroup differences was verified using the Duncan's test and SAS software.

Results

CRP and Hp levels

In group I, mean serum levels of CRP and Hp on day 0 were low (Fig. 1); a significant increase in CRP ($P < 0.01$) was observed between post-vaccination day 1 and 7 as compared to baseline values, with the highest mean value (18.1 ± 1.7) found on post-vaccination day 1. Mean CRP values at the final two measurement points were significantly lower ($P < 0.01$) than baseline values. The statistically significant ($P < 0.01$) and highest increase in serum Hp levels was noted on post-vaccination day 3. Mean Hp levels at the final four measurement points were comparable to baseline values (Fig. 1).

In group II, a statistically significant ($P < 0.01$) CRP increase was observed between day 1 and 14 after experimentally induced inflammation and vaccination (Fig. 2). The highest mean values of CRP were noted on day 1, 2 and 3, i.e. 80.4 ± 3.2, 81.4 ± 1.9 and 79.7 ± 2.2 μg/ml, respectively. At the final two measurement points, mean concentrations of CRP were comparable to baseline values. Mean values of Hp in this group were comparable to baseline ones for 3 consecutive days to increase significantly ($P < 0.05$) on day 7 (Fig. 2). On day 14, Hp reached the maximum value (1.9 ± 0.1 mg/ml) and subsequently gradually decreased, yet remained higher throughout the experiment compared to day 0.

In the group with experimentally induced inflammation (group III), the mean CRP value on day 0 was found to be low – 5.1 ± 0.4 μg/ml (Fig. 3). The maximum and statistically significant CRP level ($P < 0.01$) compared to the

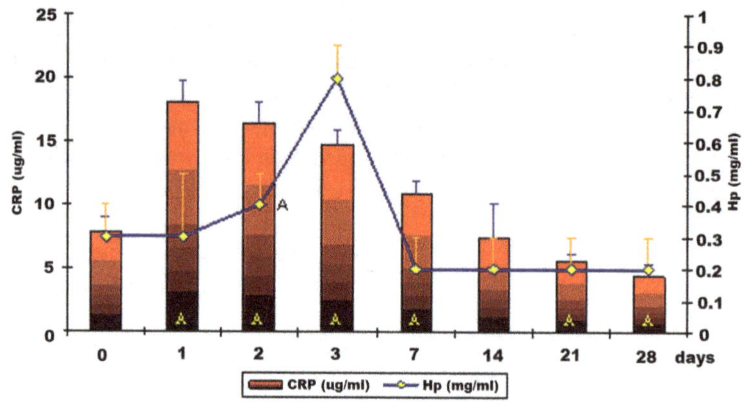

Fig. 1 Serum levels of CRP and Hp in dogs vaccinated with Nobivac® DHP (α+/− SD) (group I). A – statistically significant differences compared to baseline values ($P < 0.01$)

baseline one was observed on post-induction day 1 (106.3 ± 7.8 μg/ml). Subsequently, its mean concentration gradually decreased and on the last observation day it was lower than the baseline value. Furthermore, a significant increase in Hp ($P < 0.01$) in this group was noticed on post-induction day 2 reaching its highest mean value at the next measurement point (2.1 ± 0.1 mg/ml). Subsequently, mean Hp values decreased albeit remained significantly higher ($P < 0.01$) than baseline values (Fig. 3) at each measurement point.

SN and HA titres

Positive titres of antibodies neutralising distemper and inhibiting haemagglutination of parvovirus were observed on post-Nobivac® DHP day 7 in all dogs of both experimental groups; at the next measurement points they further gradually increased (Figs. 4 and 5). However, there were significant differences in positive SN and HI results between group I and II at all measurement points; their magnitude was correlated with serum levels of CRP and Hp. During the entire observation period, the highest SN and HI titres in group I and II were found on post-vaccination day 28. The kinetics of increases in titres of SN and HI antibodies in both experimental groups was similar yet their mean values were significantly lower ($P < 0.01$) in group II at each measurement point (Figs. 4 and 5).

Discussion

Our study demonstrated that serum levels of CRP and Hp could reflect the degree of activation of the immune system in dogs with induced inflammation or with inflammation and after vaccination. It is however difficult to compare the obtained results as the literature lacks any data regarding the usefulness of determinations of acute phase proteins (APPs) as sensitive markers of the severity of asymptomatic inflammation in dogs. Low mean levels of CRP and Hp, within the physiological range, in dogs before Nobivac® DHP administration (day 0) indicate that dogs in the period preceding vaccinations were healthy and their immune system was not activated. A twofold increase in mean serum levels

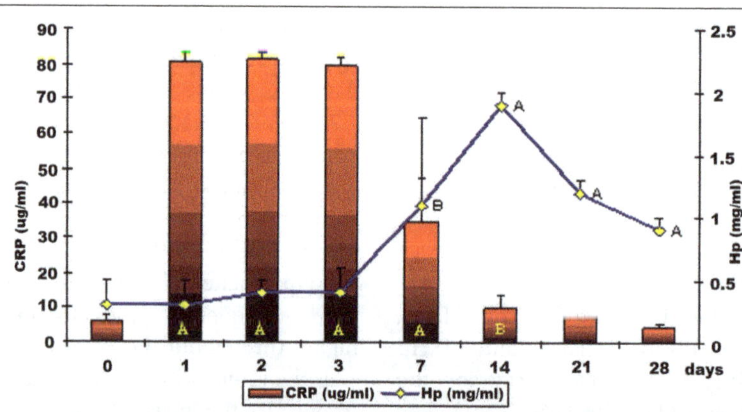

Fig. 2 Serum levels of CRP and Hp in dogs with subclinical inflammation and vaccinated with Nobivac® DPH (α+/− SD) (group II). A – statistically significant differences compared to baseline values ($P < 0.01$). B – statistically significant differences compared to baseline values ($P < 0.05$)

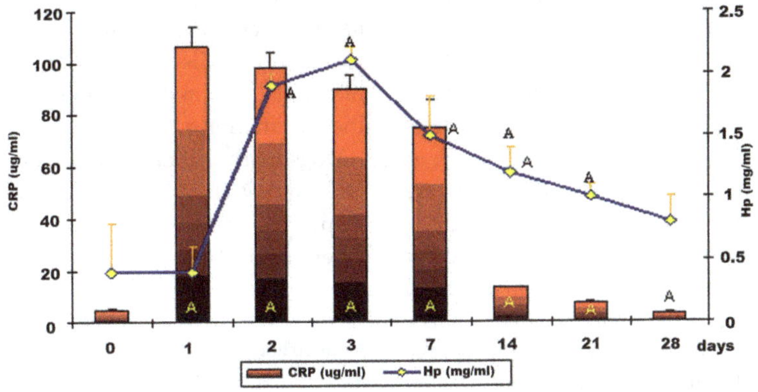

Fig. 3 Serum levels of CRP and Hp in dogs with subclinical inflammation (group III) (α+/− SD). A – statistically significant differences compared to baseline values ($P < 0.01$)

of these proteins during the first post-vaccination week evidences the existence of immune response. The correlation of CRP and Hp changes after vaccination with the kinetics of increasing titres of antibodies reflects the enhancement of inflammatory response associated with antigenic stimulation. However, Nobivac® DHP relatively poorly induced the inflammatory immune response, showing good immunogenic properties at the same time (Figs. 1, 4 and 5). The above finding was also confirmed by Yule et al. [24]. They observed that increased CRP and Hp levels after challenge in dogs earlier immunised against parvovirus were inversely proportional to the extent of specific immunity, which either evidences poor immunogenic properties of the vaccine or presence of persisting immunosuppression which developed prior to immunisation. Thus, serum levels of CRP and Hp, reflecting the immune system activation can be the main biochemical markers to assess the dogs' health in the period preceding specific immunoprophylaxis and efficacy of the vaccine used.

The efficacy of vaccinations is likely to be markedly affected by subclinical inflammations, which is indicated by the correlation between serum CRP and Hp levels and specific humoral immunity against distemper and parvovirus. The maximum serum levels of CRP on day 1 and of Hp on day 3 after experimental induction of inflammation observed in controls demonstrate that CRP is the major whereas Hp a moderate APP in dogs [2, 3, 6, 7, 11, 13], which is additionally confirmed by the results in dogs with inflammation and after vaccination (group II, Fig. 2). In group II, significantly higher mean values of these proteins than baseline values were observed until day 14 (CRP) and 28 (Hp) whereas in group III until day 21 (CRP) and 28 (Hp), which resulted from long-term subclinical inflammation induced with administration of intramuscular turpentine oil. From Figs. 1 and 2, the conclusion could be drawn that in group I the mean values of CRP and Hp concentrations on the first and the third day of the experiment were 4 fold decreased comparing with group II values. In both groups, the kinetics of the immune response was not similar and the mean values of both Hp and CRP concentrations differed significantly between group I and II. In the final stage of the experiment the mean

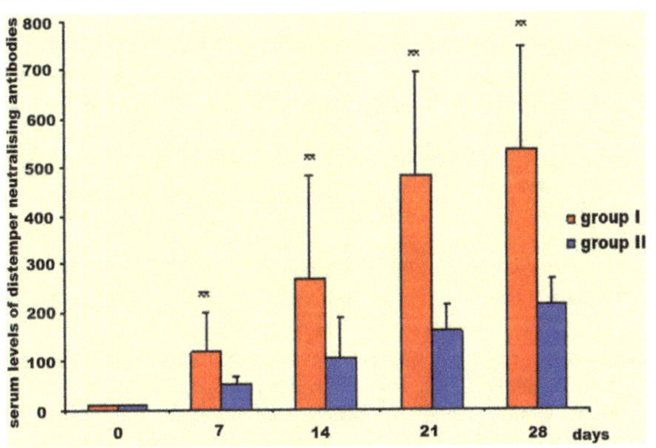

Fig. 4 Serum levels of distemper neutralising antibodies in group I and II (α ± SD). Intergroup comparison at the same time intervals. ** - $P < 0.01$

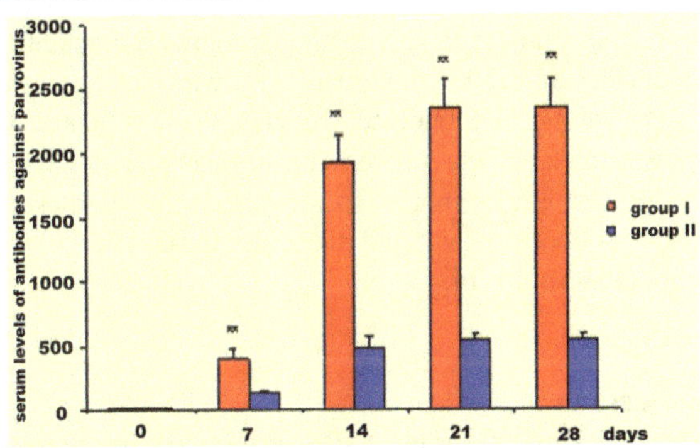

Fig. 5 Serum levels of parvovirus haemagglutination inhibiting antibodies in group I and II (α ± SD). Intergroup comparison at the same time intervals. ** - $P < 0.01$

CRP values were congenial in both group I and II. However the mean values of Hp in group II were significantly higher than in group I till the end of the study which can be connected with interference of inflammatory process caused by turpentine oil with the effect of Nobivac® DHP vaccine.

The increases in CRP and Hp in group II and III are likely to be associated with their involvement in the regulation of inflammatory immune response and repair of inflammation-injured tissues [9, 13]. Normalisation of CRP concentrations in group II, which did not occur until the final two measurement points, reflects the gradual subsidence of inflammation. Thus, monitoring of serum CRP and Hp levels in dogs with subclinical inflammation and vaccinated against distemper and parvovirus, may be helpful to assess the efficacy of biopreparations.

The induction of specific immune response in dogs with experimentally induced inflammation and immunised against distemper and parvovirus was confirmed by SN and HI titres (Figs. 4 and 5). Immunosuppression develops during inflammation due to increased percentages of TCD8$^+$ suppressor lymphocytes and direct inhibitory effects on Th1 cells producing cytokines supporting the specific humoral immunity. In the final study period, on the other hand, the SN and HI test results in group II were found to reach the highest values in the entire experiment. This can be explained by the subsidence of inflammation inhibiting the specific humoral immune response and Th2 dominance in this period, which is confirmed by the results in group I dogs which were administered the vaccine. During the subsidence of inflammation in group II dogs, there was a relatively close correlation between SN and HI results versus serum levels of CRP and Hp. The above proteins, exerting both pro- and anti-inflammatory effects, are involved in immune response regulation [13, 14]. Low levels of CRP enhance the proliferation of lymphocytes whereas its high concentrations inhibit lymphocyte blastogenesis [14]. Moreover, Hp, as an active ligand for CD11b/CD18 integrins, inhibits multinuclear cell migration and, once released due to their activation, inhibits the activity of granulocytes infiltrating the inflammatory focus. High levels of Hp inhibit lymphocyte blastogenesis, chemotaxis, phagocytosis and the process of intracellular killing in granulocytes. Furthermore, Hp modulates the synthesis of specific antibodies by regulating the proliferation of B lymphocytes [8, 10, 14].

Conclusions

Determinations of serum CRP and Hp as markers of inflammation, introduced to routine diagnostic procedures, broaden the possibilities of canine health monitoring in the period preceding specific immunoprophylaxis.

Inflammation, even subclinical, can result in the development of an immunological risk group, in which vaccination fails to provide sufficient immunity and individual vaccination schemes are required to increase the vaccination efficacy.

Dogs with subclinical inflammation vaccinated with Nobivac® DHP tend to have weakened humoral immune responses, which can lead to shortened duration and extent of post-vaccination immunity.

Abbreviations

CAV2: Canine adenovirus type 2; CDV: Canine distemper virus; CPV: Canine parvovirus; CRP: C-reactive protein; Hp: Haptoglobin

Acknowledgements

Not applicable.

Funding

No funding was obtained for this study.

Authors' contributions

PR and KK designed the experiment and drafted the manuscript; PR, KK and UL collected and analyzed samples and performed the statistical analysis of the results. All authors read and approved the final manuscript.

Consent for publication

Not applicable.

Competing interests

The authors declare that they have no competing interests.

Author details

[1]Department of Epizootiology and Clinic of Infectious Diseases, Faculty of Veterinary Medicine, University of Life Sciences in Lublin, 20-612 Lublin, Poland. [2]Animal Medical Center, 5255 York Rd, P.O. Box. 324, Holicong, PA 18928, USA.

References

1. Carpenter JW, Appel MJ, Erickson RC, Novilla MN. Fatal vaccine-induced canine distemper virus infection in black-footed ferrets. J Am Vet Med Assoc. 1976;169:961–4.
2. Ceron JJ, Eckersall PD, Martinez-Subiela S. Acute phase proteins in dogs and cats: current knowledge and future perspectives. Vet Clin Pathol. 2005;34:85–99.
3. Cray C, Zaias J, Altman NH. Acute phase response in animals: a review. Comp Med. 2009;59:517–26.
4. Dąbrowski R, Wawron W, Kostro K. Changes in CRP, SAA and haptoglobin produced in response to ovariohysterectomy in healthy bitches and those with pyometria. Theriogenology. 2007;67:321–7
5. Dąbrowski R, Kostro K, Lisiecka U, Szczubiał M, Krakowski L. Usefulness of C-reactive protein, serum amyloid a komponent, and haptoglobin determinations in bitches with pyometra for monitoring early post-ovariohysterectomy complications. Theriogenology. 2009;72:471–6.
6. Dąbrowski R, Kostro K, Szczubiał M. Concentrations of C-reactive protein, serum amyloid a, and haptoglobin in uterine arterial and peripheral blood in bitches with pyometra. Theriogenology. 2013;80:494–7.

7. Eckersall PD, Bell R. Biomarkers of infection and inflammation in veterinary medicine. Vet J. 2010;185:23–7.
8. Georgieva TM, Zapryanova D, Nikiforov I, Denev SA. Plasdma C-reactive protein concentration in dogs with experimentally-induced *Staphylococcus aureus* infection. Revue Med Vet. 2013;164:156–61.
9. Hayashi S, Jinbo T, Iguchi K, Shimizu M, Shimada T, Nomura Y, Ishida Y, Yamamoto S. A comparison of the concentrations of C-reactive protein and α1-acid glycoprotein in the serum of young and adult dogs with acute inflammation. Vet Res Comm. 2001;25:117–26.
10. Huntoon KM, Wang Y, Eppolito CA, Barbour KW, Berger FG, Shrikant PA, Baumann H. The acute phase protein haptoglobin regulates host immunity. J Leukoc Biol. 2008;84:1–12.
11. Jain S, Gautam V, Naseem S. Acute-phase proteins: as diagnostic tool. J Pharm Bioallied Sci. 2011;3:118–27.
12. Kherli ME, Burton JL, Nonnecke BJ, Lee EK. Effects of stress on leukocyte trafficking and immune responses: implications for vaccination. Adv Vet Med. 1999;41:61–81.
13. Kostro K, Gliński Z, Wojcicka-Lorenowicz K, Krakowski L. Acute-phase proteins as indicators of diseases in animals. Medycyna Wet. 2001;57:539–44.
14. Kostro K, Wojcicka-Lorenowicz K, Gliński Z, Krakowski L, Wrona Z. Acute phase proteins as ligands of cells of the immune system. Medycyna Wet. 2002;58:929–33.
15. Kurzawa H, Wysocka M, Aruga E, Chang AE, Trinchieri G, Lee WM. Recombinant interleukin 12 enhances cellular immune responses to vaccination only after a period of suppression. Cancer Res. 1998;58:491–9.
16. Miyamoto T, Taura Y, Une S, Yoshitake M, Nakama S, Watanabe S. Immunological responses after vaccination pre- and post-surgery in dogs. J Vet Med Sci. 1995;57:29–32.
17. Miyamoto T, Taura Y, Une S, Yoshitake M, Nakama S, Watanabe S. Immunological responses to polyvalent canine vaccines in dogs. J Vet Med Sci. 1995;57:347–9.
18. Pardo MC, Tanner P, Bauman J. Immunization of puppies in the presence of maternally derived antibodies against canine distemper virus. J Comp Pathol. 2007;137:572–5.
19. Phillips TR, Schultz RD. Failure of vaccine or virulent strains of canine parvovirus to induce immunosuppressive effects of the immune system of the dog. Viral Immunol. 1987;1:135–43.
20. Spibey N, Greenwood NM, Sutton D. Canine parvovirus type 2 vaccine protects against virulent challenge with type 2c virus. Vet Microbiol. 2008; 128:48–55.
21. Strasser A, May B, Teltscher A, Wistrela E, Niedermuller H. Immune modulation following immunization with polyvalent vaccines in dogs. Vet Immunol Immunopathol. 2003;94:113–21.
22. Taura Y, Ishi KS, Nagami M, Mikasa N, Nakaichi M, Nakama S. Changes in lymphocyte proliferation and DTH responses after vaccination immediately before surgery in puppies. J Vet Med Sci. 1995;57:899–904.
23. Yousfi ME, Mercier S, Breuille D, Denis F, Papet I, Mirand PP, Obled C. The inflammatory response to vaccination is altered in the elderly. Mech Ageing Dev. 2005;126:874–81.
24. Yule TD, Roth MB, Dreier K, Johnson AF, Palmer-Densmore M, Simmons K, Fanton R. Canine parvovirus vaccine elicits protection from the inflammatory and clinical consequences of the disease. Vaccine. 1997;15:720–6.

22

Transcriptomics of *Haemophilus* (*Glässerella*) *parasuis* serovar 5 subjected to culture conditions partially mimetic to natural infection for the search of new vaccine antigens

Álvaro Álvarez-Estrada, César B. Gutiérrez-Martín*, Elías F. Rodríguez-Ferri and Sonia Martínez-Martínez

Abstract

Background: *Haemophilus* (*Glässerella*) *parasuis* is the etiological agent of Glässer's disease in pigs. Control of this disorder has been traditionally based on bacterins. The search for alternative vaccines has focused mainly on the study of outer membrane proteins. This study investigates the transcriptome of *H.* (*G.*) *parasuis* serovar 5 subjected to in vitro conditions mimicking to those existing during an infection (high temperature and iron-restriction), with the aim of detecting the overexpression of genes coding proteins exposed on bacterial surface, which could represent good targets as vaccine candidates.

Results: The transcriptomic approach identified 13 upregulated genes coding surface proteins: TbpA, TbpB, HxuA, HxuB, HxuC, FhuA, FimD, TolC, an autotransporter, a protein with immunoglobulin folding domains, another large protein with a tetratricopeptide repeat and two small proteins that did not contain any known domains. Of these, the first six genes coded proteins being related to iron extraction.

Conclusion: Six of the proteins have already been tested as vaccine antigens in murine and/or porcine infection models and showed protection against *H.* (*G.*) *parasuis*. However, the remaining seven have not yet been tested and, consequently, they could become useful as putative antigens in the prevention of Glässer's disease. Anyway, the expression of this seven novel vaccine candidates should be shown in other serovars different from serovar 5.

Keywords: *Haemophilus* (*Glässerella*) *parasuis*, Glässer's disease, Vaccine antigens, RNA-sequencing, Transcriptome, Iron uptake

Background

Haemophilus (*Glässerella*) *parasuis* is a Gram-negative bacterium which forms part of the microbiota in the upper respiratory tract in pigs. Under certain conditions, such as stress or absence of prior contact, virulent strains can cause a systemic infection resulting in polyserositis, meningitis or arthritis (Glasser's disease) [1]. In addition, *H.* (*G.*) *parasuis* is involved in pneumonias as secondary agent within the porcine respiratory complex disease [2]. Each year *H.* (*G.*) *parasuis* causes significant loss to the swine industry worldwide [1].

Most vaccines used to prevent *H.* (*G.*) *parasuis* infection are bacterins although a minory of them are based on live vaccines. These traditional vaccines present several disadvantages, with the main one being the lack of cross-protection against different serotypes [3]. The use of these vaccines has been gradually replaced by subunit vaccines, whose study has been focused on outer membrane proteins (Omps) among other molecules. However, a huge variability has been still found among isolates from different countries, with substantial variations in MLST profiles, in such a manner that problems

* Correspondence: cbgutm@unileon.es
Microbiology & Immunology Section, Animal Health Department, Faculty of Veterinary Medicine, University of León, León, Spain

with cross-protection remain [4]. Recent advances in genomics, proteomics and transcriptomics have greatly enabled the search for Omps that are more likely to behave as good vaccine antigens [5].

Most bacteria remodel their coating structures inside the host since they need to adapt to new environments that could be potentially harmful to them, such as high temperature, osmolarity, pH or oxidative stress and these changes often involve the synthesis of surface structures that are important virulence factors [6]. It has been speculated that the change from a physiological temperature to a higher one (similar to that hyperthermia measured during Glässer's disease) in the host could also be used by some pathogens as a signal to enter into a persistence state in animals that leads to expression of mechanisms triggered during hyperthermia, used to avoid the host immune response. Some of them may correspond to changes in bacterial surface proteins [7].

Although iron is an essential element for organisms, being required for energy processes and DNA, protein or sugar metabolism; however, the concentration of free iron in the host is not enough to support the growth of bacteria [8]. For this reason, pathogenic bacteria have developed different mechanisms to scanvenge iron from host (siderophores, hemophores or host-molecule-binding proteins), which involve the expression of surface-exposed proteins [9]. In this respect, some reports have already concerned the expression of genes of *H.* (*G.*) *parasuis* to iron-restriction stress [10–12].

The aim of this work was to study the modifications which occur in the transcriptome of *H.* (*G.*) *parasuis* by RNA sequencing, when it is grown in vitro under culture conditions of iron-restriction and temperature stresses. These conditions were selected in order to partially mimic the host environment during natural infection. The transcriptome of bacteria grown under these conditions was compared with that of bacteria grown under optimal in vitro conditions (37 °C and non-iron-restriction stress) for detecting the overexpression of genes coding proteins exposed on the bacterial surface.

Results

Quality control of RNA samples

The RNA integrity from each sample was tested by automated electrophoresis in a Bioanalyzer Agilent 2100. The RNA integrity number (RIN) was not calculated because of the peculiar arrangement of the rRNA peaks from bacteria belonging to genus *Haemophilus* [22], in which the 23S subunit of the rRNA is fragmented in 1.2 and 1.7 kb portions. However, the graphs showed that the RNA present in each sample had A correct integrity (data not shown).

Upregulation under mimetic conditions (iron-restriction and 41 °C)

The number of genes upregulated under these conditions was 433, of which 154 had a $log_2 > 10$. Among these 154, there were eight pseudogenes, two genes encoding tRNA and 144 genes encoding proteins (Fig. 1). The amino acid sequence of the proteins encoded by the upregulated genes was obtained, and the cellular location of the proteins and their relation to pathogenesis was investigated. Four extracellular proteins (Eps), 17 Omps, 10 periplasmic proteins (Pps), 13 inner membrane proteins (Imps) and 100 cytoplasmic proteins (Cps) were found using CELLO v.2.5. As the main aim of this study was to search the proteins exposed to the cell surface, we verified individually the location of those proteins that CELLO assigned as belonging to the extracellular and Omp fractions and they were found different. Thus, two of the proteins firstly assigned to Omps were found to be Imps, while three others were Pps and two more were Cps. One of the Eps and another protein initially assigned to Omps appeared to be really the same extracellular protein but they were noted as two different proteins in the reference genome because of a point mutation involving the emergence of a stop codon. Therefore, after this correction, four proteins remained assigned to an extracellular localization (Eps), nine as Omps, 15 as Imps, 13 as Pps and 102 as Cps (Fig. 1).

A total of 31 proteins were recognized as being related to pathogenesis and therefore possibly involved in the pathogenesis of Glässer's disease (Fig. 1), and of them, four were Eps, nine were Omps, six were Imps, five were Pps and seven were Cps. All proteins predicted to be located on the bacterial surface were also predicted as being related to pathogenesis.

Table 1 shows the upregulated proteins that were predicted to be located on the bacterial surface (Omps or Eps) and/or related to pathogenesis. The proteins predicted to be located on the bacterial surface or related to pathogenes is that were not identified in GenBank and Uniprot databases were subjected to further studies of sequence homology and searched for the presence of domains of a known function. The findings are shown in Table 2. Additional file 1 summarizes the findings for genes that were upregulated under mimetic conditions with a log_2 (fold change) > 10.

Downregulation under mimetic conditions (without iron-restriction and 37 °C)

The number of genes underexpressed under control conditions was 460, of which 187 were selected for having a $log_2 > 10$. They included four pseudogenes, seven genes encoding tRNA, another gene encoding rRNA and 175 genes encoding proteins (Fig. 2). The CELLO v.2.5 program predicted six Eps, five Omps, 34 Imps, 30 Pps

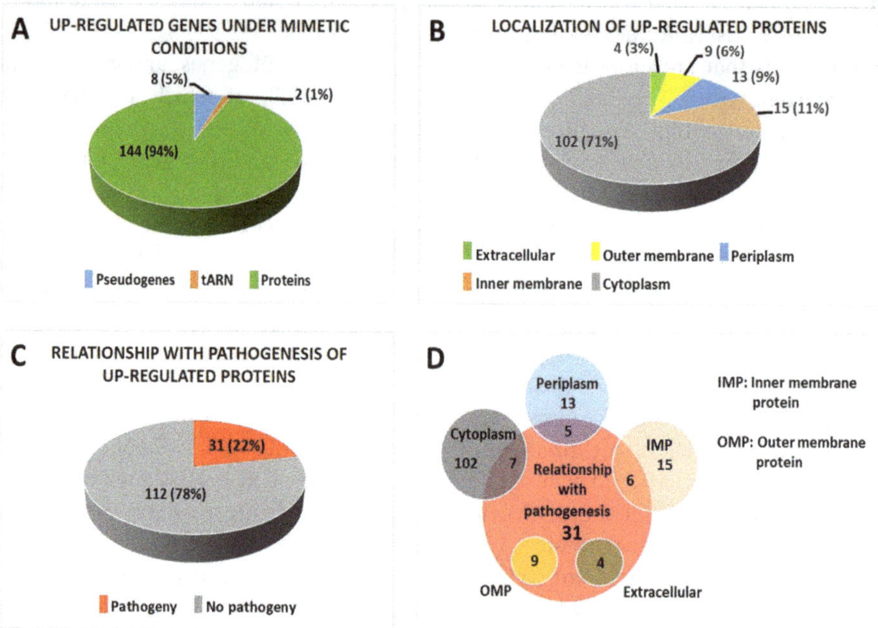

Fig. 1 Genes and proteins upregulated under mimetic conditions. **(a)**: Number of pseudogenes, tRNA and protein-coding genes indicating the percentage of the total number of upregulated genes with $\log_2$ (fold change) > 10 under mimetic conditions. **(b)**: Number of different locations of proteins upregulated under mimetic conditions and percentage of total proteins. Further corrections were taken into account. **(c)**: Number and percentage of proteins related to pathogenesis upregulated under mimetic conditions. Further corrections were considered. **(d)**: Venn diagram representing the relationship between cell localization and the pathogenesis of upregulated proteins. Further corrections were taken into account

and 100 Cps. Those assigned as Omps or Eps were individually rechecked and, after correction, four proteins remained assigned as Omps wihle the number of Cps rose to 101 (Fig. 2). The MP3 server found 34 proteins that were recognized as being related to pathogenesis (Fig. 2), of which five were Eps, three were Omps, 13 were Imps, eight were Pps and five were Cps. Additional file 2 summarizes findings for genes that were downregulated under mimetic conditions with a log2 > 10.

Gene ontology (GO) term enrichment analysis

Among the genes upregulated under mimetic conditions, only the GO term GO:0003676 (nucleic acid binding) was found to be enriched and associated with the presence in 37 upregulated genes (Table 3). With regard to genes downregulated under mimetic conditions, 31 GO terms were classified as being enriched (Table 4).

Discussion

Most bacteria reshape their coating structures inside the host since they need to adapt to a new potentially harmful environment [6]. Although the environment that a microorganism endures inside the host is much more complex than that replicated in the laboratory, the two selected conditions in this study (iron-restriction and temperature higher than 37 °C) attempted to partially simulate the infection in natural conditions. Some reports have been carried out on the changes occurring in the *H. (G.) parasuis* transcriptome when this bacterium was subjected to these two mimetic conditions of high temperature and iron scarcity [10, 12, 23]. However, the two circumstances in those studies were not tested together because these studies were focused in the understanding of both metabolism and virulence factors but not to search putative candidates that could be used as vaccine antigens.

The bacterial mechanisms used to remove iron from the host need surface-exposed proteins [9], and their expression is induced by a low iron concentration [24]. Among the genes upregulated under mimetic conditions, we detected six genes coding for Eps or Omps related to the obtaining of iron from the host (TbpA, TbpB, HxuA, HxuB, HxuC and FhuA). In a previous study of the transcriptome of *H. (G.) parasuis* exposed to the intraalveolar environment for two hours, upregulation of genes encoding membrane proteins involved in iron uptake were detected [25]. This finding reinforces our results concerning the high probability that the six above mentioned genes will be overexpressed during infection with *H. (G.) parasuis*.

TbpA and TbpB are porcine transferrin binding proteins that show different protection degrees against Glässer's disease [26, 27]. HxuA, HxuB and HxuC correspond to hemophore, transporter and receptor of the heme/hemopexin-binding protein (hxu) operon, respectively

Table 1 Upregulated proteins under mimetic conditions related to pathogenesis and located on the bacterial surface

Locus[a]	GenBank product	Access number Uniprot	Name Uniprot	Pathogenesis	Location
HAPS_RS00370	protein TolA	B8F375	|tolA|Cell envelope integrity inner membrane protein TolA	P	IM
HAPS_RS00485	TonB-dependent receptor	–	–	P	OM
HAPS_RS00735	hypothetical protein	–	–	P	OM
HAPS_RS00740[a]	autotransporter domain-containing protein	–	–	P	OM[a]
HAPS_RS00745[a]	hypothetical protein	–	–	P	EX
HAPS_RS01255	ABC transporter permease	B8F3P0	|HAPS_0253|ABC-type nitrate/sulfonate/bicarbonate transport permease	P	IM
HAPS_RS01260	ABC transporter substrate-binding protein	B8F3P1	|HAPS_0254|ABC-type nitrate/sulfonate/bicarbonate transport systems periplasmic components protein	P	CP
HAPS_RS01265	ABC transporter ATP-binding protein	B8F3P2	|HAPS_0255|ABC-type nitrate/sulfonate/bicarbonate transport system, ATPase	P	IM
HAPS_RS01400	sulfurtransferase FdhD	–	–	P	CP
HAPS_RS01435	hypothetical protein	B8F3S4	|HAPS_0289|Uncharacterized protein	P	CP
HAPS_RS01805	ABC transporter ATPase	B8F3Z5	|HAPS_0364|ATPase components of ABC transporters with duplicated ATPase domains-containing protein	P	PP
HAPS_RS01895	hypothetical protein	B8F410	|HAPS_0382|Uncharacterized protein	P	EX
HAPS_RS02610	hypothetical protein	B8F4D5	|purL|Phosphoribosylformylglycinamidine synthase	P	CP
HAPS_RS03735	fimbrial usher protein	–	–	P	OM
HAPS_RS04480	hypothetical protein	–	–	P	PP
HAPS_RS04485	hypothetical protein	B8F5E9	|HAPS_0923|Uncharacterized protein	P	EX
HAPS_RS06520	hypothetical protein	B8F6H3	|yaaH|Permease, Inner membrane protein yaaH	P	IM
HAPS_RS00370	protein TolA	B8F375	|tolA|Cell envelope integrity inner membrane protein TolA	P	IM
HAPS_RS00485	TonB-dependent receptor	–	–	P	OM
HAPS_RS00735	hypothetical protein	–	–	P	OM
HAPS_RS00740[a]	autotransporter domain-containing protein	–	–	P	OM
HAPS_RS00745[a]	hypothetical protein	–	–	P	EX
HAPS_RS06610	cell envelope protein TonB	B8F6J2	|tonB|Protein TonB	P	PP
HAPS_RS07630	iron ABC transporter permease	B8F723	|hmuU|Hemin transport system permease protein HmuU	P	IM
HAPS_RS07950	hypothetical protein	–	–	P	CP
HAPS_RS09000	hypothetical protein	B8F7Q0	|HAPS_1850|Uncharacterized protein	P	IM
HAPS_RS10195	DUF262 domain-containing protein	B8F899	|HAPS_2100|Uncharacterized protein	P	CP
HAPS_RS10530	TolC family protein tolC	B8F8F2	|tolC|RND efflux system outer membrane lipoprotein/RND superfamily resistance-nodulation-cell division antiporter	P	OM
HAPS_RS10585	ligand-gated channel	B8F8G2	|hxuC|Heme/hemopexin utilization protein C/outer membrane receptor protein, mostly Fe transport	P	OM
HAPS_RS10590	ShlB/FhaC/HecB family hemolysin secretion/activation protein	B8F8G3	|hxuB|Heme/hemopexin-binding protein B, hemolysin activation/secretion protein	P	OM
HAPS_RS10595	hypothetical protein	B8F8G4	|hxuA|Heme/hemopexin-binding protein A (Heme:hemopexin utilization protein A)	P	EX
HAPS_RS10780	membrane protein	B8F8J9	|HAPS_2219|Possible outer membrane protein/FOG: TPR repeat protein	P	OM
HAPS_RS10800	transferrin-binding protein-like solute binding protein	–	–	P	OM

Table 1 Upregulated proteins under mimetic conditions related to pathogenesis and located on the bacterial surface *(Continued)*

Locus[a]	GenBank product	Access number Uniprot	Name Uniprot	Pathogenesis	Location
HAPS_RS10805	lactoferrin/transferrin family TonB-dependent receptor	B8F8K4	|tbpA|Transferrin-binding protein 1	P	OM
HAPS_RS11010	transpeptidase	B8F8P5	|HAPS_2267|Uncharacterized protein	P	PP
HAPS_RS11030	transcriptional regulator	B8F8P9	|impA|SOS-response transcriptional repressor	P	CP

P indicates the relationship to pathogenesis; Locations are indicated by: *OM* outer membrane, *EX* extracellular, *IM* inner membrane, *PP* periplasmic, *CP* cytoplasmic. The *locus* in the reference genome (SH0165 strain) is indicated. [a] indicates that this was a single protein recognized as two different ones.

[28]. A protection of 87.5% for HxuC, 62.5% for HxuB and 37.5% for HxuA has been recently showed in mice against *H. (G.) parasuis* [29]. The upregulated gene *HAPS_RS00485*, coding for FhuA protein, a receptor for siderophores, has not been tested as vaccine antigen until date [30]. Curiously, Melnikow et al. [10] did not find *fhuA* among the genes upregulated under iron-restrictive conditions. One possible explanation for the difference between this study and ours could be that the combination of both conditions is required for upregulation of this gene.

Depending on the bacterial species, fever could cause a heat stress [31] that triggered changes involving coating structures [6]. It would be therefore expected that the reprogramming of the transcriptome undergone by the bacterium to resist heat stress could affect some genes encoding for surface-exposed proteins. The upregulated gene *tolC* found in this study encodes an Omp (TolC) lipoprotein that forms a trimeric channel and acts in the transport of several molecules [32]. Li et al. [33] observed that mice immunized with this protein and then challenged with *H. (G.) parasuis* showed a survival rate of 80%.

In addition to these well-characterized proteins in the databases, another five proteins were predicted to be located on the bacterial surface (Eps or Omps). The largest of them was an autotransporter with a serine protease domain which is annotated as two different genes (*HAPS_RS00740* and *HAPS_RS00745*) in the reference genome (SH0165 strain) because it presents a punctual mutation that triggers off the appearance of a stop codon. This long protein presents a broad sequence homology with the AasP autotransporter of *A. pleuropneumoniae*, which it is upregulated when this bacterium is grown under iron restriction stress [34]. On the other hand, a previous study performed with an *AasP* mutant *in A. pleuropneumoniae* showed that AasP protein is involved in adhesion under iron-restriction conditions [35].

The upregulated gene *HAPS_RS04485* codes a protein that harbors domains with an immunoglobulin-like fold, which are usually present in proteins related to invasion or adhesion in prokaryotes [36]. Among the three remaining surface proteins whose genes were upregulated, two of them (*HAPS_RS00735* and *HAPS_RS01895*) neither presented homology to known proteins nor harbored domains with a known function, while in the remaining one (*HAPS_RS10780*) only a β-barrel and a single tetratricopeptide repeat could be detected.

With regard to the functional enrichment analysis under mimetic conditions to natural infection, only one significant enrichment was observed in the GO term 0003676, corresponding to nucleic acid binding, which was found in 37 upregulated genes. This could be consistent with the important reprogramming, at both transcriptional and translational levels, which the bacteria

Table 2 Findings in upregulated proteins under mimetic conditions related to pathogenesis but not characterized in the databases

Locus	Access number Uniprot	Location	Findings
HAPS_RS00735	–	OM	Nothing was recognized
HAPS_RS00740[a]	–	OM[a]	Half C-terminal Carrier [a]
HAPS_RS00745[a]	–	EX[a]	Half n-terminal auto transporter [a]
HAPS_RS01435	B8F3S4	CP	Nothing was recognized
HAPS_RS01895	B8F410	EX	Nothing was recognized
HAPS_RS04480	–	PP	Domain of the superfamily Glycoside-hydrolase
HAPS_RS04485	B8F5E9	EX	Immunoglobulin-like fold domain
HAPS_RS07950	–	CP	Domain of the Thioredoxin-like superfamily
HAPS_RS09000	B8F7Q0	IM	Homology with permease
HAPS_RS10195	B8F899	CP	ParB-like and HNH nuclease domains

The locus in the reference genome (SH0165 strain) is also indicated. [a] indicates that this was a single protein recognized as two different ones

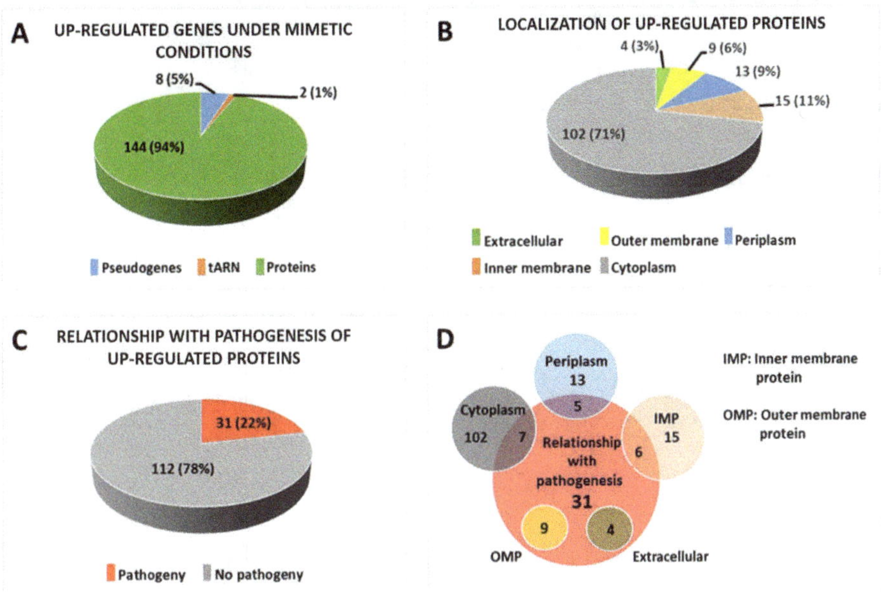

Fig. 2 Genes and proteins downregulated under mimetic conditions. **(a)**: Number of pseudogenes, tRNA and protein-coding genes indicating the percentage of the total number of genes down regulated genes with $\log_2$ (fold change) > 10 under mimetic conditions. **(b)**: Number of different locations of proteins downregulated under mimetic conditions and percentage of total proteins. Further corrections were taken into account. **(c)**: Number and percentage of proteins related to pathogenesis downregulated under mimetic conditions. Further corrections were considered. **(d)**: Venn diagram representing the relationship between cell localization and the pathogenesis of downregulated proteins. Further corrections were taken into account

Table 3 List of upregulated genes where GO term GO:0003676 (nucleic acid binding) was found

Locus	GenBank product	*Locus*	GenBank product
HAPS_RS06635	tRNA-dihydrouridine synthase	*HAPS_RS06640*	Fis family transcriptional regulator
HAPS_RS07775	30S ribosomal protein S10	*HAPS_RS07795*	50S ribosomal protein L2
HAPS_RS01040	LysR family transcriptional regulator	*HAPS_RS07785*	50S ribosomal protein L4
HAPS_RS03460	tRNA pseudouridine (65) synthase TruC	*HAPS_RS01015*	translation initiation factor IF-2
HAPS_RS07435	MurR/RpiR family transcriptional regulator	*HAPS_RS07790*	50S ribosomal protein L23
HAPS_RS02800	transcriptional regulator	*HAPS_RS10775*	ATPase AAA
HAPS_RS02140	transcriptional regulator	*HAPS_RS06525*	Holliday junction DNA helicase RuvA
HAPS_RS09580	23S rRNA (guanosine-2′-O-)-methyltransferase	*HAPS_RS07720*	RNA polymerase, beta subunit
HAPS_RS08560	restriction endonuclease	*HAPS_RS01010*	transcription termination factor NusA
HAPS_RS09560	30S ribosomal protein S7	*HAPS_RS07780*	50S ribosomal protein L3
HAPS_RS09565	elongation factor G	*HAPS_RS01395*	elongation factor Ts
HAPS_RS08275	endonuclease	*HAPS_RS02855*	single-stranded DNA-binding protein
HAPS_RS10985	Fur family transcriptional regulator	*HAPS_RS00670*	transposase
HAPS_RS02340	RNA helicase	*HAPS_RS10560*	transcriptional regulator
HAPS_RS04055	DNA polymerase III subunit epsilon	*HAPS_RS03180*	50S ribosomal protein L25
HAPS_RS01380	lysine tRNA synthetase	*HAPS_RS04045*	heat-shock protein
HAPS_RS08565	restriction endonuclease	*HAPS_RS01070*	tRNA s (4) U8 sulfurtransferase
HAPS_RS08440	transcriptional regulator	*HAPS_RS04180*	formamidopyrimidine-DNA glycosylase
HAPS_RS05455	DNA-binding protein		

The locus in the reference genome (SH0165 strain) and GenBank product are indicated

Table 4 GO terms found to be enriched among downregulated genes under mimetic conditions

GO term	GO domain	Number of genes
GO:0008643 *carbohydrate transport*	BP	16
GO:0015980 *energy derivation by oxidation of organic compounds*	BP	17
GO:0055114 *oxidation-reduction process*	BP	21
GO:0009401 *phosphoenolpyruvate-dependent sugar phosphotransferase system*	BP	13
GO:0009401 *phosphoenolpyruvate-dependent sugar phosphotransferase system*	BP	13
GO:0006091 *generation of precursor metabolites and energy*	BP	19
GO:0045333 *cellular respiration*	BP	14
GO:0006099 *tricarboxylic acid cycle*	BP	10
GO:0006099 *tricarboxylic acid cycle*	BP	10
GO:0009060 *aerobic respiration*	BP	10
GO:0044712 *single-organism catabolic process*	BP	17
GO:0044699 *single-organism process*	BP	73
GO:0005975 *carbohydrate metabolic process*	BP	25
GO:0044724 *single-organism carbohydrate catabolic process*	BP	11
GO:0044282 *small molecule catabolic process*	BP	12
GO:0016052 *carbohydrate catabolic process*	BP	11
GO:1901575 *organic substance catabolic process*	BP	18
GO:1901476 *carbohydrate transporter activity*	MF	8
GO:0015144 *carbohydrate transmembrane transporter activity*	MF	8
GO:0044765 *single-organism transport*	BP	23
GO:0009056 *catabolic process*	BP	18
GO:0005996 *monosaccharide metabolic process*	BP	10
GO:1902578 *single-organism localization*	BP	23
GO:0071702 *organic substance transport*	BP	17
GO:0044723 *single-organism carbohydrate metabolic process*	BP	17
GO:0006810 *transport*	BP	26
GO:0019318 *hexose metabolic process*	BP	8
GO:0051179 *localization*	BP	26
GO:0051234 *establishment of localization*	BP	26
GO:0044710 *single-organism metabolic process*	BP	49
GO:0046365 *monosaccharide catabolic process*	BP	5

The number of genes where each GO term was found is indicated. The gene ontology domain (GO domain) to which each GO term belongs is also indicated, *BP* biological process, *MF* molecular function

undergo when exposed to environmental stress [37]. Among these genes, six coded ribosomal subunit binding proteins, four coded rRNA-related enzymes (translational level) and eight coded transcriptional regulators (transcriptional level). Within the upregulated transcriptional regulators, the iron uptake regulatory protein (Fur) must be highlighted. This protein forms a dimer in the presence of Fe^{2+} that represses the expression of genes related to iron uptake. However, when available iron is scarce, this dimer breaks down and transcription of genes related to iron uptake is allowed [38]. The upregulation of a negative regulator of iron acquisition under iron-restricted conditions may be paradoxical effect; however, different findings have been shown over the last years that the role of Fur is not as simple as it had been previously stated although it remains fully valid. There are positively regulated genes for Fe-induced Fur dimers and other positively or negatively regulated genes for Fur when this protein does not form a complex with Fe^{2+}. Some of the genes that are regulated in these ways are related to the response to stressful conditions or to virulence [38]. Therefore, it was not unusual to find *Fur* gene among those upregulated under our stress conditions.

Concerning functional enrichment analysis of downregulated genes under mimetic conditions, the most enriched terms were related to energy metabolism, redox reactions, or to both of them. Relative to energy metabolism, this finding would make sense with slowing of growth braking expected in a stressful environment, which should result in a general decrease in the metabolism. In the case of redox processes, it might simply be a reflection of the decrease in bacterial growth and/or it could be that the microorganism, when detecting iron deficiency, prefers not to waste energy in the production of compounds that cannot perform their function since the iron is the main limiting factor [9].

As previously mentioned, microorganisms have to face a number of stressors during infection, such as unfavorable temperatures, pH changes or free radicals, which trigger the expression of several proteins known as cellular stress proteins [39]. These proteins behave as chaperones promoting the assembly of other macromolecules and are often called heat shock proteins (Hsp) since it was previously believed that they acted alone against heat stress [40]. Several genes encoding different Hsp were upregulated in our study, such as DnaJ, DnaK, HslO and HslR. Several Hsp behaving as surface antigens were observed, which might seem a contradiction considering that the role played as chaperones should imply an intracellular location. However, many of these proteins, in addition to act as chaperones, also present functions related to pathogenesis that may imply a superficial location [40]. Accordingly, it would be reasonable to study these proteins as vaccine antigens; however, it would not be appropriate to do because Hsp have been highly conserved throughout evolution and there is a high homology between the Hsp from bacterial and those from mammalian origin. For this reason, the use of Hsp as vaccine antigens could trigger autoimmune diseases [39].

Conclusion

Slowing of growth expected in stressful conditions have given rise to the upregulation of 13 *H.* (*G.*) *parasuis* genes coding for proteins located on the bacterial surface. Among them, seven proteins untested to date were detected as vaccine antigens: FhuA (encoded by *HAPS_RS00485*), a fimbrial usher protein (encoded by *HAPS_RS03735*), a long autotransporter (encoded by *HAPS_RS00740* and *HAPS_RS00745*), a protein containing domains with an Ig-like fold (encoded by *HAPS_RS04485*) and other three surface proteins without known function (encoded by *HAPS_RS10780*, *HAPS_RS00735* and *HAPS_RS01895*). These seven novel vaccine candidates could provide protection against Glässer disease, but their effectiveness have to be tried in future studies. Anyway, their expression must be sustained in other serovars different from serovar 5.

Methods

Bacterial strain and growth conditions

H. (*G.*) *parasuis* was grown under (i) in vitro optimal culture conditions (control conditions) and (ii) under in vitro growth conditions partially mimicking the host environment encountered during infection (iron-restriction and temperature stress by raising incubation temperature above 37 °C). The transcriptomes from both growths were compared by RNA sequencing to detect overexpressed genes coding proteins exposed on the bacterial surface.

For control culture conditions (without iron-restriction and 37 °C), *H.* (*G.*) *parasuis* Nagasaki strain (reference strain of serovar 5 kindly supplied by Kielstein P., Federal Institute for Health Protection of Consumers and Veterinary Medicine, Jena, Germany) was inoculated into 30 ml of PPLO broth (Conda Laboratories, Spain) with 150 μM nicotinamide adenine dinucleotide (NAD, Sigma-Aldrich, Spain) and 0.075% glucose (Sigma-Aldrich), and it was cultured at 37 °C until reaching an optical density of 0.5 at 600 nm (OD_{600}). Three replicates were made under these conditions. For mimetic conditions (iron-restriction and 41 °C), *H.* (*G.*) *parasuis* Nagasaki strain was inoculated into 30 ml of the same broth and was cultured at 41 °C until reaching an OD_{600} of 0.3. Then, iron was restricted by adding 200 μM 2 2′-dipyridyl, and the culture was grown again at 41 °C to an OD_{600} of 0.5. Three replicates were also made.

RNA extraction and sample preparation

When the appropriate OD_{600} was reached for each replicate, the culture was centrifuged at 7000×*g* and 4 °C for 7 min. The supernatants were removed and the pellets were preserved on ice. RNA extraction was performed using the High Pure RNA Isolation kit (Sigma-Aldrich) following the manufacturer's specifications. The DNA-free kit (Thermo-Fisher) was used to remove the contaminating DNA, which was verified by species-specific PCR [13], testing the absence of amplification in samples treated with DNAse. Finally, RNA concentrations were measured in a NanoDrop 1000 (Thermo-Fisher), and samples were stored at − 80 °C. The RNA integrity checking was tested using a Bioanalyzer Agilent 2100 (Agilent Technologies, Spain) from the Laboratory of Instrumental Techniques (University of León, Spain).

Library preparation and Illumina sequencing

Ribosomal RNA (rRNA) was removed from the samples using a Ribo-Zero Magnetic Kit Bacteria (Illuminia, Portugal). Libraries were then prepared following the instructions of the NEBNext Ultra Directional RNA Library Prep kit for Illumina (New England Biolabs, USA). The input of ribosome-depleted RNA to start the protocol was 10 ng quantified by an Agilent 2100 Bioanalyzer using a RNA 6000 nano LabChip kit (Agilent Technologies, Germany). The fragmentation time used was 15 min. The cDNA libraries obtained were validated and quantified by an Agilent 2100 Bioanalyzer using a DNA7500 LabChip kit (Agilent Technologies). An equimolecular pool of libraries were titrated by quantitative PCR using the Kapa-SYBR FAST qPCR kit for LightCycler480 (Kapa BioSystems, USA), and a reference standard for quantification. The pool of libraries was denatured prior to be seeded on a flowcell at a density of 2 2 pM, where clusters were formed and sequenced with a depth of 10 M using a NextSeq 500 High Output Kit (Illumin) in a 1×75 single-read sequencing run on a NextSeq 500 sequencer (Illumin).

Bioinformatic analysis of differential gene expression

Bioinformatic analysis for the RNAseq data was performed by Era7 bioinformatics (Spain) following the protocol described by Trapnell et al. [14]. Quality control of raw readings was performed with the FastQC tool (http://www.bioinformatics.babraham.ac.uk/projects/fastqc/). Alignment to the reference genome was performed using TopHat2 software, but since the genome of the Nagasaki strain has not been completely sequenced, the SH0165 strain genome (GenBank accession nr NC_011852.1), also belonging to serovar 5, was used as the reference genome. Transcripts assembly was performed with the Cufflinks tool and transcripts merge with the Cuffmerge tool. Analysis of differences in gene expression was performed with Cuffdiff. Statistical significance was considered for $p < 0.05$ (corrected by the multiple testing Benjamini-Hochberg method). Only genes with a $\log_2$ (fold change) being > 10 were considered for further analyses.

Studies of differentially expressed genes

Differentially expressed genes were subjected to search in the GenBank database to discard pseudogenes and tRNA genes. GenBank [15] and Uniprot [16] annotation was obtained to genes and proteins differentially expressed. The sequences of the proteins encoded by differentially expressed genes were obtained using QuickGo [17]. Prediction of the protein cellular location was carried out using the CELLO v 2.5 web tool (http://cello.life.nctu.edu.tw/) [18]. Proteins predicted to be related to pathogenesis were searched for using the MP3 web tool (http://metagenomics.iiserb.ac.in/mp3/index.php) [19]. Proteins that were not identified in the GenBank or Uniprot databases but were considered of interest (predicted to be found on the bacterial surface or related to pathogenesis) were subjected to a study using BLASTp in order to find orthologous proteins in related species and using GenBank or InterproScan databases [20] to find domains of a known function. Databases and BLASTp were also used to verify the protein location that CELLO assigned as belonging to the extracellular and Omp fractions.

Genes upregulated under culture mimetic conditions are referred to as "upregulated under mimetic conditions", while those genes upregulated under control conditions are referred to as "downregulated under mimetic conditions". Only genes with $\log_2$ (fold change) was > 10 blank were considered in the analysis of data.

Gene ontology (GO) term enrichment analysis

Functional enrichment analysis in terms of gene ontology (GO) of differentially expressed genes was conducted using the DAVID v 6.7 web server (https://david.ncifcrf.gov/home.jsp) [21]. Only the GO terms containing a minimum of five differentially expressed genes were considered and the GO terms that showed a $p < 0.05$ (corrected by the multiple testing Benjamini-Hochberg method) were considered significantly enriched.

Additional files

Additional file 1: Summary of genes that were upregulated under mimetic conditions with a $\log_2$ (fold change) > 10. Indicated findings in GenBank and Uniprot databases of genes that were upregulated under mimetic conditions with a $\log_2$ (fold change) > 10. P indicates that the encoded protein is related to pathogenesis, and NP indicates that there is no relationship with pathogenesis. The location of the protein is indicated with EX (extracellular), OM (outer membrane), PP (periplasmic), IM (inner membrane) or CP (cytoplasmic). * indicates that they are the same protein (PDF 117 kb).

Additional file 2: Summary of genes that were downregulated under mimetic conditions with a $\log_2$ (fold change) > 10. Indicated findings in GenBank and Uniprot databases of genes that were downregulated under mimetic conditions with a $\log_2$ (fold change) > 10. P indicates that the encoded protein is related to pathogenesis, and NP indicates that there is no relationship with pathogenesis. The location of the protein is indicated with EX (extracellular), OM (outer membrane), PP (periplasmic), IM (inner membrane) or CP (cytoplasmic). * indicates that they are the same protein (PDF 127 kb).

Abbreviations

Cps: Cytoplasmic proteins; Eps: Extracellular proteins; Fur: Ferric uptake regulatory protein; GO: Gene ontology; Hsp: Heat shock proteins; Imps: Inner membrane proteins; Omps: Outer membrane proteins; Pps: Periplasmic proteins; RNAseq: RNA-sequencing

Funding

This work was supported by project AGL2011-23195 from the Spanish Ministry of Economy and Competitivity. AAE was a recipient of long-predoctoral fellowships from this Ministry financed by the project AGL2011-23195.

Authors' contributions

AAE and SMM performed the bacterial cultures and the RNA sampling; AAE performed the study of the differentially expressed genes; AAE wrote the paper; SMM, CBGM and EFRF contributed to critical review of the manuscript. All authors read and approved the final manuscript.

Consent for publication
Not applicable.

Competing interests
The authors declare that they have no competing interests.

References

1. Nedbalcova K, Satran P, Jaglic R, Sondirasova R, Kucerova Z. *Haemophilus parasuis* and Glässer's disease in pigs: a review. Veterinar Med. 2006;51:168–79.
2. Li J, Wang S, Li C, Wang C, Liu Y, Wang G, He X, Hu L, Liu Y, Cui M, Bi C, Shao Z, Wang X, Xiong T, Cai X, Huang L, Weng C. Secondary *Haemophilus parasuis* infection enhances highly pathogenic porcine reproductive and respiratory syndrome virus (HP-PRRSV) infection-mediated inflammatory responses. Vet Microbiol. 2017;204:35–42. https://doi.org/10.1016/j.vetmic.2017.03.035.
3. Liu H, Xue Q, Zeng Q, Zhao Z. *Haemophilus parasuis* vaccines. Vet Immunol Immunopathol. 2016;180:53–8. https://doi.org/10.1016/j.vetimm.2016.09.002.
4. Ruiz A, Oliveira S, Torremorell M, Pijoan C. Outer membrane proteins and DNA profiles in strains of *Haemophilus parasuis* recovered from systemic and respiratory sites. J Clin Microbiol. 2001;39:1757–62.
5. Sette A, Rappuoli R. Reverse vaccinology: developing vaccines in the era of genomics. Immunity. 2010;33:530–41. https://doi.org/10.1016/j.immuni.2010.09.017.
6. Darwin AJ. Stress relief during host infection: the phage shock protein response supports bacterial virulence in various ways. PLoS Pathog. 2013;9:e1003388. https://doi.org/10.1371/journal.ppat.1003388.
7. González Plaza JJ, Hulak N, Zhumadilov Z, Akilzhanova A. Fever as an important resource for infectious diseases research. Intractable Rare Dis Res. 2016;5:97–102. https://doi.org/10.5582/irdr.2016.01009.
8. del Río ML, Gutiérrez Martín CB, Rodríguez Barbosa JI, Navas J, Rodríguez Ferri EF. Identification and characterization of the TonB region and its role in transferrin-mediated iron acquisition in *Haemophilus parasuis*. FEM Immunol Med Immunopathol. 2005;45:75–86.
9. Parrow NL, Fleming RE, Minnick MF. Sequestration and scavenging of iron in infection. Infect Immun. 2013;81:3503–14. https://doi.org/10.1128/IAI.00602-13.
10. Melnikow E, Dornan S, Sargent C, Duszenko M, Evans G, Gunkel N, Selzer PM, Ullrich HJ. Microarray analysis of *Haemophilus parasuis* gene expression under *in vitro* conditinos mimicking the *in vivo* environment. Vet Microbiol. 2005;110:255–63.
11. Metcalf DS, MacInnes JI. Differential expression of *Haemophilus parasuis* genes in response to iron restriction and cerebrospinal fluid. Can J Vet Res. 2007;71:181–8.
12. Xie Q, Jin H, Luo R, Wan Y, Chu J, Zhou H, Shi B, Chen H, Zhou R. Transcriptional responses of *Haemophilus parasuis* to iron-restriction stress *in vitro*. Biometals. 2009;22:907–16.
13. Oliveira S. Diagnostic notes *Haemophilus parasuis*. J Swine Health Prod J Swine Health Prod. 2007;15:99–103 http://www.aasv.org/shap.html. Accessed 21 Nov 2017.
14. Trapnell C, Hendrickson DG, Sauvageau M, Goff L, Rinn JL, Pachter L. Differential analysis of gene regulation at transcript resolution with RNA-seq. Nat Biotechnol. 2012;31:46–53. https://doi.org/10.1038/nbt.2450.
15. Benson DA, Karsch-Mizrachi I, Lipman DJ, Ostell J, Wheeler DL. GenBank. Nucleic Acids Res. 2005;33(Database issue):D34–8. https://doi.org/10.1093/nar/gki063.
16. The UniProt Consortium. UniProt: the universal protein knowledgebase. Nucleic Acids Res. 2017;45:D158–69. https://doi.org/10.1093/nar/gkw1099.
17. Binns D, Dimmer E, Huntley R, Barrell D, O'Donovan C, Apweiler R. QuickGO: a web-based tool for gene ontology searching. Bioinformatics. 2009;25:3045–6. https://doi.org/10.1093/bioinformatics/btp536.
18. Lee S, Lee B, Kim D. Prediction of protein secondary structure content using amino acid composition and evolutionary information. Prot Struct Funct Bioinform. 2005;62:1107–14. https://doi.org/10.1002/prot.20821.
19. Gupta A, Kapil R, Dhakan DB, Sharma VK. MP3: a software tool for the prediction of pathogenic proteins in genomic and metagenomic data. PLoS One. 2014;9:e93907. https://doi.org/10.1371/journal.pone.0093907.
20. Finn RD, Attwood TK, Babbitt PC, Bateman A, Bork P, Bridge AJ, et al. InterPro in 2017-beyond protein family and domain annotations. Nucleic Acids Res. 2017;45:D190–9. https://doi.org/10.1093/nar/gkw1107.
21. Huang DW, Sherman BT, Lempicki RA. Systematic and integrative analysis of large gene lists using DAVID bioinformatics resources. Nat Protoc. 2009;4:44–57. https://doi.org/10.1038/nprot.2008.211.
22. Song XM, Forsgren A, Janson H. Fragmentation heterogeneity of 23S ribosomal RNA in *Haemophilus* species. Gene. 1999;230:287–93 http://www.ncbi.nlm.nih.gov/pubmed/ 10216268. Accessed 21 Nov 2017.
23. Hill CE, Metcalf DS, JI MI. A search for virulence genes of Haemophilus parasuis using differential display RT-PCR. Vet Microbiol. 2003;96:189–202 http://www.ncbi.nlm.nih.gov/pubmed/14519336. Accessed 21 Nov 2017.
24. Goethe R, Gonzáles OF, Lindner T, Gerlach GF. A novel strategy for protective Actinobacillus pleuropneumoniae subunit vaccines: detergent extraction of cultures induced by iron restriction. Vaccine. 2000;19:966–75 http://www.ncbi.nlm.nih.gov/pubmed/11115723. Accessed 21 Nov 2017.
25. Bello-Ortí B, Howell KJ, Tucker AW, Maskell DJ, Aragon V. Metatranscriptomics reveals metabolic adaptation and induction of virulence factors by *Haemophilus parasuis* during lung infection. Vet Res. 2015;46:102.
26. Frandoloso R, Martínez S, Rodríguez-Ferri EF, García-Iglesias MJ, Pérez-Martínez C, Martínez-Fernández B, Gutiérrez Martín CB. Development and characterization of protective *Haemophilus parasuis* subunit vaccines based on native proteins with affinity to porcine transferrin and comparison with other subunit and commercial vaccines. Clin Vaccine Immunol. 2011;18:50–8. https://doi.org/10.1128/CVI.00314-10.
27. Frandoloso R, Martínez-Martínez S, Calmettes C, Fegan J, Costa E, Curran D, Yu RH, Gutiérrez-Martín CB, Rodríguez-Ferri EF, Moraes TF, Schryvers AB. Nonbinding site-directed mutants of transferrin binding protein B exhibit enhanced immunogenicity and protective capabilities. Infect Immun. 2015;83:1030–8. https://doi.org/10.1128/IAI.02572-14.
28. Morton DJ, Seale TW, Madore LL, VanWagoner TM, Whitby PW, Stull TL. The haem-haemopexin utilization gene cluster (hxuCBA) as a virulence factor of *Haemophilus influenzae*. Microbiology. 2007;153(Pt 1):215–24. https://doi.org/10.1099/mic.0.2006/000190-0.
29. Wen Y, Yan X, Wen Y, Cao S, He L, Ding L, Zhang L, Zhou P, Huang X, Wu R, Wen X. Immunogenicity of the recombinant HxuCBA proteins encoded by *hxuCBA* gene cluster of *Haemophilus parasuis* in mice. Gene. 2016;591:478–83. https://doi.org/10.1016/j.gene.2016.07.001.
30. Mikael LG, Pawelek PD, Labrie J, Sirois M, Coulton JW, Jacques M. Molecular cloning and characterization of the ferric hydroxamate uptake (fhu) operon in *Actinobacillus pleuropneumoniae*. Microbiology. 2002;148(Pt 9):2869–82. https://doi.org/10.1099/00221287-148-9-2869.
31. Hasday JD, Singh IS. Fever and the heat shock response: distinct, partially overlapping processes. Cell Stress Chaperones. 2000;5:471–80 http://www.ncbi.nlm.nih.gov/ pubmed/11189454. Accessed 21 Nov 2017.
32. Koronakis V, Sharff A, Koronakis E, Luisi B, Hughes C. Crystal structure of the bacterial membrane protein TolC central to multidrug efflux and protein export. Nature. 2000;405:914–9. https://doi.org/10.1038/35016007.
33. Li M, Cai R-J, Song S, Jiang Z-Y, Li Y, Gou H-C, Chu PP, Li CL, Qiu HJ. Evaluation of immunogenicity and protective efficacy of recombinant outer membrane proteins of *Haemophilus parasuis* serovar 5 in a murine model. PLoS One. 2017;12:e0176537. https://doi.org/10.1371/journal.pone.0176537.
34. Deslandes V, Nash JHE, Harel J, Coulton JW, Jacques M. Transcriptional profiling of *Actinobacillus pleuropneumoniae* under iron-restricted conditions. BMC Genomics. 2007;8:72. https://doi.org/10.1186/1471-2164-8-72.
35. Tegetmeyer HE, Fricke K, Baltes N. An isogenic *Actinobacillus pleuropneumoniae* AasP mutant exhibits altered biofilm formation but retains virulence. Vet Microbiol. 2009;137:392–6. https://doi.org/10.1016/j.vetmic.2009.01.026.
36. Bodelón G, Palomino C, Fernández LÁ. Immunoglobulin domains in *Escherichia coli* and other enterobacteria: from pathogenesis to applications in antibody technologies. FEMS Microbiol Rev. 2013;37:204–50. https://doi.org/10.1111/j.1574-6976.2012.00347.x.
37. Starosta AL, Lassak J, Jung K, Wilson DN. The bacterial translation stress response. FEMS Microbiol Rev. 2014;38:1172–201. https://doi.org/10.1111/1574-6976.12083.
38. Carpenter BM, Whitmire JM, Merrell DS. This is not your mother's repressor: the complex role of fur in pathogenesis. Infect Immun. 2009;77:2590–601. https://doi.org/10.1128/IAI.00116-09.

PERMISSIONS

All chapters in this book were first published in VR, by BioMed Central; hereby published with permission under the Creative Commons Attribution License or equivalent. Every chapter published in this book has been scrutinized by our experts. Their significance has been extensively debated. The topics covered herein carry significant findings which will fuel the growth of the discipline. They may even be implemented as practical applications or may be referred to as a beginning point for another development.

The contributors of this book come from diverse backgrounds, making this book a truly international effort. This book will bring forth new frontiers with its revolutionizing research information and detailed analysis of the nascent developments around the world.

We would like to thank all the contributing authors for lending their expertise to make the book truly unique. They have played a crucial role in the development of this book. Without their invaluable contributions this book wouldn't have been possible. They have made vital efforts to compile up to date information on the varied aspects of this subject to make this book a valuable addition to the collection of many professionals and students.

This book was conceptualized with the vision of imparting up-to-date information and advanced data in this field. To ensure the same, a matchless editorial board was set up. Every individual on the board went through rigorous rounds of assessment to prove their worth. After which they invested a large part of their time researching and compiling the most relevant data for our readers.

The editorial board has been involved in producing this book since its inception. They have spent rigorous hours researching and exploring the diverse topics which have resulted in the successful publishing of this book. They have passed on their knowledge of decades through this book. To expedite this challenging task, the publisher supported the team at every step. A small team of assistant editors was also appointed to further simplify the editing procedure and attain best results for the readers.

Apart from the editorial board, the designing team has also invested a significant amount of their time in understanding the subject and creating the most relevant covers. They scrutinized every image to scout for the most suitable representation of the subject and create an appropriate cover for the book.

The publishing team has been an ardent support to the editorial, designing and production team. Their endless efforts to recruit the best for this project, has resulted in the accomplishment of this book. They are a veteran in the field of academics and their pool of knowledge is as vast as their experience in printing. Their expertise and guidance has proved useful at every step. Their uncompromising quality standards have made this book an exceptional effort. Their encouragement from time to time has been an inspiration for everyone.

The publisher and the editorial board hope that this book will prove to be a valuable piece of knowledge for researchers, students, practitioners and scholars across the globe.

LIST OF CONTRIBUTORS

Ioannis Arsenakis, Luca Panzavolta, Annelies Michiels, Rubén Del Pozo Sacristán and Dominiek Maes
Porcine Health Management Unit, Department of Reproduction, Obstetrics & Herd Health, Faculty of Veterinary Medicine, Ghent University, Salisburylaan 133, Merelbeke 9820, Belgium

Filip Boyen and Freddy Haesebrouck
Department of Pathology, Bacteriology and Avian Diseases, Faculty of Veterinary Medicine, Ghent University, Salisburylaan 133, Merelbeke 9820, Belgium

Giovanni Loris Alborali, Jessica Ruggeri and Nicola Martinelli
Istituto Zooprofilattico Sperimentale della Lombardia e dell'Emilia Romagna [Experimental Zooprophylactic Institute of Lombardy and Emilia Romagna], 25124 Brescia, Italy

Michele Pesciaroli
FAO Reference Center for Veterinary Public Health, Department of Veterinary Public Health and Food Safety, Istituto Superiore di Sanità, 00161 Rome, Italy
UCM-UPM, Campus Moncloa, Madrid, Spain

Barbara Chirullo and Paolo Pasquali
FAO Reference Center for Veterinary Public Health, Department of Veterinary Public Health and Food Safety, Istituto Superiore di Sanità, 00161 Rome, Italy

Serena Ammendola and Andrea Battistoni
Department of Biology, Università di Roma Tor Vergata, 00133 Rome, Italy

Maria Cristina Ossiprandi and Attilio Corradi
Department of Veterinary Sciences, University of Parma, Parma, Italy

Declan O'Brien and Morgane Delavergne
International Federation for Animal Health Europe, Avenue de Tervueren 168, Brussels, Belgium

Jim Scudamore
Institute of Infection and Global Health, University of Liverpool, Liverpool, UK

Johannes Charlier
Avia-GIS, Risschotlei 33, 2980 Zoersel, Belgium

Andrea M. Spiri and Regina Hofmann-Lehmann
Clinical Laboratory, Vetsuisse Faculty, University of Zurich, Winterthurerstr. 260, 8057 Zurich, Switzerland
Center for Clinical Studies, Vetsuisse Faculty, University of Zurich, Winterthurerstr. 260, 8057 Zurich, Switzerland

Sabrina Rodriguez-Campos
Institute of Veterinary Bacteriology, Vetsuisse Faculty, University of Bern, Länggassstr. 122, 3001 Bern, Switzerland

José M. Matos, Tony M. Glaus and Claudia E. Reusch
Clinic for Small Animal Internal Medicine, Vetsuisse Faculty, University of Zurich, Winterthurerstr. 260, 8057 Zurich, Switzerland

Barbara Riond
Clinical Laboratory, Vetsuisse Faculty, University of Zurich, Winterthurerstr. 260, 8057 Zurich, Switzerland

Barbara Willi
Clinical Laboratory, Vetsuisse Faculty, University of Zurich, Winterthurerstr. 260, 8057 Zurich, Switzerland
Clinic for Small Animal Internal Medicine, Vetsuisse Faculty, University of Zurich, Winterthurerstr. 260, 8057 Zurich, Switzerland

Gaby Hirsbrunner and Adrian Steiner
Clinic for Ruminants, Vetsuisse Faculty, University, of Berne, Bremgartenstrasse 109a, CH-3012 Berne, Switzerland

Sarah Rigert
Tierarztpraxis Arche, CH-3952 Susten, Switzerland

Fredi Janett
Department of Farm Animals, Vetsuisse-Faculty, University of Zurich, Winterthurerstrasse 260, CH-8057 Zurich, Switzerland

Jürg Hüsler
Institute of Mathematical Statistics and Actuarial Science, Sidlerstrasse 5, CH-3012 Berne, Switzerland

Philipp Schnydrig
Institut for Veterinary Bacteriology, Länggassstrasse 122, CH-3012 Berne, Switzerland

Ester Lopez and Sue Amatayakul-Chantler
Zoetis Research and Manufacturing, 45 Poplar Road, Parkville, VIC A-3052, Australia

M. S. Ismail and M. Firdaus-Nawi
Department of Veterinary Laboratory Diagnosis, Faculty of Veterinary Medicine, Universiti Putra Malaysia, 43400 Serdang, Malaysia

A. Siti-Zahrah and M. R. M. Syafiq
National Fish Research and Disease Diagnosis, Fisheries Research Institute, 11960 BatuMaung, Penang, Malaysia

M. N. A. Amal
Department of Biology, Faculty of Science, Universiti Putra Malaysia, 43400 Serdang, Malaysia

M. Zamri-Saad
Department of Veterinary Laboratory Diagnosis, Faculty of Veterinary Medicine, Universiti Putra Malaysia, 43400 Serdang, Malaysia
Institute of Bioscience, Universiti Putra Malaysia, 43400 Serdang, Malaysia

Tobias Theuß, Thomas Lindner and Sven Springer
IDT Biologika GmbH, Business Unit Animal Health, Research and Development, Am Pharmapark, 06861 Dessau-Rosslau, Germany

Elke Ueberham and Jörg Lehmann
Fraunhofer Institute for Cell Therapy and Immunology, Perlickstraße 1, 04103 Leipzig, Germany

Zhijie Lin, Peipei Tang, Yang Jiao, Xilong Kang, Qiuchun Li, Zhiming Pan and Xinan Jiao
Jiangsu Key Laboratory of Zoonosis, Jiangsu Co-Innovation Center for Prevention and Control of Important Animal Infectious Diseases and Zoonosis, MOA Key Laboratory of Prevention and Control of Biological Hazard Factors (Animal Origin) for Agrifood Safety and Quality, MOE Joint International Research Laboratory of Agriculture and Agri-product Safety, Yangzhou University, Yangzhou 225001, China

Xiulong Xu
Jiangsu Key Laboratory of Zoonosis, Jiangsu Co-Innovation Center for Prevention and Control of Important Animal Infectious Diseases and Zoonosis, MOA Key Laboratory of Prevention and Control of Biological Hazard Factors (Animal Origin) for Agrifood Safety and Quality, MOE Joint International Research Laboratory of Agriculture and Agri-product Safety, Yangzhou University, Yangzhou 225001, China
Center for Comparative Medicine, Animal Infectious Disease Laboratory, College of Veterinary Medicine, Yangzhou University, Yangzhou 225001, China
Department of Anatomy and Cell Biology, Rush University Medical Center, Chicago 60612, USA

Jun Sun
Jiangsu Key Laboratory of Zoonosis, Jiangsu Co-Innovation Center for Prevention and Control of Important Animal Infectious Diseases and Zoonosis, MOA Key Laboratory of Prevention and Control of Biological Hazard Factors (Animal Origin) for Agrifood Safety and Quality, MOE Joint International Research Laboratory of Agriculture and Agri-product Safety, Yangzhou University, Yangzhou 225001, China
Division of Gastroenterology and Hepatology, College of Medicine, University of Illinois at Chicago, Chicago 60612, USA

Gui-sheng Wang
Shandong Provincial Center for Animal Disease Control and Prevention, Jinan, China
School of Life Sciences, Shandong University, 27 Shanda Road South, Jinan 250100, China

Yijun Du and Jia-qiang Wu
Shandong Key Laboratory of Animal Disease Control and Breeding, Institute of Animal Science and Veterinary Medicine, Shandong Academy of Agricultural Sciences, Jinan, China

Fu-lin Tian
Shandong Provincial Center for Animal Disease Control and Prevention, Jinan, China

Xue-jie Yu
School of Health Science, Wuhan University, Wuhan, China

Jin-bao Wang
School of Life Sciences, Shandong University, 27 Shanda Road South, Jinan 250100, China

Jacopo Guccione, Luigi D'Andrea, Angela De Rosa and Paolo Ciaramella
Department of Veterinary Medicine and Animal Productions, University of Napoli "Federico II", Via Delpino 1, 80137 Naples, Italy

Antonella Pesce and Caterina Salzano
Istituto Zooprofilattico del Mezzogiorno, Via A. Jervolino 19, 81100, Tuoro, Caserta District, Italy

Massimo Pascale
Veterinary practitioner, Caserta District 81100, Italy

Gianni Tedeschi
Hipra Italia s.r.l., Via Franciacorta 74, 25038 Rovato, Italy

Reta D. Abdi
Clinical Studies Department, College of Veterinary Medicine and Agriculture, Addis Ababa University, Bishoftu, Ethiopia
Department of Animal Science, University of Tennessee, 2506 River Drive, Knoxville, USA

Kasahun Amsalu
College of Veterinary Science, Mekelle University, Mekelle, Ethiopia

Olana Merera
College of Veterinary Medicine and Agriculture, Samara University, Samara, Ethiopia

Yilkal Asfaw and Teshale Sori
Clinical Studies Department, College of Veterinary Medicine and Agriculture, Addis Ababa University, Bishoftu, Ethiopia

Eseyas Gelaye and Marta Yami
National Veterinary Institute, Bishoftu, Ethiopia

Sergi Segarra, Daniel Costa and Natàlia Coyo
Departament de Medicina i Cirurgia Animals, Facultat de Veterinària, Bellaterra, Spain

Marta Leiva and Teresa Peña
Departament de Medicina i Cirurgia Animals, Facultat de Veterinària, Bellaterra, Spain
Fundació Hospital Clínic Veterinari, UAB, Bellaterra, Spain

Maria Sabés-Alsina
Department of Animal Health and Anatomy, Facultat de Veterinària, UAB, Bellaterra, Spain

José Río
Medical Statistics Core Facility, IDIBAPS, Hospital Clínic Barcelona, Barcelona, Spain
Biostatistics Unit, Faculty of Medicine, UAB, Bellaterra, Spain

J. Manyweathers
Centre for Health Research, Western Sydney University, Sydney, Australia
School of Animal Biology, University of Western Australia, Tathra, NSW, Australia

H. Field
Eco Health Alliance, New York, NY, USA

N. Longnecker
School of Animal Biology, University of Western Australia, Tathra, NSW, Australia
Centre for Science Communication, University of Otago, Dunedin, New Zealand

K. Agho
School of Science and Health, Western Sydney University, Sydney, Australia

C. Smith
Department of Agriculture and Fisheries, Queensland Centre for Emerging Infectious Diseases, Biosecurity Queensland, Coopers Plains, QLD, Australia

M. Taylor
Centre for Health Research, Western Sydney University, Sydney, Australia
Department of Psychology, Macquarie University, Sydney, Australia

Juan M. Pacheco, Ethan J. Hartwig, George R. Smoliga, Mary A. Kenney, William T. Golde, Luis L. Rodriguez and Jonathan Arzt
United States Department of Agriculture (USDA), Plum Island Animal Disease Center (PIADC), Foreign Animal Disease Research Unit (FADRU), Agricultural Research Service (ARS), Greenport, NY 11944, USA

Michael Eschbaumer, Carolina Stenfeldt and Steven I. Rekant
United States Department of Agriculture (USDA), Plum Island Animal Disease Center (PIADC), Foreign Animal Disease Research Unit (FADRU), Agricultural Research Service (ARS), Greenport, NY 11944, USA
Oak Ridge Institute for Science and Education, PIADC Research Participation Program, Oak Ridge, TN, USA

Susanne M. Koehler
Department of Infectiology and Animal Hygiene, University of Hohenheim, Institute of Animal Science, 70593 Stuttgart, Germany
Robert-Koch-Institut, 13353 Berlin, Germany

Fatih Buyuk, Ozgur Celebi, Mitat Sahin and Salih Otlu
Faculty of Veterinary Medicine, Department of Microbiology, Kafkas University, 36300 Kars, Turkey

Hayati Demiraslan and Mehmet Doganay
Faculty of Medicine, Department of Infectious Diseases, Erciyes University, 38039 Kayseri, Turkey

Jens Moehring
Institute for Crop Science, University of Hohenheim, Biostatistical Unit, 70593 Stuttgart, Germany

Okechukwu C. Ndumnego
Department of Veterinary Tropical Diseases, University of Pretoria, Onderstepoort 0110, South Africa
Africa Health Research Institute, Durban 4013, South Africa

Henriette van Heerden
Department of Veterinary Tropical Diseases, University of Pretoria, Onderstepoort 0110, South Africa

Wolfgang Beyer
Department of Infectiology and Animal Hygiene, University of Hohenheim, Institute of Animal Science, 70593 Stuttgart, Germany

Jichun Wang, Rongli Guo, Yongfeng Qiao, Mengwei Xu, Zhisheng Wang, Yamei Liu and Jibo Hou
National Research Center of Engineering and Technology for Veterinary Biologicals/Institute of Veterinary Medicine, Jiangsu Academy of Agricultural Sciences, Nanjing, Jiangsu 210014, China
Jiangsu Co-innovation Center for Prevention and Control of Important Animal Infectious Diseases and Zoonoses, Yangzhou, China

Yiqi Gu and Chang Liu
National Research Center of Engineering and Technology for Veterinary Biologicals/Institute of Veterinary Medicine, Jiangsu Academy of Agricultural Sciences, Nanjing, Jiangsu 210014, China
College of Veterinary Medicine, Nanjing Agricultural University, Nanjing 210095, China

Wenlong Nan, Lide Qin, Yueyong Zhang and Yiping Chen
Laboratory of Diagnositics Development, China Animal Health and Epidemiology Center, 369 Nanjing Road, Qingdao, Shandong 266032, China

Yong Wang and Pengfei Tan
Laboratory of Diagnositics Development, China Animal Health and Epidemiology Center, 369 Nanjing Road, Qingdao, Shandong 266032, China
College of Veterinary Medicine, Yangzhou University, 12 East Wenhui Road, Yangzhou, Jiangsu 225009, China

Yuqi Chen
Xi'an Jiaotong-Liverpool University, 111 Ren'ai Road, Suzhou, Jiangsu Province 215123, China

Kairong Mao
China Institute of Veterinary Drug Control, 8 Zhongguanchun South Street, Beijing 100081, China

Deborah A Grosenbaugh, Bradley Feilmeier, Kristopher DeWitt and Frederic David
Merial Inc., Boehringer Ingelheim, Athens, GA, USA

Karelle De Luca, Pierre-Yves Durand, Cecile Sigoillot-Claude and Marie-Line Sajous
MERIAL S.A.S., Boehringer Ingelheim, Lyon, France

Michael J Day
Bristol Veterinary School, University of Bristol, Langford, UK

Haiyun Jin, Wan Wang, Xueqin Yang, Hailong Su, Jiawen Fan, Rui Zhu, Huoying Shi and Xiufan Liu
College of Veterinary Medicine, Yangzhou University, Yangzhou, Jiangsu 225009, People's Republic of China
Jiangsu Co-innovation Center for the Prevention and Control of Important Animal Infectious Diseases and Zoonoses, Yangzhou 225009, China

Shifeng Wang
Department of Infectious Diseases and Pathology, College of Veterinary Medicine, University of Florida, Gainesville, FL 32611-0880, USA

Jean Artois
Spatial Epidemiology Lab. (SpELL), Université Libre de Bruxelles, Brussels, Belgium

Carla Ippoliti and Annamaria Conte
Istituto Zooprofilattico Sperimentale dell'Abruzzo e del Molise 'G. Caporale', Teramo, Italy

Madhur S. Dhingra
Spatial Epidemiology Lab. (SpELL), Université Libre de Bruxelles, Brussels, Belgium
Food and Agriculture Organization of the United Nations, Rome, Italy

Pastor Alfonso
National Center for Animal and Plant Health (CENSA), OIE Collaborating Center for Reduction of the Risk of Disasters in Animal Health, 32700 San José de las Lajas, Mayabeque, Cuba

Abdelgawad El Tahawy, Ahmed Elbestawy and Hany F. Ellakany
Faculty of Veterinary Medicine, Damanhour University, Damanhour, Egypt

Marius Gilbert
Spatial Epidemiology Lab. (SpELL), Université Libre de Bruxelles, Brussels, Belgium
Fonds National de la Recherche Scientifique, Brussels, Belgium

Melinda Hergert
Department of Paraclinical Sciences, Faculty of Veterinary Science, University of Pretoria, Onderstepoort 0110, South Africa

Kevin Le Roux
KwaZulu-Natal Department of Environment, Agriculture and Rural Development, Government Veterinary Services, 458 Townbush Road, Pietermaritzburg 3202, South Africa

Louis H. Nel
Department of Biochemistry, Genetics and Microbiology, Faculty of Natural and Agricultural Sciences University of Pretoria, Pretoria 0002, South Africa
Global Alliance for Rabies Control, 529 Humboldt St., Suite 1, Manhattan, KS 66502, USA

Przemysław Romiszewski
Animal Medical Center, 5255 York Rd, Holicong, PA 18928, USA

Krzysztof Kostro and Urszula Lisiecka
Department of Epizootiology and Clinic of Infectious Diseases, Faculty of Veterinary Medicine, University of Life Sciences in Lublin, 20-612 Lublin, Poland

Álvaro Álvarez-Estrada, César B. Gutiérrez-Martín, Elías F. Rodríguez-Ferri and Sonia Martínez-Martínez
Microbiology & Immunology Section, Animal Health Department, Faculty of Veterinary Medicine, University of León, León, Spain

Index

www.ingramcontent.com/pod-product-compliance
Lightning Source LLC
LaVergne TN
LVHW080654210926
848485LV00003B/375